See also Index of *DSM-IV* Psychiatric Diagnoses on page xvii.

Nursing Diagnoses in Psychiatric Nursing:
CARE PLANS AND PSYCHOTROPIC MEDICATIONS

Fifth Edition

MARY C. TOWNSEND, RN, MN, CS
Clinical Nurse Specialist
Private Practice
Adult Psychiatric/Mental Health Nursing
Oklahoma City, Oklahoma

Former Assistant Professor and
Coordinator, Mental Health Nursing
Oklahoma City University
Oklahoma City, Oklahoma

F. A. Davis Company • Philadelphia

F. A. Davis Company
1915 Arch Street
Philadelphia, PA 19103

Printed in the United States of America

Last digit indicates print number: 10 9 8 7 6 5 4 3

Publisher, Nursing: Robert G. Martone
Cover Designer: Louis J. Forgione

As new scientific information becomes available through basic and clinical research, recommended treatments and drug therapies undergo changes. The author and publisher have done everything possible to make this book accurate, up to date, and in accord with accepted standards at the time of publication. The author, editors, and publisher are not responsible for errors or omissions or for consequences from application of the book, and make no warranty, expressed or implied, in regard to the contents of the book. Any practice described in this book should be applied by the reader in accordance with professional standards of care used in regard to the unique circumstances that may apply in each situation. The reader is advised always to check product information (package inserts) for changes and new information regarding dose and contraindications before administering any drug. Caution is especially urged when using new or infrequently ordered drugs.

Library of Congress Cataloging-in-Publication Data

Townsend, Mary C., 1941–
Nursing diagnoses in psychiatric nursing : care plans and psychotropic medications / Mary C. Townsend.—5th ed.
p. cm.
Previous eds. published with the subtitle: a pocket guide for care plan construction.
Includes bibliographical references and index.
ISBN 0-8036-0703-2 (pbk.)
1. Psychiatric nursing—Diagnosis—Handbooks, manuals, etc. 2. Mental illness—Handbooks, manuals, etc. 3. Nursing diagnosis—Handbooks, manuals, etc. I. Title.

RC440 .T69 2000
610.73′68—dc21

00-056953

This Book Is Dedicated:

To my husband, Jim, who has encouraged and supported me throughout this project and whose love continues to nurture and sustain me, even after 39 years.

To my daughters, Kerry and Tina, who have brought joy that only a parent could understand, frustrations that only a parent could tolerate, happiness that only a parent could appreciate, and tears that only a parent could endure. You are truly loved.

To my faithful and beloved companions, Affic and Bucky, whose warm, furry bodies at my feet helped to make the long hours of writing more tolerable and enjoyable.

And finally, to my father and mother, Francis and Camalla Welsh, who reared my sister Francie and me without knowledge of psychology or developmental theories but with the kind of unconditional love I have come to believe is so vital to the achievement and maintenance of emotional wellness.

MCT

Acknowledgments

My special thanks and appreciation:

To Bob Martone, who patiently provided essential editorial assistance and guidance throughout the project.

To the editorial and production staffs of the F. A. Davis Company, who are always willing to provide assistance when requested and whose consistent excellence in publishing makes me proud to be associated with them.

To the gracious individuals who read and critiqued the original manuscript, providing valuable input into the final product.

And finally, a special acknowledgment to the nurses who staff the psychiatric units of the clinical agencies where nursing students go to learn about psychiatric nursing. To those of you who willingly share your knowledge and expertise with, and act as role models for, these nursing students. If this book provides you with even a small amount of nursing assistance, please acknowledge it as my way of saying, "thanks."

MCT

Consultants

Maude H. Alston, RN, PhD
Assistant Professor of Nursing
University of North Carolina at Greensboro
Greensboro, North Carolina

Betty J. Carmack, RN, EdD
Assistant Professor
University of San Francisco
School of Nursing
San Francisco, California

Doris K. DeVincenzo, PhD
Professor
Lienhard School of Nursing
Pace University
Pleasantville, New York

Mary Jo Gorney-Fadiman, RN, PhD
Assistant Professor
San Jose State University
School of Nursing
San Jose, California

Mary E. Martucci, RN, PhD
Associate Professor and Chairman
Saint Mary's College
Notre Dame, Indiana

Sheridan V. Mc Cabe, BA, BSN, MSN, PhD
Assistant Professor of Nursing
University of Virginia
School of Nursing
Charlottesville, Virginia

Elizabeth Anne Rankin, PhD
Psychotherapist and Consultant
The University of Maryland
School of Nursing
Baltimore, Maryland

Judith M. Saunders, DNS, FAAN
Postdoctoral Research Fellow
University of Washington
School of Nursing
Seattle, Washington

Gail Stuart, RN, CS, PhD
Associate Professor
Medical University of South Carolina
College of Nursing
Charleston, South Carolina

Contents

Index of DSM-IV *Psychiatric Diagnoses*

Page numbers followed by a "t" indicate tabular material.

How to Use This Book

In an attempt to standardize clinical nursing practice, the North American Nursing Diagnosis Association (NANDA) has published a list of nursing diagnoses that have been approved through the 13th National Conference on Classification of Nursing Diagnosis in 1998. Standardization of nursing actions and common terminology is important in the provision of consistent care over time, among nurses, across shifts, and even between different health-care agencies.

There are those individuals who believe that NANDA's list is incomplete. My intent is not to judge the completeness of this list but to suggest the need for clinical testing of what is available. NANDA encourages nurses to submit new nursing diagnoses for consideration by the group after conducting testing and research of that diagnosis in the clinical setting.

There are three essential components in a nursing diagnosis, which have been referred to as the *PES format* (Gordon, 1987). The "P" identifies the health problem, the "E" represents the etiology (or cause) of the problem, and the "S" describes a cluster of signs and symptoms, or what has come to be known as "defining characteristics." These three parts are combined into one statement by the use of "connecting words." The diagnosis would then be written in this manner: Problem "related to" etiology "evidenced by" signs and symptoms (defining characteristics).

The problem can be identified as the human response to actual or potential health problems as assessed by the nurse. The etiology may be represented by past experiences of the individual, genetic influences, current environmental factors, or pathophysiological changes. The defining characteristics describe what the client says and what the nurse observes that indicate the existence of a particular problem.

Nursing diagnoses, then, become the basis for the care

plan. This book may be used as a guide in the construction of care plans for various psychiatric clients. The concepts are presented in such a manner that they may be applied to several types of health-care settings: inpatient hospitalization, outpatient clinic, home health, partial hospitalization, and private practice, to name a few. Major divisions in the book have been identified by psychiatric diagnostic categories, according to the order in which they appear in the *Diagnostic and Statistical Manual of Mental Disorders, 4th Edition* (*DSM-IV,* 1994). The use of this format is not to imply that nursing diagnoses are based on, or flow from, medical diagnoses, but is meant only to enhance the usability of the book. In addition, I am not suggesting that those nursing diagnoses presented with each psychiatric category are all-inclusive.

It is valid, however, to state that certain nursing diagnoses are indeed common to individuals with specific psychiatric disorders. The diagnoses presented in this book are meant to be used as guidelines for construction of care plans that must be individualized for each client, based on the nursing assessment. The interventions can also be used in areas in which interdisciplinary treatment plans take the place of the nursing care plan.

Each chapter in Unit II begins with an overview of information related to the medical diagnostic category, which may be useful to the nurse as background assessment data. This section includes:

1. **The Disorder:** A definition and common types or categories that have been identified.
2. **Predisposing Factors:** Information regarding theories of etiology, which the nurse may use in formulating the "related to" portion of the nursing diagnosis, as it applies to the client.
3. **Symptomatology:** Subjective and objective data identifying behaviors common to the disorder. These behaviors, as they apply to the individual client, may be pertinent to the "evidenced by" portion of the nursing diagnosis.

Information presented with each nursing diagnosis includes the following:

1. **Definition:** The approved NANDA definition is used with those nursing diagnoses for which a NANDA definition exists. I have suggested definitions for clarification of the other nursing diagnoses, and these are identified by brackets [ ].

2. **Possible Etiologies ("related to"):** This section suggests possible causes for the problem identified. Those not approved by NANDA are identified by brackets [ ]. **Related/Risk Factors** are given for diagnoses for which the client is at risk. ***Note:* Defining characteristics are replaced by "related/risk factors" for the "Risk for" diagnoses.**
3. **Defining Characteristics ("evidenced by"):** This section includes signs and symptoms that may be evident to indicate that the problem exists. Again, as with definitions and etiologies, those not approved by NANDA are identified by brackets [ ].
4. **Goals:** These statements are made in client behavioral objective terminology. They are measurable, short- and long-term goals, to be used in evaluating the effectiveness of the nursing interventions in alleviating the identified problem. There may be more than one short-term goal, and they may be considered "stepping stones" to fulfillment of the long-term goal. For purposes of this book, "long-term," in most instances, is designated as "by discharge," whether the client is in an inpatient or outpatient setting.
5. **Interventions with *Selected Rationales:*** Only those interventions that are appropriate to a particular nursing diagnosis within the context of the psychiatric setting are presented. Rationales for selected interventions are included to provide clarification beyond fundamental nursing knowledge and to assist in the selection of appropriate interventions for individual clients.
6. **Outcome Criteria:** These are behavioral changes that can be used as criteria to determine the degree to which the nursing diagnosis has been resolved.

To use this book in the preparation of psychiatric nursing care plans, find the section in the text applicable to the client's psychiatric diagnosis. Review background data pertinent to the diagnosis, if needed. Complete a biopsychosocial history and assessment on the client. Select and prioritize nursing diagnoses appropriate to the client. Using the list of NANDA-approved nursing diagnoses, be sure to include those that are client specific and not just those that have been identified as "common" to this particular medical diagnosis. Select nursing interventions and outcome criteria appropriate to the client for each nursing diagnosis identified. Write all of this information on the care plan, with a date for evaluating the status of each problem. On the evaluation date, document success of the nursing interventions in achieving the goals of care, using the desired client outcomes as criteria. Modify the plan as required.

Several new chapters, as well as an entire new unit, have been added to this edition. New chapters in Unit III discuss HIV Disease, Homelessness, Psychiatric Home Nursing Care, Forensic Nursing, and Complementary Therapies. Unit IV, Psychotropic Medications, is new to this edition. Each chapter in this unit is devoted to a specific category of psychotropic medication. Within each chapter, the categories are identified by chemical class. Information is presented related to indications, actions, contraindications and precautions, and adverse reactions and side effects. Examples of medications in each chemical class are presented by generic and trade name, along with information about half-life, controlled categories, daily adult dosage range, and available forms of the medication. Therapeutic plasma level ranges are provided, where appropriate. Nursing diagnoses related to each category, along with nursing interventions, and client and family education are included in each chapter.

An additional new feature to this edition is the table in Appendix N, which lists some client behaviors commonly observed in the psychiatric setting and the most appropriate nursing diagnosis for each. It is hoped that this information will broaden the understanding of use of a variety of nursing diagnoses in preparation of the client treatment plan.

This book helps to familiarize the nurse with the current NANDA-approved nursing diagnoses and provides suggestions for their use within the psychiatric setting. It is designed to be used as a quick reference in the preparation of care plans, with the expectation that additional information will be required under each nursing diagnosis as the nurse individualizes care for psychiatric clients.

■ NURSING DIAGNOSES ACCEPTED BY NANDA (Through 14th Conference—April 2000)*

Activity intolerance
Activity intolerance, risk for
Adaptive capacity, intracranial, decreased
Adjustment, impaired
Airway clearance, ineffective
Anxiety [specify level]
Anxiety, death
Aspiration, risk for

Body image disturbance
Body temperature, altered, risk for
Breastfeeding, effective
Breastfeeding, ineffective
Breastfeeding, interrupted
Breathing pattern, ineffective

Cardiac output, decreased
Caregiver role strain
Caregiver role strain, risk for
Communication, impaired verbal
Confusion, acute
Confusion, chronic
Constipation
Constipation, perceived
Constipation, risk for
Coping, community, ineffective
Coping, community, potential for enhanced
Coping, defensive
Coping, family, ineffective, compromised
Coping, family, ineffective, disabling
Coping, family, potential for growth
Coping, individual, ineffective

Decisional conflict
Denial, ineffective
Dentition, altered
Development, risk for altered

---

*SOURCE: Adapted from and used with permission of the North American Nursing Diagnosis Association: Definitions and Classification 1999–2000. NANDA, Philadelphia, 1999.

Diarrhea
Disuse syndrome, risk for
Diversional activity deficit
Dysreflexia
Dysreflexia, risk for autonomic

Energy field disturbance
Environmental interpretation syndrome, impaired

Failure to thrive, adult
Falls, risk for
Family process, altered
Family processes, altered: alcoholism
Fatigue
Fear
Fluid volume deficit
Fluid volume deficit, risk for
Fluid volume excess
Fluid volume imbalance, risk for

Gas exchange, impaired
Grieving, anticipatory
Grieving, dysfunctional
Growth, risk for altered
Growth and development, altered

Health maintenance, altered
Health-seeking behaviors
Home maintenance management, impaired
Hopelessness
Hyperthermia
Hypothermia

Incontinence, bowel
Incontinence, urinary, functional
Incontinence, urinary, reflex
Incontinence, urinary, stress
Incontinence, urinary, total
Incontinence, urinary, urge
Incontinence, urinary, risk for urge
Infant behavior, disorganized
Infant behavior, disorganized, risk for
Infant behavior, organized, potential for enhanced
Infant feeding pattern, ineffective
Infection, risk for
Injury, risk for

Knowledge deficit

Latex allergy response
Latex allergy response, risk for
Loneliness, risk for

Management of therapeutic regimen: community, ineffective
Management of therapeutic regimen: families, ineffective
Management of therapeutic regimen: individual, effective
Management of therapeutic regimen: individual ineffective
Memory, impaired
Mobility, bed, impaired
Mobility, physical, impaired
Mobility, wheelchair, impaired

Nausea
Noncompliance
Nutrition, altered: less than body requirements
Nutrition, altered: more than body requirements
Nutrition, altered: risk for more than body requirements

Oral mucous membrane, altered

Pain
Pain, chronic
Parent-infant attachment, risk for insecure
Parent/infant/child attachment, altered, risk for
Parental role conflict
Parenting, altered
Parenting, altered, risk for
Perioperative positioning injury, risk for
Peripheral neurovascular dysfunction, risk for
Personal identity disturbance
Poisoning, risk for
Posttrauma syndrome
Posttrauma syndrome, risk for
Powerlessness
Powerlessness, risk for
Protection, altered

Rape-trauma syndrome
Rape-trauma syndrome: compound reaction

Rape-trauma syndrome: silent reaction
Relocation stress syndrome
Relocation stress syndrome, risk for
Role performance, altered

Self-care deficit (specify): feeding, bathing/hygiene, dressing/grooming, toileting
Self-esteem, chronic low
Self-esteem, disturbance
Self-esteem, situational low
Self-esteem, risk for situational low
Self-mutilation
Self-mutilation, risk for
Sensory-perceptual alterations [specify: visual, auditory, kinesthetic, gustatory, tactile, olfactory]
Sexual dysfunction
Sexuality patterns, altered
Skin integrity, impaired
Skin integrity, impaired, risk for
Sleep deprivation
Sleep pattern disturbance
Social interaction, impaired
Social isolation
Sorrow, chronic
Spiritual distress
Spiritual distress, risk for
Spiritual well-being, potential for enhanced
Suffocation, risk for
Surgical recovery, delayed
Suicide, risk for
Swallowing, impaired

Thermoregulation, ineffective
Thought processes, altered
Tissue integrity, impaired
Tissue perfusion, altered (specify): cerebral, cardiopulmonary, gastrointestinal, peripheral, renal
Transfer ability, impaired
Trauma, risk for

Unilateral neglect
Urinary elimination, altered
Urinary retention

Ventilation, inability to sustain spontaneous
Ventilatory weaning response, dysfunctional

Violence, risk for: directed at others
Violence, risk for: self-directed

Walking, impaired
Wandering (specify sporadic or continual)

■ INTERNET REFERENCES

- http://www.apna.org
- http://www.nursecominc.com

UNIT ONE

THE FOUNDATION FOR PLANNING PSYCHIATRIC NURSING CARE

CHAPTER 1

Nursing Process: One Step to Professionalism

Nursing has struggled for many years to achieve recognition as a profession. Out of this struggle has emerged an awareness of the need to do the following:

1. Define the boundaries of nursing. (What is nursing?)
2. Identify a scientific method for the delivery of nursing care.

In its statement on social policy, the American Nurses Association (ANA) has presented the following definition: "Nursing is the diagnosis and treatment of human responses to actual or potential health problems" (ANA, 1980).

The nursing process has been identified as nursing's scientific methodology for the delivery of nursing care. The curricula of most nursing schools include nursing process as a component of their conceptual frameworks. The National Council of State Boards of Nursing (NCSBN) uses the nursing process as the basis for the Registered Nurse State Board Test Pool Examination (Schmitt, 1996). Questions that relate to nursing behaviors in a variety of client situations are presented according to the steps of the nursing process:

1. **Assessment:** Establishing a database about a client
2. **Diagnosis:** Identifying the client's health-care needs and selecting goals of care
3. **Outcome Identification:** Establishing criteria for measuring achievement of desired outcomes
4. **Planning:** Designing a strategy to achieve the goals established for client care

5. **Implementation:** Initiating and completing actions necessary to accomplish the defined goals
6. **Evaluation:** Determining the extent to which the goals of care have been achieved

By following these six steps, the nurse has a systematic framework for decision making and problem solving in the delivery of nursing care. The nursing process is dynamic, not static. It is an ongoing process that continues for as long as the nurse and client have interactions directed toward change in the client's physical or behavioral responses. Figure 1–1 presents a schematic of the ongoing nursing process.

Nursing diagnosis is an integral part of the nursing process. In this step, the nurse identifies the "human responses to actual or potential health problems." In some states, diagnosing is identified within the Nurse Practice Acts as a legal responsibility of the professional nurse. Shoemaker has stated, "Nursing diagnosis provides the basis for prescriptions for definitive therapy for which the nurse is accountable" (Kim et al., 1984).

As an inherent part of the nursing process, nursing diagnosis is also reflected in the ANA Standards of Practice. These standards provide one broad basis for evaluating

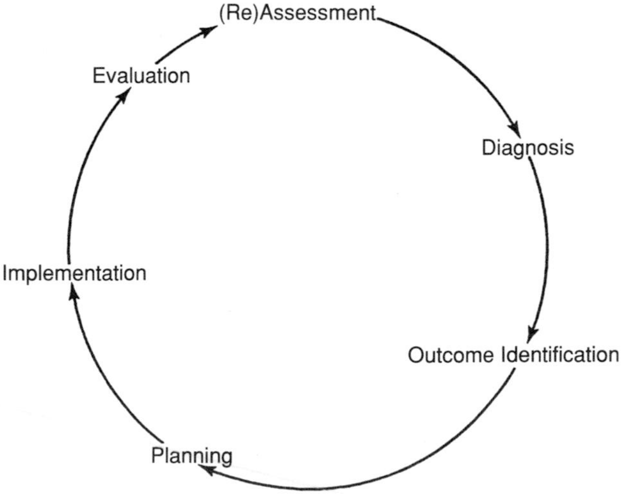

Figure 1–1. The ongoing nursing process.

practice and reflect a recognition of the rights of the person receiving nursing care (ANA, 1998).

Nursing diagnosis can no longer be recognized as part of nursing's future. Nursing diagnosis is now. This provides a challenge for nursing educators and administrators to assist not only the nursing students of today but also those registered nurses currently staffing health-care agencies who were never introduced to nursing diagnosis in their basic educational programs and who are now being told they must conform. The purpose of this book is to provide that assistance to students and staff nurses as they endeavor to provide high-quality nursing care to their psychiatric clients.

This chapter includes one example of a nursing history and assessment tool that may be used to gather information about the client during the assessment phase of the nursing process. Also presented is a sample case study using this assessment tool to formulate the client database, followed by a care plan developed from the assessment information.

■ NURSING HISTORY AND ASSESSMENT TOOL*

General Information

Client name: ___________
Room number: ________
Doctor: _______________
Age: __________________
Gender: _______________
Race: _________________
Dominant language: _____
Marital status: _________
Chief complaint: _______
____
____

Allergies: _____________
Diet: _________________
Height/weight: _________
Vital signs: TPR/BP _____
Name and phone no. of significant other: _____
____
City of residence: ______
Diagnosis (admitting and current:) ___________
____

Conditions of Admission

Date: _________________ Time: _______________
Accompanied by: ______________________________
Route of admission (wheelchair, ambulatory, cart): ____
Admitted from: ________________________________

Predisposing Factors

Genetic Influences

Family configuration (use genograms):
Family of origin: Present family:

Family dynamics (describe significant relationships between family members): ______________________
____
____
____
____

Medical/Psychiatric History: ____________________
Client: ____
____
____
Family Members: ________________________________
____
____

Other GENETIC influences affecting present adaptation. (This might include effects specific to gender, race, appearance [such as genetic physical defects], or any other factor related to genetics that is affecting the client's adaptation that has not been mentioned elsewhere in this assessment.)

____
____
____
____
____

Past Experiences

CULTURAL AND SOCIAL HISTORY

Environmental factors (family living arrangements, type of neighborhood, special working conditions): ________
____
____

Health beliefs and practices (personal responsibility for health; special self-care practices): ________________
____
____

Religious beliefs and practices: ______________________
____
____

Educational background: ___________________________
____
____

Significant losses/changes (include dates): ____________
____
____

Peer/friendship relationships: ________________________
____
____

Occupational history: ______________________________
____
____

Previous pattern of coping with stress: ______________
____
____

Other lifestyle factors contributing to present adaptation:
____
____

Existing Conditions

STAGE OF DEVELOPMENT (Erikson)
Theoretically: ______________________________
Behaviorally: ______________________________
Rationale: ______________________________
____
Support systems: ______________________________
____
Economic security: ______________________________
____
Avenues of productivity/contribution: ______________
Current job status: ______________________________
____
Role contributions and responsibility for others: ______
____

Precipitating Event

Describe the situation or events that precipitated this illness/hospitalization: ______________________________
____
____

Client's Perception of the Stressor

Client's and/or family member's understanding or description of stressor/illness and expectations of hospitalization/treatment: ______________________________
____
____
____

Adaptation Responses

Psychosocial

ANXIETY LEVEL (circle the level and check the behaviors that apply):

Mild Moderate Severe Panic
Calm _____ Friendly _____ Passive _____ Alert _____
Perceives environment correctly _____ Cooperative _____
Impaired attention _____ "Jittery" _____
Unable to concentrate _____ Hypervigilant _____
Tremors _____ Rapid speech _____ Withdrawn _____
Confused _____ Disoriented _____ Fearful _____

Hyperventilating _____ Misinterpreting the environment (hallucinations/delusions) _____ Depersonalization _____ Obsessions _____ Compulsions _____ Somatic complaints _____ Excessive hyperactivity _____
Other ____
____
____

MOOD/AFFECT (circle as many as apply):
Happiness Sadness Dejection Despair
Elation Euphoria Suspiciousness
Apathy (little emotional tone) Anger/Hostility

EGO DEFENSE MECHANISMS (describe how used by client:)
Projection: ________________________________
Suppression: ________________________________
Undoing: ________________________________
Displacement: ________________________________
Intellectualization: ________________________________
Rationalization: ________________________________
Denial: ________________________________
Repression: ________________________________
Isolation: ________________________________
Regression: ________________________________
Reaction formation: ________________________________
Splitting: ________________________________
Religiosity: ________________________________
Sublimation: ________________________________
Compensation: ________________________________

LEVEL OF SELF-ESTEEM (circle one):
Low Moderate High
Things client likes about self: ____________________
____
Things client would like to change about self: __________
____
Objective assessment of self-esteem: ______________
Eye contact: ________________________________
General appearance: __________________________
____
Personal hygiene: ____________________________
Participation in group activities and interactions with others: ________________________________
____
____

STAGE AND MANIFESTATIONS OF GRIEF (circle one):
Denial Anger Bargaining Depression
Acceptance
Describe client's behaviors that are associated with this stage of grieving in response to loss or change: ________
____
____
____

THOUGHT PROCESSES (circle as many as apply):
Clear Logical Easy to follow Relevant
Confused Blocking Delusional Rapid flow of thoughts Slowness in thought association
Suspicious
Memory: Recent (circle one): Loss Intact
Remote (circle one): Loss Intact
Other:____
____

COMMUNICATIONS PATTERNS (circle as many as apply):
Clear Coherent Slurred speech Incoherent
Neologisms Loose associations Flight of ideas
Aphasic Perseveration Rumination
Tangential speech Loquaciousness
Slow, impoverished speech
Speech impediment (describe):____________________
Other:____
____

INTERACTION PATTERNS (describe client's pattern of interpersonal interactions with staff and peers on the unit, e.g., manipulative, withdrawn, isolated, verbally or physically hostile, argumentative, passive, assertive, aggressive, passive-aggressive, other):_______________
____
____
____
____

REALITY ORIENTATION (check those that apply):
Oriented to: Time _______ Person _______________
Place _______ Situation _____________

IDEAS OF DESTRUCTION TO SELF/OTHERS? Yes No
If yes, consider plan; available means: _______________
____
____
____

Physiological

PSYCHOSOMATIC MANIFESTATIONS (describe any somatic complaints that may be stress-related): ________
____
____
____

Drug History and Assessment

Use of prescribed drugs:

Name	*Dosage*	*Prescribed for*	*Results*

Use of over-the-counter drugs:

Name	*Dosage*	*Used for*	*Results*

Use of street drugs and/or alcohol:

Name	*Amount Used*	*How Often Used*	*When Last Used*	*Effects Produced*

Pertinent Physical Assessments

RESPIRATIONS Normal: _____ Labored: _____
Rate: _____ Rhythm: _____

SKIN Warm: _____ Dry: _____ Moist: _____ Cool: _____
Clammy: _____ Pink: _____ Cyanotic: _____
Poor turgor: _____ Edematous: _____
Evidence of: Rash: _____ Bruising: _____

Needle tracks: _____ Hirsutism: _____ Loss of hair: _____
Other: ____

MUSCULOSKELETAL STATUS Weakness: __ Tremors: __
Degree of range of motion (describe limitations): ______
____
Pain (describe): ____________________________________
Skeletal deformities (describe): ________________________
Coordination (describe limitations): ___________________

NEUROLOGICAL STATUS
History of (check all that apply): Seizures: _____________
(describe method of control): _________________________
Headaches (describe location and frequency): _________
____
Fainting spells: _________ Dizziness: _____________
Tingling/numbness (describe location): _______________

CARDIOVASCULAR BP: _____ Pulse: _____
History of (check all that apply):
Hypertension: _____ Palpitations: ___________________
Heart murmur: _____ Chest pain: ___________________
Shortness of breath: _____ Pain in legs: _______________
Phlebitis: _____ Ankle/leg edema: ___________________
Numbness/tingling in extremities: ___________________
Varicose veins: ____________________________________

GASTROINTESTINAL
Usual diet pattern: _________________________________
Food allergies: ____________________________________
Dentures? _____ Upper: _____ Lower: ________________
Any problems with chewing or swallowing? ___________
Any recent change in weight? _______________________
Any problems with:
Indigestion/heartburn? _____________________________
Relieved by: ____________________________________
Nausea/vomiting? _________________________________
Relieved by: ____________________________________
Loss of appetite? _________________________________
History of ulcers? __________________________________
Usual bowel pattern: ________________________________
Constipation: _____ Diarrhea: _______________________
Type of self-care assistance provided for either of the above problems: _____________________________________

GENITOURINARY/REPRODUCTIVE
Usual voiding pattern: ______________________________
Urinary hesitancy: _____ Frequency: __________________

Nocturia: _____ Pain/burning: ________________________
Incontinence: ________________________________
Genital lesions: ______________________________
Discharge: _____ Odor: ______________________
History of venereal disease: _____ If yes, explain: _______
____
Any concerns about sexuality/sexual activity: _________
____
____
Method of birth control used: ____________________

Females:
Date of last menstrual cycle: ___________________
Length of cycle: _____________________________
Problems associated with menstruation: __________
____
Breasts: Pain/tenderness: ______________________
Swelling: _____ Discharge: ____________________
Lumps: _____ Dimpling: _______________________
Practice self–breast examination: _______________
Frequency: __________________________________

Males:
Penile discharge: ______________________________
Prostate problems: _____________________________

Eyes:	*Yes*	*No*	*Explain*
Glasses	_____	_____	____________
Contacts	_____	_____	____________
Swelling	_____	_____	____________
Discharge	_____	_____	____________
Itching	_____	_____	____________
Blurring	_____	_____	____________
Double vision	_____	_____	____________

Ears:	*Yes*	*No*	*Explain*
Pain	_____	_____	____________
Drainage	_____	_____	____________
Difficulty hearing	_____	_____	____________
Hearing aid	_____	_____	____________
Tinnitus	_____	_____	____________

MEDICATION SIDE EFFECTS Symptoms that may be attributed to current medication usage: ______________
____
____

ALTERED LABORATORY VALUES AND POSSIBLE SIGNIFICANCE

____

____

ACTIVITY/REST PATTERNS

Exercise (amount, type, frequency):________________

____

Leisure time activities:___________________________

____

Patterns of sleep: Number of hours per night:________
Use of sleep aids:________________
Pattern of awakening during the night: ______________________
____
Feeling rested on awakening:______

PERSONAL HYGIENE/ACTIVITIES OF DAILY LIVING

Patterns of self-care: Independent ________________
Requires assistance with: Mobility ________________
Hygiene ________________
Toileting ________________
Feeding ________________
Dressing ________________
Other ________________

Statement describing personal hygiene and general appearance:________________________________

____

OTHER PERTINENT PHYSICAL ASSESSMENTS ____

____

____

Summary of Initial Psychosocial/Physical Assessment

Knowledge Deficits Identified

Nursing Diagnoses Indicated

---

*Modified with permission from Nursing Faculty, Butler County Community College, El Dorado, KS, who formulated this tool in August 1984 based on the concept of stress adaptation.

SAMPLE: NURSING HISTORY, ASSESSMENT, AND CARE PLAN

■ GENERAL INFORMATION

Sam is a 45-year-old white male admitted to the psychiatric unit of a general medical center by his family physician, Dr. Jones, who reported that Sam had become increasingly despondent over the last month. His wife reported that he had made statements such as, "Life is not worth living," and "I think I could just take all those pills Dr. Jones prescribed at one time; then it would all be over." He was admitted at 6:40 PM via wheelchair from admissions and accompanied by his wife. He reports no known allergies. Vital signs upon admission were temperature, 97.9°F; P, 80; respirations, 16; and BP, 132/77. He is 5 feet 11 inches tall and weighs 160 lb. He was referred to Dr. Smith, the psychiatrist on call. Orders include suicide precautions, level I; regular diet; chemistry profile and routine urinalysis in AM; Desyrel, 200 mg tid; Dalmane, 30 mg hs prn for sleep.

■ PREDISPOSING FACTORS

Genetic Influences

Family Configuration

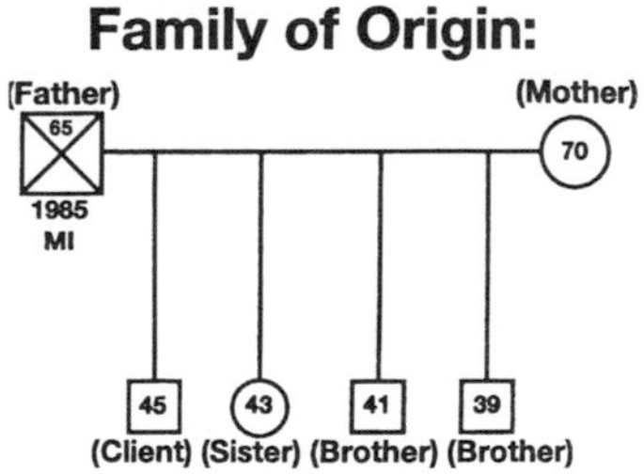

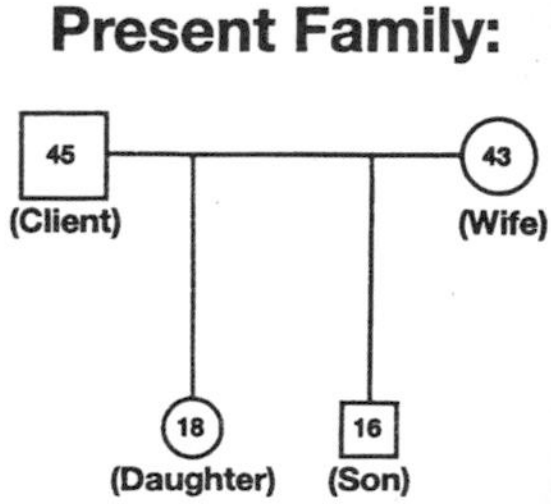

DYNAMICS Sam says he loves his wife and children and does not want to hurt them but feels they no longer need him. He states, "They would probably be better off without me." His wife appears to be very concerned about his condition, though in his despondency, he seems oblivious to her feelings. His mother lives in a neighboring state, and he sees her infrequently. He admits that he is somewhat bitter toward her for allowing him and his siblings to "suffer from the physical and emotional brutality of their father." His siblings and their families live in distant states, and he sees them rarely, during holiday gatherings. He feels closest to the older of the two brothers.

Medical/Psychiatric History

Sam's father died 5 years ago of a myocardial infarction at age 65. Sam and both his brothers have a history of high cholesterol and triglycerides from approximately age 30. During his regular physical examination 1 month ago, Sam's family doctor recognized symptoms of depression and prescribed Elavil. Sam's mother has a history of depressive episodes. She was hospitalized once about 7 years ago for depression, and she has taken various antidepressant medications over the years. Her family physician has also prescribed Valium for her on numerous occasions for her "nerves." No other family members have a history of psychiatric problems.

Past Experiences

Sam was the first child in a family of four. He is 2 years older than his sister and 4 years older than the third child, a brother. He was 6 years old when his youngest sibling, also a boy, was born. Sam's father was a career Army man, who moved his family many times during their childhood years. Sam attended 15 schools from the time he entered kindergarten until he graduated from high school.

Sam reports that his father was very autocratic and had many rules that he expected his children to obey without question. Infraction resulted in harsh discipline. Because Sam was the oldest child, his father believed Sam should assume responsibility for the behavior of his siblings. Sam describes the severe physical punishment he received from his father when he or his siblings allegedly violated one of the rules. It was particularly intense when Sam's father had been drinking, which he did most evenings and weekends.

Sam's mother was very passive. Sam believes she was afraid of his father, particularly when he was drinking, so she quietly conformed to his lifestyle and offered no resistance, even though she did not agree with his disciplining of the children. Sam reports that he observed his father physically abusing his mother on a number of occasions, most often when he had been drinking.

Sam states that he had very few friends when he was growing up. With all the family moves, he gave up trying to make new friends because it became too painful to give them up when it was time to leave. He took a paper route when he was 13 years old and then worked in fast food restaurants from age 15 on. He was a hard worker and never seemed to have difficulty finding work in any of the family's relocations. He states that he appreciated the independence and being away from home as much as his job would allow. "I guess I can honestly say I hated my father, and working was my way of getting away from all the stress that was going on in that house. I guess my dad hated me, too, because he never was satisfied with anything I did. I never did well enough for him in school, on the job, or even at home. When I think of my dad now, my memories are of being criticized and beaten with a belt."

On graduation from high school, Sam joined the Navy, where he learned a skill that he used after discharge to obtain a job in a large aircraft plant. He also attended the local university at night, where he earned his accounting degree. When he completed his degree, he was reassigned to the administration department of the aircraft company, and he has been in the same position for 12 years without a promotion.

Sam says he believes in God but does not attend a church. He drinks socially but does not smoke. He has regular physical, dental, and eye examinations.

Significant losses include loss of self-esteem due to being passed over for promotion and loss of a satisfactory father-son relationship.

His previous pattern of coping with stress was to develop a migraine headache, to escape into sleep, to use suppression excessively, or to become mildly depressed and withdrawn until the stressor was relieved.

Existing Conditions

Stage of Development

Sam is in the generativity versus self-absorption stage. Most of the time he is fulfilling the tasks of generativity (successful at work and in community; rearing children).

However, when depressed, he becomes very self-absorbed and his behaviors are focused inward.

Sam has a strong support system in his wife and children. He is currently holding a position of responsibility in the aircraft company, his wife teaches elementary school, and they have sufficient insurance to cover medical expenses. He has fulfilled his responsibilities on the job and in the home until recently, when his despondency began to interfere with social and occupational functioning.

■ PRECIPITATING EVENT

Over the last 12 years, Sam has watched while a number of his peers were promoted to management positions. Sam has been considered for several of these positions but has never been selected. Last month a management position became available for which Sam felt he was qualified. He applied for this position, believing he had a good chance of being promoted. However, when the announcement was made, the position had been given to a younger man who had been with the company only 5 years. Sam seemed to accept the decision, but over the last few weeks he has become more and more withdrawn. He speaks to very few people at the office and is becoming more and more behind in his work. At home, he eats very little, talks to family members only when they ask a direct question, withdraws to his bedroom very early in the evening, and does not come out until time to leave for work the next morning. Today, he refused to get out of bed or to go to work. His wife convinced him to talk to their family doctor, who admitted him to the hospital.

■ CLIENT'S PERCEPTION OF THE STRESSOR

Sam states that all his life he has "not been good enough at anything. I could never please my father. Now I can't seem to please my boss. What's the use of trying? I came to the hospital because my wife and my doctor are afraid I might try to kill myself. I must admit the thought has crossed my mind more than once. I seem to have very little motivation for living. I just don't care any more."

■ ADAPTATION RESPONSES

Psychosocial

1. Anxiety level is moderate. Client is alert and cooperative, though attention seems to be impaired at times and client has difficulty concentrating. No misinterpretation of the environment noted.
2. Mood is one of dejection and despair. Affect is sad, flat, with little emotional tone.
3. Ego defense mechanisms employed:
   a. ***Displacement:*** Client is displacing anger at parents and boss onto self.
   b. ***Regression:*** Client is withdrawing into self and becoming socially isolated.
4. Level of self-esteem is very low. Client speaks of himself as never having been able to please the important people in his life. Feels as though family would be better off without him. Eye contact is poor. Client looks at hands in lap while talking. Hygiene appears to be appropriate, but general appearance is disheveled. Clothes are wrinkled, hair is uncombed. Interaction with others is virtually nil.
5. Regarding stage of grief, client appears to be fixed in the anger stage of the grieving process, and the anger is turned inward on the self. Manifestations include feelings of low self-esteem and despair at what he perceives as a lack of accomplishment in his life.
6. Thought processes are clear and logical, though there is some slowness in thought association.
7. Communication patterns are clear and coherent, but with some ruminations regarding his inability to please his parents and boss.
8. Interaction patterns: withdrawn; isolated; passive; no attempt to interact with others.
9. Client is oriented to time, person, place, and situation.
10. Client admits to having thoughts of killing self at this time. He had previously considered taking an overdose of Elavil, which had been prescribed by his family physician. He does not have the Elavil with him in the hospital.

Physiological

1. Sam states that he sometimes experiences migraine headaches (HA). He has not noticed whether they occur more often during periods of stress.

2. **Drug History and Assessment**
   a. ***Use of Prescribed Drugs***
      - Elavil, 50 mg bid, for depression. No improvement.
      - Fiorinal #3, 1 capsule q 8 hr as needed for headache pain. Relief obtained.
      - Robaxin, 750 mg prn for back pain. Relief obtained.
   b. ***Use of Over-the-Counter Drugs***
      - Aspirin, 2 tablets prn for headache. Relief obtained.
      - Actifed, 1 tablet prn for sinus drainage. Relief obtained.
      - Mylanta, 2 tablets prn for heartburn. Relief obtained.
   c. ***Use of Street Drugs and/or Alcohol***
      - Denies use of street drugs. Social drinking and two beers or glasses of wine in the evenings. Last consumed two nights ago. "Relaxes me and helps me sleep."
3. **Pertinent Physical Assessments**
   a. ***Respirations:*** Normal; rate, 16; rhythm regular.
   b. ***Skin:*** Warm and dry; pink; diminished turgor; no noticeable edema; 3-inch scar on right thigh from childhood injury.
   c. ***Range of Motion:*** Full.
   d. ***Neurological Status:*** Migraine headache about once a month; pain is usually unilateral, behind eye, in temple, and at base of skull. Fiorinal #3 provides some relief, but he usually has to sleep until pain subsides.
   e. ***Cardiovascular:*** BP, 132/77; P, 80. Denies pain or any numbness or tingling.
   f. ***Gastrointestinal:*** Usually eats a light breakfast and lunch with heaviest meal in the evening. Lately, has been able to eat very little. Has no desire to eat. Has lost about 10 lb in the last 3 weeks. Denies any food allergies. Experiences heartburn 3 to 4 times per week, which is relieved by two Mylanta tablets. No history of peptic ulcers. Denies problems with constipation. Reports daily bowel movement; however, with loss of appetite, has a bowel movement every 2 to 3 days.
   g. ***Genitourinary/Reproductive:*** Denies any problems with voiding. Denies concerns about sexuality; however, reports decrease in libido with feelings of depression. Vasectomy performed when client was 32 years old.

h. ***Eyes:*** Wears bifocal glasses for both close and distant vision. Complained of occasional blurred vision.
i. ***Ears:*** Denies problems with ears or hearing. Reports occasional mild tinnitus with aspirin use.
j. ***Medication Side Effects:*** Client complains of dry mouth and blurred vision (both common side effects of Elavil).
k. ***Altered Laboratory Values and Possible Significance:***
   Serum albumin, 3.3 g/dL (normal, 3.5 to 5), possibly caused by malnourished condition
   BUN, 16 mg/100 mL (normal, 10 to 15); may be caused by mild dehydration
   Cholesterol, 275 mg/dL (150 to 250), familial hyper-cholesterolemia
   Sodium, 143 mEq/L (normal, 136 to 142), possible dehydration and insufficient water intake
l. ***Activity/Rest Patterns:*** Exercises very little; enjoys walking but does not seem to have the energy lately. Used to play bridge in leisure time but has not socialized much in last couple of months. Sleeps at least 8 hours per night. Lately, since depressed, some nights falls asleep right after dinner (or even before) and sleeps till morning. Still has very little energy.
m. ***Personal Hygiene/Activities of Daily Living (ADLs):*** Functions independently in ADLs. Client is clean, with no noticeable body odor. Clothes are clean but wrinkled (as though they had been slept in). Hair is not combed. Has about 2 days' growth of beard.

■ SUMMARY OF INITIAL PSYCHOSOCIAL/PHYSICAL ASSESSMENT

A 45-year-old gentleman admitted to the psychiatric unit by family physician after expressing suicidal ideations. He is very despondent and admits to having thoughts of suicide. He is lethargic and unkempt. He maintains minimal eye contact. There is no evidence of psychotic behaviors. Thinking process is slow but intact. Client is withdrawn, with minimal verbalizations, but he is cooperative with admission process.

■ KNOWLEDGE DEFICITS IDENTIFIED

Client needs to learn:

- Available resources when feeling suicidal
- Ways to increase self-esteem
- Side effects of Desyrel
- Methods of relaxation
- Assertiveness techniques
- More appropriate ways of coping with stress

■ NURSING DIAGNOSES INDICATED

1. Risk for suicide related to depressed mood and expressions of having nothing to live for.
2. Dysfunctional grieving related to unresolved losses (promotion and satisfactory father-son relationship) evidenced by anger turned inward on self and desire to end life.
3. Chronic low self-esteem related to lack of positive feedback and learned helplessness evidenced by a sense of worthlessness, lack of eye contact, social isolation, and negative/pessimistic outlook.
4. Social isolation related to depressed mood and feelings of worthlessness evidenced by withdrawal and desire to be alone; uncommunicative.
5. Powerlessness related to lack of positive feedback evidenced by apathy, passivity, and statements: "I was never able to please my father; now I can't please my boss. What's the use of trying? I just don't care anymore."
6. Alteration in nutrition, less than body requirements related to decreased food intake because of depressed mood and loss of appetite evidenced by loss of weight (10 lb in 3 weeks), diminished skin turgor, decreased serum albumin, increased serum sodium.

Nursing Diagnoses and Interventions for Sam

■ RISK FOR SUICIDE

Related/Risk Factors ("related to")

Depressed mood
Expressions of having nothing to live for

Goals/Objectives

Short-Term Goal

Client will seek out staff when ideas of suicide occur.

Long-Term Goal

Client will not harm self during hospitalization.

Interventions with *Selected Rationales*

1. Ask client directly: "Have you thought about killing yourself? If so, what do you plan to do? Do you have the means to carry out this plan?" ***The risk of suicide is greatly increased if the client has developed a plan, and particularly if means exist for the client to execute the plan.***
2. Create a safe environment for the client. Remove all potentially harmful objects from client's access (sharp objects, straps, belts, ties, glass items). ***Client safety is a nursing priority.***
3. Formulate a short-term verbal contract with the client that he will not harm himself during next 24 hours. When that contract expires, make another, and so forth. ***Discussion of suicidal feelings with a trusted individual provides a degree of relief to the client. A contract gets the subject out in the open and places some of the responsibility for his safety with the client. An attitude of acceptance of the client as a worthwhile individual is conveyed.***
4. Secure a promise from the client that he will seek out a staff member if thoughts of suicide emerge. ***Suicidal clients are often very ambivalent about their feelings. Discussion of feelings with a trusted individual may provide assistance before the client experiences a crisis situation.***
5. Encourage verbalizations of honest feelings. Through exploration and discussion, help client to identify symbols of hope in his life (participating in activities he finds satisfying outside of his job).
6. Allow client to express angry feelings within appropriate limits. Encourage use of exercise room and punching bag each day. Help client to identify true source of anger, and work on adaptive coping skills for use outside the hospital (e.g., jogging, exercise club available to employees of his company). ***Depression and suicidal behaviors may be viewed as anger turned inward on the self. If this anger can be verbalized in a nonthreatening environment, the client may be able to resolve these feelings, regardless of the discomfort involved. Physical activities relieve pent-up tension.***

7. Identify community resources that the client may use as a support system and from whom he may request help if feeling suicidal (e.g., suicidal or crisis hotline; psychiatrist or social worker at community mental health center; hospital "HELP" line). ***Having a concrete plan for seeking assistance during a crisis may discourage or prevent self-destructive behaviors.***
8. Introduce client to support and education groups for adult children of alcoholics (ACOA). ***The purpose of these ACOA groups is to help members overcome the guilt, depression, low self-esteem, and other characteristics common to adults who grew up in homes with an alcohol-dependent parent.***
9. Most important, spend time with the client. ***This provides a feeling of safety and security, while also conveying the message, "I want to spend time with you because I think you are a worthwhile person."***

Outcome Criteria

1. Client verbalizes no thoughts of suicide and expresses some hope for the future.
2. Client is able to verbalize names of resources outside the hospital from whom he may request help if feeling suicidal.

DYSFUNCTIONAL GRIEVING

Possible Etiologies ("related to")

Unresolved losses (job promotion and satisfactory father-son relationship)

Defining Characteristics ("evidenced by")

Anger turned inward on self and desire to end life

Goals/Objectives

Short-Term Goal

Client will verbalize anger toward boss and parents within 1 week.

Long-Term Goal

Client will verbalize own position in grief process and begin movement in the progression toward resolution by discharge.

Interventions with *Selected Rationales*

1. Client is fixed in anger stage of grieving process. Discuss with him behaviors associated with this stage. ***Accurate***

baseline assessment data are necessary to effectively plan care for the grieving client.

2. Develop trusting relationship with client. Show empathy and caring. Be honest and keep all promises. ***Trust is the basis for a therapeutic relationship.***
3. Convey an accepting attitude—one in which client is not afraid to express feelings openly. ***An accepting attitude conveys to the client that you believe he is a worthwhile person. Trust is enhanced.***
4. Allow client to verbalize feelings of anger. Initial expression of anger may be displaced on nurse or therapist. Do not become defensive if this should occur. Assist client to explore angry feelings so that they may be directed toward the intended persons. ***Verbalization of feelings in a nonthreatening environment may help client come to terms with unresolved issues.***
5. Assist client to discharge pent-up anger through participation in large motor activities (brisk walks, jogging, physical exercises, volleyball, punching bag, exercise bike, or other equipment. ***Physical exercise provides a safe and effective method for discharging pent-up tension.***
6. Explain normal stages of grief and the behaviors associated with each stage. Help client to understand that feelings such as guilt and anger toward boss and parents are appropriate and acceptable during this stage of the grieving process. Help him also to understand that he must work through these feelings and move past this stage to eventually feel better. ***Knowledge of acceptability of the feelings associated with normal grieving may help to relieve some of the guilt that these responses generate. Knowing why he is experiencing these feelings may also help to resolve them.***
7. Encourage client to review relationship with his parents. With support and sensitivity, point out reality of the situation in areas in which misrepresentations are expressed. Explain common roles and behaviors of members in an alcoholic family. ***Client must give up desire for idealized family and accept the reality of his childhood situation and the effect it has had on his adult life before the grief process can be completed.***
8. Assist client in problem solving as he attempts to determine methods for more adaptive coping. Suggest alternatives to anger turned inward on the self when negative thinking sets in (e.g., thought-stopping techniques). Provide positive feedback for strategies identified and decisions made. ***Positive feedback increases self-esteem and encourages repetition of desirable behaviors.***

9. Encourage client to reach out for spiritual support during this time in whatever form is desirable to him. Assess spiritual needs of client, and assist as necessary in the fulfillment of those needs.

Outcome Criteria

1. Client is able to verbalize normal stages of grief process and behaviors associated with each stage.
2. Client is able to identify own position within the grief process and express honest feelings related to loss of job promotion and satisfactory parent-child relationship.
3. Client is no longer manifesting exaggerated emotions and behaviors related to dysfunctional grieving and is able to carry out ADLs independently.

CHRONIC LOW SELF-ESTEEM

Possible Etiologies ("related to")

Lack of positive feedback and learned helplessness

Defining Characteristics ("evidenced by")

A sense of worthlessness, lack of eye contact, social isolation and negative, pessimistic outlook.

Goals/Objectives

Short-Term Goal

Client will discuss feelings about self, and when these feelings were developed, with staff nurse by 1 week.

Long-Term Goal

Client will exhibit increased feelings of self-worth by discharge, as evidenced by verbal expression of positive aspects about self, past accomplishments, and future prospects.

Interventions with *Selected Rationales*

1. Be accepting of client and his negativism. *An attitude of acceptance enhances feelings of self-worth.*
2. Spend time with client *to convey acceptance and contribute toward feelings of self-worth.*
3. Help client to recognize and focus on strengths, accomplishments, and experiences that create good feelings about himself. Minimize attention given to past (real or perceived) failures. *Self-esteem is enhanced by recog-*

nition and discussion of positive aspects of self. Lack of attention to negative ruminations may help to eliminate them.

4. Encourage participation in group activities from which client may receive positive feedback and support from peers. *Recognition and acceptance increase self-esteem.*
5. Help client identify realistic aspects he would like to change about himself and assist with problem solving toward this effort. *Low self-worth may interfere with client's perception of own problem-solving ability. Assistance may be required.*
6. Ensure that client is not becoming increasingly dependent and that he is accepting responsibility for his own behaviors. *Client must be able to function independently if he is to be successful within the less-structured community environment.*
7. Ensure that therapy groups offer client simple methods of achievement within a short time period. Offer recognition and positive feedback for actual accomplishments. *Successes and recognition increase self-esteem.*
8. Teach assertiveness techniques: The ability to recognize the differences among passive, assertive, and aggressive behaviors; the importance of respecting the human rights of others while protecting one's own basic human rights. *Self-esteem is enhanced by the ability to interact with others in an assertive manner.*
9. Teach effective communication techniques, such as the use of "I" messages and placing emphasis on ways to avoid making judgmental statements.
10. Assist client to perform aspects of self-care where required. Offer positive feedback for tasks performed independently. *Successful accomplishments and positive feedback enhance self-esteem and encourage repetition of desirable behaviors.*

Outcome Criteria

1. Client is able to verbalize positive aspects about self.
2. Client is able to communicate assertively with others.
3. Client expresses some optimism and hope for the future.

SOCIAL ISOLATION

Possible Etiologies ("related to")

Depressed mood and feelings of worthlessness

Defining Characteristics ("evidenced by")

Withdrawal and desire to be alone; uncommunicative

Goals/Objectives

Short-Term Goal

Client will develop trusting relationship with one staff nurse by end of first week of hospitalization.

Long-Term Goal

Client will voluntarily spend time with other clients and staff members in group activities on the unit by discharge.

Interventions with *Selected Rationales*

1. Spend time with client. This may mean just sitting in silence for a while. ***Presence of the nurse will help improve client's perception of self as a worthwhile person.***
2. Develop a therapeutic nurse-client relationship through frequent, brief contacts and an accepting attitude. Show unconditional positive regard. ***The nurse's presence, acceptance, and conveyance of positive regard will enhance the client's feelings of self-worth.***
3. After client feels comfortable in one-to-one relationship, encourage attendance in group activities. May need to attend with him the first few times to offer support. Accept client's decision to remove himself from group situation if anxiety becomes too great. ***The presence of a trusted individual provides emotional security for the client.***
4. Verbally acknowledge client's absence from any group activities. ***Knowledge that his absence was noticed may reinforce the client's feelings of self-worth.***
5. Teach client assertiveness techniques. Interactions with others may be discouraged by client's use of passive or aggressive behaviors. ***Knowledge and use of assertive techniques may increase self-confidence and improve client's relationships with others.***
6. Provide lots of structure in client's daily activities. Devise a time schedule of therapeutic activities and provide client with a written copy. Try to schedule most of his activities for afternoon and early evening. ***Depressed clients must have considerable structure in their lives because of impairment in decision-making and problem-solving abilities. The written schedule provides a concreteness from which the client can derive some security. Severely depressed clients feel their worst early in the morning and feel better as the day progresses.***

7. Teach skills that client may use to approach others in a socially acceptable manner. Practice these skills with client through role playing.
8. Provide positive reinforcement for client's voluntary interactions with others. ***Positive reinforcement enhances self-esteem and encourages repetition of desirable behaviors.***

Outcome Criteria

1. Client demonstrates willingness or desire to socialize with others.
2. Client voluntarily attends group activities.
3. Client approaches others in appropriate manner for one-to-one interaction.

POWERLESSNESS

Possible Etiologies ("related to")

Lack of positive feedback

Defining Characteristics ("evidenced by")

"I could never please my father. Now I can't seem to please my boss. What's the use of trying? . . . I just don't care anymore."

Goals/Objectives

Short-Term Goal

Client will take charge of own ADL within 1 week.

Long-Term Goal

Client will be able to effectively problem-solve ways to take control of own life situation by discharge, thereby decreasing feelings of powerlessness.

Interventions with *Selected Rationales*

1. Allow client to take as much responsibility as possible for own self-care practices. ***Providing client with choices will increase his feelings of control.*** Examples:
   a. Include client in setting the goals of care he wishes to achieve.
   b. Allow client to establish own schedule for self-care activities.
   c. Provide client with privacy as need is determined.
   d. Provide positive feedback for decisions made. Respect client's right to make those decisions independently,

and refrain from attempting to influence him toward those that may seem more logical.

2. Assist client to set realistic goals for himself. ***Goals that are unrealistic set the client up for failure, reinforcing feelings of powerlessness.***
3. Help client identify areas of life situation that he can control (employment situation). ***Client's emotional condition interferes with his ability to problem-solve. Assistance is required to accurately perceive the benefits and consequences of available alternatives.***
4. Help client identify areas of life situation that are not within his ability to control (loss of satisfactory father-son relationship). Encourage verbalization of feelings related to this inability ***in an effort to deal with unresolved issues and accept what cannot be changed.***
5. Identify ways in which client can achieve. Encourage participation in these activities and provide positive reinforcement for participation, as well as achievement. ***Positive reinforcement enhances self-esteem and encourages repetition of desirable behaviors.***

Outcome Criteria

1. Client verbalizes choices he has made in a plan to maintain control over his own life situation.
2. Client verbalizes honest feelings about life situations over which he has no control.
3. Client is able to verbalize system for problem solving as required for adequate role performance.

ALTERED NUTRITION, LESS THAN BODY REQUIREMENTS

Possible Etiologies ("related to")

Decreased food intake because of depressed mood and loss of appetite

Defining Characteristics ("evidenced by")

Loss of weight (10 lb in 3 weeks), diminished skin turgor, decreased serum albumin, increased serum sodium

Goals/Objectives

Short-Term Goal

By third hospital day, client will eat regular meals and snacks as provided on each shift.

Long-Term Goal

By discharge, client will exhibit no signs or symptoms of malnutrition.

Interventions with *Selected Rationales*

1. In collaboration with dietitian, determine number of calories required to provide adequate nutrition and realistic weight gain.
2. Ensure that diet includes foods high in fiber content to prevent constipation. Encourage client to increase fluid consumption and physical exercise to promote normal bowel functioning. Fluid is also required to correct mildly dehydrated condition. ***Depressed clients are particularly vulnerable to constipation brought on by psychomotor retardation. Abnormal laboratory values indicate possible mild dehydration.***
3. Perform strict documentation of intake, output, calorie count. ***This information is necessary to make an accurate nutritional assessment and maintain client safety.***
4. Weigh client daily. ***Weight loss or gain is important assessment information.***
5. Determine client's likes and dislikes and collaborate with dietitian to provide favorite foods. Encourage wife to bring in foods that he has enjoyed in the past. ***Client is more likely to eat foods that he particularly enjoys.***
6. If client continues to experience loss of appetite, it may be desirable to provide small, frequent feedings, including a bedtime snack, rather than three larger meals. ***Large amounts of food may be objectionable, or even intolerable, to an anorectic client.***
7. Stay with client during meals to assist as needed and to offer support and encouragement. ***Mealtime is a social time, and the presence of a trusted individual can provide needed security.***
8. Monitor laboratory values, and report significant changes to physician. Monitor serum albumin, sodium, and blood urea nitrogen for return to normal levels. ***Laboratory values provide objective data regarding nutritional status.***
9. Teach the importance of adequate nutrition and fluid intake. ***Client may have inadequate or inaccurate knowledge regarding the contribution of good nutrition to overall wellness.***

Outcome Criteria

1. Client has shown a slow, progressive weight gain during hospitalization.

2. Vital signs, blood pressure, and all laboratory serum studies are within normal limits.
3. Client is able to verbalize importance of adequate nutrition and fluid intake.

■ INTERNET REFERENCES

- http://www.nursingworld.org
- http://www.sciencekomm.at/journals/medicine/nurse.html

CHAPTER 2

Concepts of Psychobiology

■ INTRODUCTION

The 101st legislature of the United States designated the 1990s as the "decade of the brain." With this legislation came the challenge of studying the biological basis of behavior. In keeping with this "neuroscientific revolution," greater emphasis has been placed on the study of the organic basis for psychiatric illness. Certain mental illnesses are now looked upon as "physical illnesses characterized by, or resulting from, malfunctions and/or malformations of the brain" (Peschel and Peschel, 1991).

This is not to imply that psychosocial and sociocultural influences are totally discounted. The systems of biology, psychology, and sociology are not mutually exclusive but are interacting systems. This is clearly indicated by the fact that individuals experience biological changes in response to various environmental events. Indeed, each of these disciplines may at various times be most appropriate for explaining behavioral phenomena.

This chapter presents an overview of neurophysiological, neurochemical, and endocrine influences on psychiatric illness. Various diagnostic procedures used to detect alterations in biological function that may contribute to psychiatric illness are identified.

■ NEUROPHYSIOLOGICAL INFLUENCES

The Brain

Following is a summary of the major structures of the brain and their primary functions. Diagrams of these structures are presented in Figures 2–1, 2–2, and 2–3.

1. **The Forebrain:** The forebrain is composed of the cerebrum and the diencephalon.
   a. ***Cerebrum:*** The cerebrum is composed of two hemispheres separated by a deep groove that houses a band of 200 million neurons called the *corpus callosum*. The outer shell is called the *cortex*. It is extensively folded and consists of billions of neurons. The left hemisphere appears to be dominant in most

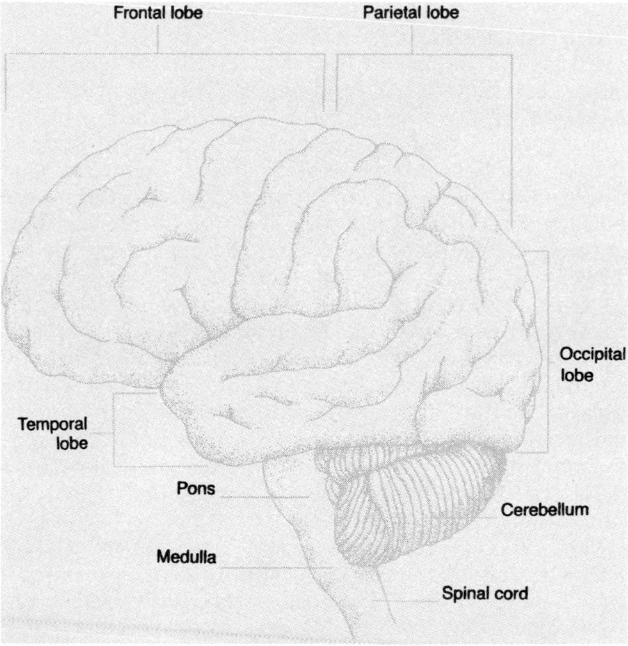

Figure 2–1. The human brain: cerebral lobes, cerebellum, and brain stem. (Adapted from Scanlon VC and Sanders T: Essentials of Anatomy and Physiology, ed. 3. FA Davis, Philadelphia, 1999, p 165, with permission.)

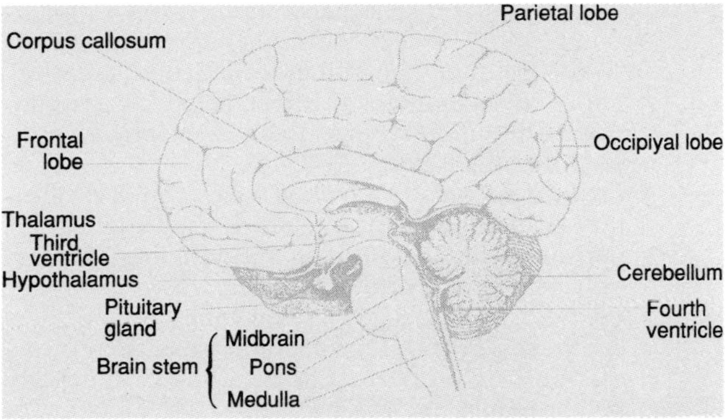

Figure 2–2. The human brain: midsagittal surface. (Adapted from Scanlon VC and Sanders T: Essentials of Anatomy and Physiology, ed. 3. FA Davis, Philadelphia, 1999, p 165, with permission.)

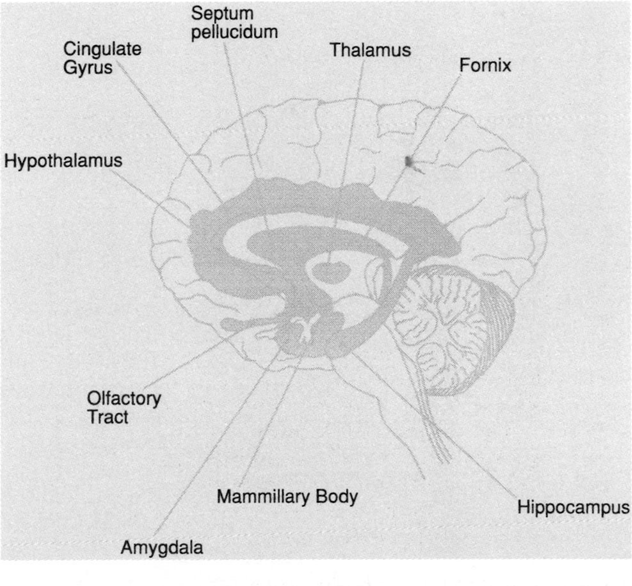

Figure 2–3. Structures of the limbic system. (Adapted from Scanlon VC and Sanders T: Essentials of Anatomy and Physiology, ed. 3. FA Davis, Philadelphia, 1999, p 165, with permission.)

people. It controls speech, comprehension, rationality, and logic. The right hemisphere is nondominant in most people. Sometimes called the "creative" brain, it is associated with affect, behavior, and spacial perceptual functions. Each hemisphere is divided into four lobes.

- ***Frontal Lobes:*** The frontal lobes control voluntary body movement, including movements that permit speaking, thinking and judgment formation, and expression of feelings.
- ***Parietal Lobes:*** The parietal lobes control perception and interpretation of most sensory information (including touch, pain, taste, and body position).
- ***Temporal Lobes:*** The temporal lobes are concerned with hearing, short-term memory, sense of smell, and expression of emotions through connection with the limbic system.
- ***Occipital Lobes:*** The occipital lobes are the primary area of visual reception and interpretation.

b. ***Diencephalon:*** The diencephalon connects the cerebrum with lower brain structures. Its major structures include the thalamus, hypothalamus, and limbic system.

- ***Thalamus:*** The thalamus integrates all sensory input (except smell) on its way to the cortex. The thalamus also has some involvement with emotions and mood.
- ***Hypothalamus:*** The hypothalamus regulates the anterior and posterior lobes of the pituitary gland. It exerts control over the actions of the autonomic nervous system and regulates appetite and temperature.
- ***Limbic System:*** The limbic system consists of medially placed cortical and subcortical structures and the fiber tracts connecting them with one another and with the hypothalamus. These structures include the hippocampus, mammillary body, amygdala, olfactory tract, hypothalamus, cingulate gyrus, septum pellucidum, thalamus, and fornix. The limbic system, which is sometimes called the "emotional brain," is associated with feelings of fear and anxiety; anger and aggression; love, joy, and hope; and with sexuality and social behavior.

2. **The Midbrain:** The main structures of the midbrain are called the mesencephalon.

a. ***Mesencephalon:*** Structures of major importance in the mesencephalon include nuclei and fiber tracts. They extend from the pons to the hypothalamus and are responsible for the integration of visual, auditory, and balance ("righting") reflexes.

3. **The Hindbrain:** The hindbrain consists of the pons, the medulla, and the cerebellum.
   a. ***Pons:*** The pons is responsible for regulation of respiration and skeletal muscle tone. Ascending and descending fiber tracts of the pons connect the brain stem with the cerebellum and cortex.
   b. ***Medulla:*** The medulla provides a pathway for all ascending and descending fiber tracts. It contains vital centers that regulate heart rate, blood pressure, and respiration, and reflex centers for swallowing, sneezing, coughing, and vomiting.
   c. ***Cerebellum:*** The cerebellum regulates muscle tone and coordination and maintains posture and equilibrium.

Nerve Tissue

The tissue of the central nervous system (CNS) consists of nerve cells called neurons that generate and transmit electrochemical impulses. The structure of a neuron is composed of a cell body, an axon, and dendrites. The cell body contains the nucleus and is essential for the continued life of the neuron. The dendrites are processes that transmit impulses toward the cell body, and the axon transmits impulses away from the cell body. Cells called *afferent* (or *sensory*) *neurons* carry impulses from the periphery to the CNS, where they are interpreted into various sensations. The *efferent* (or *motor*) *neurons* carry impulses from the CNS to the muscles and glands of the periphery. A third type of cell, called *interneurons*, exists entirely within the CNS. Ninety-nine percent of all nerve cells belong to this group. They may carry only sensory or motor impulses, or they may serve as integrators in the pathways between afferent and efferent neurons. They account in large part for thinking, feelings, learning, language, and memory.

Some messages may be processed through only a few neurons, while others may require thousands of neuronal connections. The neurons that transmit the impulses do not actually touch each other. The junction between two neurons is called a *synapse*. The small space between the axon terminals of one neuron and the cell body or dendrites of another is called the *synaptic cleft*.

Chemicals called *neurotransmitters* are stored in the axon terminals of presynaptic neurons. Electrical impulses cause the release of these chemicals into the synaptic cleft. The neurotransmitter combines with receptor sites on the postsynaptic neuron, resulting in a determination of whether another electrical impulse is generated.

■ NEUROCHEMICAL INFLUENCES

Neurotransmitters

Neurotransmitters are responsible for essential functions in the role of human emotion and behavior. They are also the target for the mechanism of action of many of the psychotropic medications.

After a neurotransmitter has performed its function in the synaptic cleft, it either returns to the vesicles in the axon terminals to be stored and used again, or it is inactivated and dissolved by enzymes. The process of being stored for reuse is called *reuptake*, a function that holds significance for understanding the mechanism of action of certain psychotropic medications.

Many neurotransmitters exist within the central and peripheral nervous systems, but only a limited number have implications for psychiatry. Major categories include the cholinergics, monoamines, amino acids, and neuropeptides. The location, function, and implications of these neurotransmitters are described in Table 2–1.

■ ENDOCRINE INFLUENCES

Human endocrine functioning has a strong foundation in the CNS, under the direction of the hypothalamus, which has direct control over the pituitary gland. The pituitary gland has two major lobes—the anterior lobe (also called the *adenohypophysis*) and the posterior lobe (also called the *neurohypophysis*). The pituitary gland is only about the size of a pea. However, despite its size and because of the powerful control it exerts over endocrine functioning in humans, it is sometimes called the "master gland." Many of the hormones subject to hypothalamus-pituitary regulation may have implications for behavioral functioning. Discussion of these hormones is summarized in Table 2–2.

TABLE 2–1 **Neurotransmitters in the Central Nervous System**

Neurotransmitter	Location/Function	Possible Implications for Mental Illness
I. Cholinergics		
A. Acetylcholine	Autonomic nervous system (ANS): Sympathetic and parasympathetic presynaptic nerve terminals; parasympathetic postsynaptic nerve terminals. CNS:Cerebral cortex, hippocampus, limbic structures, and basal ganglia. Functions: Sleep, arousal, pain perception, movement, memory.	Increased levels: Depression. Decreased levels: Alzheimer's disease, Huntington's Chorea, Parkinson's disease.
II. Monoamines		
A. Norepinephrine	ANS: Sympathetic postsynaptic nerve terminals. CNS: Thalamus, hypothalamus, limbic system, hippocampus, cerebellum, cerebral cortex. Functions: Mood, cognition, perception, locomotion, cardiovascular functioning, and sleep and arousal.	Decreased levels: Depression. Increased levels: Mania, anxiety states, schizophrenia.
B. Dopamine	Frontal cortex, limbic system, basal ganglia, thalamus, posterior pituitary, and spinal cord.	Decreased levels: Parkinson's disease and depression.

Table continued on following page

TABLE 2–1 **Neurotransmitters in the Central Nervous System (*Continued*)**

Neurotransmitter	Location/Function	Possible Implications for Mental Illness
	Functions: Movement and coordination, emotions, voluntary judgment, release of prolactin.	Increased levels: Mania and schizophrenia.
C. Serotonin	Hypothalamus, thalamus, limbic system, cerebral cortex, cerebellum, spinal cord.	Decreased levels: Depression.
	Functions: Sleep and arousal, libido, appetite, mood, aggression, pain perception, coordination, judgment.	Increased levels: Anxiety states.
D. Histamine	Hypothalamus.	Decreased levels: Depression.
III. Amino Acids		
A. Gamma aminobutyric acid (GABA)	Hypothalamus, hippocampus, cortex, cerebellum, basal ganglia, spinal cord, retina. Functions: Slowdown of body activity.	Decreased levels: Huntington's chorea, anxiety disorders, schizophrenia, and various forms of epilepsy.
B. Glycine	Spinal cord and brain stem. Functions: Recurrent inhibition of motor neurons.	Toxic levels: "Glycine encephalopathy," decreased levels are correlated with spastic motor movements.
C. Glutamate and aspartate	Pyramidal cells of the cortex, cerebellum, and the primary sensory afferent systems; hippocampus, thalamus, hypothalamus, spinal cord. Functions: Relay of sensory information and regulation of various motor and spinal reflexes.	Increased levels: Huntington's chorea, temporal lobe epilepsy, spinal cerebellar degeneration.

IV. Neuropeptides		
A. Endorphins and enkephalins	Hypothalamus, thalamus, limbic structures, midbrain, and brain stem. Enkephalins are also found in the gastrointestinal tract. Functions: Modulation of pain and reduced peristalsis (enkephalins).	Modulation of dopamine activity by opioid peptides may indicate some link to the symptoms of schizophrenia.
B. Substance P	Hypothalamus, limbic structures, midbrain, brain stem, thalamus, basal ganglia, and spinal cord; also found in gastrointestinal tract and salivary glands. Function: Regulation of pain.	Decreased levels: Huntington's chorea.
C. Somatostatin	Cerebral cortex, hippocampus, thalamus, basal ganglia, brain stem, and spinal cord. Function: Inhibits release of norepinephrine; stimulates release of serotonin, dopamine, and acetylcholine.	Decreased levels: Alzheimer's disease. Increased levels: Huntington's chorea.

Source: From Townsend, 2000, p 60, with permission.

TABLE 2–2 **Hormones of the Neuroendocrine System**

Hormone	Location and Stimulation of Release	Target Organ	Function	Possible Behavioral Correlation to Altered Secretion
Antidiuretic hormone (ADH)	Posterior pituitary; release stimulated by dehydration, pain, stress	Kidney (causes increased reabsorption)	Conservation of body water and maintenance of blood pressure	Polydipsia; Altered pain response; modified sleep pattern
Oxytocin	Posterior pituitary; release stimulated by end of pregnancy; stress; sexual arousal	Uterus; breasts	Contraction of the uterus for labor; release of breast milk	May play role in stress response by stimulation of ACTH
Growth hormone (GH)	Anterior pituitary; release stimulated by growth hormone–releasing hormone from hypothalamus	Bones and tissues	Growth in children; protein synthesis in adults	Anorexia nervosa
Thyroid-stimulating hormone (TSH)	Anterior pituitary; release stimulated by thyrotropin-releasing hormone from hypothalamus	Thyroid gland	Stimulation of secretion of thyroid hormones needed for metabolism of food and regulation of temperature	Increased levels: Insomnia, anxiety, emotional lability Decreased levels: Fatigue, depression

Adrenocorticotropic hormone (ACTH)	Anterior pituitary; release stimulated by corticotropin-releasing hormone from hypothalamus	Adrenal cortex	Stimulation of secretion of cortisol, which plays a role in response to stress	Increased levels: Mood disorders, psychosis Decreased levels: Depression, apathy, fatigue
Prolactin	Anterior pituitary; release stimulated by prolactin-releasing hormone from hypothalamus	Breasts	Stimulation of milk production	Increased levels: Depression, anxiety, decreased libido, irritability
Gonadotropic hormones	Anterior pituitary; release stimulated by gonadotropin-releasing hormone from hypothalamus	Ovaries and testes	Stimulation of secretion of estrogen, progesterone, and testosterone; role in ovulation and sperm production	Decreased levels: Depression and anorexia nervosa Increased testosterone: Increased sexual behavior and aggressiveness
Melanocyte-stimulating hormone (MSH)	Anterior pituitary; release stimulated by onset of darkness	Pineal gland	Stimulation of secretion of melatonin	Increased levels: Depression

Source: From Townsend, 2000, p 63, with permission.

TABLE 2–3 **Biological Implications of Psychiatric Disorders**

Anatomic Brain Structures Involved	Neurotransmitter Hypothesis	Possible Endocrine Correlation	Possible Genetic Link
Schizophrenia			
Frontal cortex, temporal lobes, limbic system	Dopamine hyperactivity	Decreased prolactin levels	Twin, familial, and adoption studies suggest a genetic link.
Depressive Disorders			
Frontal lobes, limbic system, temporal lobes	Decreased levels of norepinephrine, dopamine, and serotonin	Increased cortisol levels; thyroid hormone hyposecretion; increased melatonin	Twin, familial, and adoption studies suggest a genetic link.
Bipolar Disorder			
Frontal lobes, limbic system, temporal lobes	Increased levels of norepinephrine, dopamine, and serotonin in acute mania	Some indication of elevated thyroid hormones in acute mania	Twin, familial, and adoption studies suggest a genetic link.
Panic Disorder			
Limbic system, midbrain	Increased levels of norepinephrine; decreased GABA activity	Elevated levels of thyroid hormones	Twin and familial studies suggest a genetic link.

Anorexia Nervosa			
Limbic system, particularly the hypothalamus	Decreased levels of norepinephrine, serotonin, and dopamine	Decreased levels of gonadotropins and growth hormone; increased cortisol levels	Twin and familial studies suggest a genetic link.
Obsessive-Compulsive Disorder			
Limbic system, basal ganglia (specifically caudate nucleus)	Decreased levels of serotonin	Increased cortisol levels	Twin studies suggest a possible genetic link.
Alzheimer's Disease			
Temporal, parietal and occipital regions of cerebral cortex; hippocampus	Decreased levels of acetylcholine, norepinephrine, serotonin, and somatostatin	Decreased corticotropin-releasing hormone	Familial studies suggest a genetic predisposition; early onset disorder linked to marker on chromosome 21.

Source: From Townsend, 2000, p 69, with permission.

A summary of various psychiatric disorders and the possible biological influences discussed in this chapter (with the addition of possible genetic influences) is presented in Table 2–3.

■ DIAGNOSTIC PROCEDURES USED TO DETECT ALTERED BRAIN FUNCTIONING

A number of diagnostic procedures are used to detect alteration in biological functioning that may contribute to psychiatric disorders. Following is an explanation of various examinations, the technique used, the purpose of the examination, and possible findings.

1. **Electroencephalography (EEG)**
   a. ***Technique:*** Electrodes are placed on the scalp in a standardized position. Amplitude and frequency of beta, alpha, theta, and delta brain waves are graphically recorded on paper by ink markers for multiple areas of the brain surface.
   b. ***Purpose/Possible Findings:*** Measures brain electrical activity; identifies dysrhythmias, asymmetries, or suppression of brain rhythms; used in the diagnosis of epilepsy, neoplasm, stroke, metabolic, or degenerative disease.
2. **Computerized EEG Mapping**
   a. ***Technique:*** EEG tracings are summarized by computer-assisted systems in which various regions of the brain are identified and functioning is interpreted by color coding or gray shading.
   b. ***Purpose/Possible Findings:*** Measures brain electrical activity; used largely in research to represent statistical relationships between individuals and groups or between two populations of subjects (e.g., clients with schizophrenia vs. control subjects).
3. **Computed Tomographic (CT) Scan**
   a. ***Technique:*** May be used with or without contrast medium. X-rays are taken of various transverse planes of the brain while a computerized analysis produces a precise reconstructed image of each segment.
   b. ***Purpose/Possible Findings:*** Measures accuracy of brain structure to detect possible lesions, abscesses, areas of infarction, or aneurysm. CT has

also identified various anatomic differences in clients with schizophrenia, organic mental disorders, and bipolar disorder.

4. **Magnetic Resonance Imaging (MRI)**
   a. ***Technique:*** Within a strong magnetic field, the nuclei of hydrogen atoms absorb and re-emit electromagnetic energy that is computerized and transformed into image information. No radiation or contrast medium is used.
   b. ***Purpose/Possible Findings:*** Measures anatomic and biochemical status of various segments of the brain; detects brain edema, ischemia, infection, neoplasm, trauma, and other changes such as demyelination. Morphologic differences have been noted in brains of clients with schizophrenia as compared with control subjects.
5. **Positron Emission Tomography (PET)**
   a. ***Technique:*** The client receives an intravenous injection of a radioactive substance (type dependent on brain activity to be visualized). The head is surrounded by detectors that relay data to a computer that interprets the signals and produces the image.
   b. ***Purpose/Possible Findings:*** Measures specific brain functioning, such as glucose metabolism, oxygen utilization, blood flow, and, of particular interest in psychiatry, neurotransmitter-receptor-interaction.
6. **Single Photon Emission Computed Tomography (SPECT)**
   a. ***Technique:*** The technique is similar to PET, but a longer-acting radioactive substance must be used to allow time for a gamma camera to rotate about the head and gather the data, which are then computer assembled into a brain image.
   b. ***Purpose/Possible Findings:*** Measures various aspects of brain functioning, as with PET; has also been used to image activity or cerebrospinal fluid circulation.

■ SUMMARY

The "medicalization of psychiatry" necessitates that nurses be cognizant of the interaction between physical and mental factors in the development and management of psychiatric illness. These current trends have made it essential for nurses to increase their knowledge about the structure and functioning of the brain. This includes the processes and neurotransmission and the function of various neurotransmitters. This is especially important in light of the increasing role of psychotropic medication in the treatment of psychiatric illness. Because the mechanism of action of many of these drugs occurs at synaptic transmission, nurses must understand this process so that they may predict outcomes and safely manage the administration of psychotropic medications.

The endocrine system plays an important role in human behavior through the hypothalamic-pituitary axis. Hormones influence a number of physiological and psychological life-cycle phenomena, such as moods, sleep-arousal, stress response, appetite, libido, and fertility.

It is also important for nurses to keep abreast of the expanding diagnostic technologies available for detecting alterations in physical functioning. These technologies are facilitating the growth of knowledge linking mental illness to disorders of the brain.

■ INTERNET REFERENCES

- http://neuro.med.cornell.edu/VL
- http://www.neuroguide.com

UNIT TWO

ALTERATIONS IN PSYCHOSOCIAL ADAPTATION

CHAPTER 3

Disorders Usually First Diagnosed in Infancy, Childhood, or Adolescence

BACKGROUND ASSESSMENT DATA

Several common psychiatric disorders may arise or become evident during infancy, childhood, or adolescence. Essential features of many disorders are identical, regardless of the age of the individual. Examples include the following:

- Cognitive Disorders
- Schizophrenia
- Schizophreniform Disorder
- Adjustment Disorders
- Sexual Disorders
- Personality Disorders
- Substance-Related Disorders
- Mood Disorders
- Somatoform Disorders
- Psychological Factors Affecting Medical Conditions

There are, however, several disorders that appear during the early developmental years and are identified according to the child's ability or inability to perform age-appropriate tasks or intellectual functions. Selected disorders are presented here. It is essential that the nurse working with these clients understand normal behavior patterns characteristic of the infant, childhood, and adolescent years.

■ MENTAL RETARDATION

Defined

Mental retardation is defined by deficits in general intellectual functioning and adaptive functioning, and identified by an intelligence quotient (IQ) of approximately 70 or below on an individually administered IQ examination (APA, 1994). Mental retardation is coded on Axis II in the *DSM-IV* Classification. Codes include:

317	Mild Mental Retardation (IQ of 50–70)
318.0	Moderate Mental Retardation (IQ of 35–49)
318.1	Severe Mental Retardation (IQ of 20–34)
318.2	Profound Mental Retardation (IQ below 20)
319	Mental Retardation, Severity Unspecified

Predisposing Factors

1. **Physiological**
   a. About 5 percent of cases of mental retardation are caused by hereditary factors, such as Tay-Sachs disease, phenylketonuria, and hyperglycemia. Chromosomal disorders, such as Down syndrome and Klinefelter's syndrome, have also been implicated.
   b. Events that occur during the prenatal period, such as maternal ingestion of alcohol or other drugs, maternal infections, toxemia, and uncontrolled diabetes, and the perinatal period, such as birth trauma or premature separation of the placenta, can result in mental retardation.
   c. Mental retardation can occur as an outcome of childhood illnesses, such as encephalitis or meningitis, or can be the result of poisoning or physical trauma in childhood.
2. **Psychosocial**
   a. Fifteen to 20 percent of cases of mental retardation are attributed to deprivation of nurturance and social, linguistic, and other stimulation, and to severe mental disorders, such as autistic disorder (APA, 1994).

Symptomatology (Subjective and Objective Data)

1. At the mild level (IQ of 50–70), the individual can live independently, but with some assistance. He or she is capable of sixth-grade-level work and can learn a vocational skill. Social skills are possible, but the indi-

vidual functions best in a structured, sheltered setting. Coordination may be slightly affected.

2. At the moderate level (IQ of 35–49), the individual can perform some activities independently but requires supervision. Academic skill can be achieved to about the second-grade level. The individual may experience some limitation in speech communication and in interactions with others. Motor development may be limited to gross motor ability.
3. The severe level of mental retardation (IQ of 20–34) is characterized by the need for complete supervision. Systematic habit training may be accomplished, but the individual does not have the ability for academic or vocational training. Verbal skills are minimal and psychomotor development is poor.
4. The profoundly mentally retarded individual (IQ of less than 20) has no capacity for independent living. Constant aid and supervision are required. No ability exists for academic or vocational training. There is a lack of ability for speech development, socialization skills, and fine or gross motor movements. The individual requires constant supervision and care.

Common Nursing Diagnoses and Interventions

(Interventions are applicable to various health-care settings, such as inpatient and partial hospitalization, community outpatient clinic, home health, and private practice.)

RISK FOR INJURY

Definition: A state in which the individual is at risk of injury as a result of environmental conditions interacting with the individual's adaptive and defensive resources.

Related/Risk Factors ("related to")

Altered physical mobility
Aggressive behavior

Goals/Objectives

Short-/Long-Term Goal

Client will not experience injury.

Interventions with *Selected Rationales*

1. *To ensure client safety:*
   a. Create a safe environment for the client. Remove small items from the area where the client will be ambulating and move sharp items out of his or her reach.
   b. Store items that client uses frequently within easy reach.
   c. Pad side rails and headboard of client with history of seizures.
   d. Prevent physical aggression and acting-out behaviors by learning to recognize signs that client is becoming agitated.

Outcome Criteria

1. Client has experienced no physical harm.
2. Client responds to attempts to inhibit agitated behavior.

SELF-CARE DEFICIT

Definition: A state in which the individual experiences an impaired ability to perform or complete [activities of daily living] independently.

Possible Etiologies ("related to")

Altered physical mobility
Lack of maturity

Defining Characteristics ("evidenced by")

[Unwillingness or inability to keep self clean]
[Uncombed hair; offensive body and breath odor]
[Inability to obtain adequate nutrition without assistance]
[Inability to dress or groom self without assistance]
[Inability to toilet self without assistance]
[Incontinence]

Goals/Objectives

Short-Term Goal

Client will be able to participate in aspects of self-care.

Long-Term Goal

Client will have all self-care needs met.

Interventions with *Selected Rationales*

1. Identify aspects of self-care that may be within the client's capabilities. Work on one aspect of self-care at a time. Pro-

vide simple, concrete explanations. ***Because clients' capabilities vary so widely, it is important to know each one individually and to ensure that no client is set up to fail.***

2. Offer positive feedback for efforts at assisting with own self-care. ***Positive reinforcement enhances self-esteem and encourages repetition of desirable behaviors.***
3. When one aspect of self-care has been mastered to the best of the client's ability, move on to another. Encourage independence but intervene when client is unable to perform. ***Client comfort and safety are nursing priorities.***

Outcome Criteria

1. Client assists with self-care activities to the best of his or her ability.
2. Client's self-care needs are being met.

IMPAIRED VERBAL COMMUNICATION

Definition: The state in which an individual experiences a decreased, delayed, or absent ability to receive, process, transmit, and use a system of symbols [to communicate].

Possible Etiologies ("related to")

[Developmental alteration]

Defining Characteristics ("evidenced by")

Speaks or verbalizes with difficulty
Difficulty forming words or sentences
Difficulty expressing thought verbally
Inappropriate verbalizations
Does not or cannot speak

Goals/Objectives

Short-Term Goal

Client will establish trust with caregiver and a means of communication of needs.

Long-Term Goals

1. Client's needs are being met through established means of communication.
2. If client cannot speak or communicate by other means, needs are met by caregiver's anticipation of client's needs.

Interventions with *Selected Rationales*

1. Maintain consistency of staff assignment over time. ***This***

facilitates trust and the ability to understand client's actions and communication.

2. Anticipate and fulfill client's needs until satisfactory communication patterns are established. Learn (from family, if possible) special words client uses that are different from the norm.
3. Identify nonverbal gestures or signals that client may use to convey needs if verbal communication is absent. Practice these communication skills over and over. ***Some mentally retarded children, particularly at the severe level, can learn only by systematic habit training.***

Outcome Criteria

1. Client is able to communicate with consistent caregiver.
2. (For client who is unable to communicate): Client's needs, as anticipated by caregiver, are being met.

IMPAIRED SOCIAL INTERACTION

Definition: The state in which an individual participates in an insufficient or excessive quantity or ineffective quality of social exchange.

Possible Etiologies ("related to")

Speech deficiencies
Difficulty adhering to conventional social behavior (because of delayed maturational development)

Defining Characteristics ("evidenced by")

Observed use of unsuccessful social interaction behaviors
Dysfunctional interaction with peers, family, and/or others
Observed discomfort in social situations

Goals/Objectives

Short-Term Goal

Client will attempt to interact with others in the presence of trusted caregiver.

Long-Term Goal

Client will be able to interact with others using behaviors that are socially acceptable and appropriate to developmental level.

Interventions with *Selected Rationales*

1. Remain with client during initial interactions with others on the unit. *The presence of a trusted individual provides a feeling of security.*

2. Explain to other clients the meaning behind some of the client's nonverbal gestures and signals. ***Others may be more accepting of the client's differentness if they have a better understanding of his or her behavior.***
3. Use simple language to explain to client which behaviors are acceptable and which are not. Establish a procedure for behavior modification that offers rewards for appropriate behaviors and renders an aversive reinforcement in response to the use of inappropriate behaviors. ***Positive, negative, and aversive reinforcements can contribute to desired changes in behavior. The privileges and penalties are individually determined as staff learns the likes and dislikes of the client.***

Outcome Criterion

1. Client interacts with others in a socially appropriate manner.

■ 299.00 AUTISTIC DISORDER*

Defined

Autistic disorder is characterized by a withdrawal of the child into the self and into a fantasy world of his or her own creation. Activities and interests are restricted and may be considered somewhat bizarre. The disorder is rare, but it occurs 4 to 5 times more often in males than in females. Onset of symptoms is prior to age 3. The course is chronic and often persists into adulthood.

Predisposing Factors

1. **Physiological**
   a. ***Genetics:*** An increased risk of autistic disorder exists among siblings of individuals with the disorder (APA, 1994). Some studies suggest an increased risk as high as 50 times greater than the general population.
   b. ***Neurological Factors:*** Certain developmental problems, such as postnatal neurological infections, congenital rubella, phenylketonuria, and fragile X syndrome, have also been implicated.

---

*Reprinted with permission from the *Diagnostic and Statistical Manual of Mental Disorders, Fourth Edition.* Copyright 1994 American Psychiatric Association, 1994.

2. **Psychosocial**
   a. ***Psychodynamic Theory:*** Mahler and coworkers (1975) have suggested that the autistic child is fixed in the presymbiotic phase of development. The child does not achieve a symbiotic relationship with, nor differentiates self from, mother. Ego development is delayed; the child does not communicate or form relationships.
   b. ***Theory of Family Dynamics:*** Very early interaction patterns have been suggested as important in the predisposition to autistic disorder. In this theory, parents of autistic children were described as aloof and distant, with little emotional attachment to the child. Kanner (1973) coined the term *refrigerator parents* to describe their lack of warmth and affectionate behavior.

NOTE: These older psychosocial theories have lost much credibility through years of research. Many of their claims about the cause of autism have been proved false. Most clinicians now believe that autism is not caused by bad parenting, and no known psychological factors in the development of the child have been shown to be the primary cause of autism (Johnson and Dorman, 1998).

Symptomatology (Subjective and Objective Data)

1. Failure to form interpersonal relationships, characterized by unresponsiveness to people; lack of eye contact and facial responsiveness; indifference or aversion to affection and physical contact. In early childhood, there is a failure to develop cooperative play and friendships.
2. Impairment in communication (verbal and nonverbal) characterized by absence of language or, if developed, often an immature grammatical structure, incorrect use of words, echolalia, or inability to use abstract terms. Accompanying nonverbal expressions may be inappropriate or absent.
3. Bizarre responses to environment, characterized by resistance or extreme behavioral reactions to minor occurrences; abnormal, obsessive attachment to peculiar objects; ritualistic behaviors.
4. Extreme fascination for objects that move (e.g., fans, trains). Special interest in music, playing with water, buttons, or parts of the body.
5. Unreasonable insistence on following routines in pre-

cise detail (e.g., insisting that exactly the same route always be followed when shopping).
6. Marked distress over changes in trivial aspects of environment (e.g., when a vase is moved from its usual position).
7. Stereotyped body movements (e.g., hand flicking or twisting, spinning, head banging, complex whole-body movements).

Common Nursing Diagnoses and Interventions

(Interventions are applicable to various health-care settings, such as inpatient and partial hospitalization, community outpatient clinic, home health, and private practice.)

RISK FOR SELF-MUTILATION

Definition: A state in which an individual is at risk to perform an act upon the self to injure, not kill, which produces tissue damage and tension relief.

Related/Risk Factors ("related to")

[Neurological alterations]
[History of self-mutilative behaviors in response to increasing anxiety]
[Obvious indifference to environment or hysterical reactions to changes in the environment]

Goals/Objectives

Short-Term Goal

Client will demonstrate alternative behavior (e.g., initiating interaction between self and nurse) in response to anxiety within specified time. (Length of time required for this objective will depend on severity and chronicity of disorder.)

Long-Term Goal

Client will not inflict harm on self.

Interventions with *Selected Rationales*

1. Intervene to protect child when self-multilative behaviors, such as head banging or other hysterical behaviors, become evident. *The nurse is responsible for ensuring client safety.*

2. A helmet may be used to protect against head banging, hand mitts to prevent hair pulling, and appropriate padding to protect extremities from injury during hysterical movements.
3. Try to determine whether self-mutilative behaviors occur in response to increasing anxiety and, if so, to what the anxiety may be attributed. ***Mutilative behaviors may be averted if the cause can be determined.***
4. Work on one-to-one basis with child ***to establish trust.***
5. Offer self to child during times of increasing anxiety, ***to decrease need for self-mutilative behaviors and provide feelings of security.***

Outcome Criteria

1. Anxiety is maintained at a level at which client feels no need for self-mutilation.
2. When feeling anxious, client initiates interaction between self and nurse.

IMPAIRED SOCIAL INTERACTION

Definition: The state in which an individual participates in an insufficient or excessive quantity or ineffective quality of social exchange.

Possible Etiologies ("related to")

Self-concept disturbance
Absence of available significant others
[Unfulfilled tasks of trust vs. mistrust]
[Neurological alterations]

Defining Characteristics ("evidenced by")

[Lack of responsiveness to, or interest in, people]
[Failure to cuddle]
[Lack of eye contact and facial responsiveness]
[Indifference or aversion to affection and physical contact]
[Failure to develop cooperative play and peer friendships]

Goals/Objectives

Short-Term Goal

Client with demonstrate trust in one caregiver (as evidenced by facial responsiveness and eye contact) within specified time (depending on severity and chronicity of disorder).

Long-Term Goal

Client will initiate social interactions (physical, verbal, nonverbal) with caregiver by discharge from treatment.

Interventions with *Selected Rationales*

1. Function in a one-to-one relationship with the child. *Consistency of staff-client interaction enhances the establishment of trust.*
2. Provide child with familiar objects (favorite toys, blanket). *These items will offer security during times when the child feels distressed.*
3. Convey a manner of warmth, acceptance, and availability as client attempts to fulfill basic needs. *These characteristics enhance establishment and maintenance of a trusting relationship.*
4. Go slowly. Do not force interactions. Begin with positive reinforcement for eye contact. Gradually introduce touch, smiling, hugging. *The autistic client may feel threatened by an onslaught of stimuli to which he or she is unaccustomed.*
5. Support client with your presence as he or she endeavors to relate to others in the environment. *The presence of an individual with whom a trusting relationship has been established provides a feeling of security.*

Outcome Criteria

1. Client initiates interactions between self and others.
2. Client uses eye contact, facial responsiveness, and other nonverbal behaviors in interactions with others.
3. Client does not withdraw from physical contact.

IMPAIRED VERBAL COMMUNICATION

Definition: The state in which an individual experiences a decreased, delayed, or absent ability to receive, process, transmit, and use a system of symbols [to communicate].

Possible Etiologies ("related to")

[Inability to trust]
[Withdrawal into the self]
[Neurological alterations]

Defining Characteristics ("evidenced by")

Does not or cannot speak

[Immature grammatical structure]
[Echolalia]
[Pronoun reversal]
[Inability to name objects]
[Inability to use abstract terms]
[Absence of nonverbal expression (e.g., eye contact, facial responsiveness, gestures)]

Goals/Objectives

Short-Term Goal

Client will establish trust with one caregiver (as evidenced by facial responsiveness and eye contact) by specified time (depending on severity and chronicity of disorder).

Long-Term Goal

Client will have established a means for communicating (verbally or nonverbally) needs and desires to staff by discharge from treatment.

Interventions with *Selected Rationales*

1. Maintain consistency of staff assignment over time. ***This facilitates trust and the ability to understand client's actions and communication.***
2. Anticipate and fulfill client's needs until satisfactory communication patterns are established
3. Use the techniques of CONSENSUAL VALIDATION AND SEEKING CLARIFICATION to decode communication patterns. (Examples: "I think you must have meant . . ." or "Did you mean to say that . . . ?" ***These techniques work to verify the accuracy of the message received or to clarify any hidden meanings within the message. Take caution not to "put words into the client's mouth."***
4. Use "en face" approach (face-to-face, eye-to-eye) to convey correct nonverbal expressions by example. ***Eye contact expresses genuine interest in, and respect for, the individual.***

Outcome Criteria

1. Client is able to communicate in a manner that is understood by others.
2. Client's nonverbal messages are congruent with verbalizations.
3. Client initiates verbal and nonverbal interaction with others.

PERSONAL IDENTITY DISTURBANCE

Definition: Inability to distinguish between self and non-self.

Possible Etiologies ("related to")

[Unfulfilled tasks of trust vs. mistrust]
[Neurological alternations]
[Inadequate sensory stimulation]

Defining Characteristics ("evidenced by")

[Inability to separate own physiological and emotional needs from those of others]
[Increased levels of anxiety resulting from contact with others]
[Inability to differentiate own body boundaries from those of others]
[Repeating words he or she hears others say or mimicking movements of others]

Goals/Objectives

Short-Term Goal

Client will name own body parts and body parts of caregiver within specified time (depending on severity and chronicity of disorder).

Long-Term Goal

Client will develop ego identity (evidenced by ability to recognize physical and emotional self as separate from others) by discharge from treatment.

Interventions with Selected Rationales

1. Function in a one-to-one relationship with the child. *Consistency of staff-client interaction enhances the establishment of trust.*
2. Assist child to recognize separateness during self-care activities, such as dressing and feeding. *These activities increase child's awareness of self as separate from others.*
3. Point out, and assist child in naming, own body parts. *This activity may increase the child's awareness of self as separate from others.*
4. Gradually increase amount of physical contact, using touch to point out differences between client and nurse. Be cautious with touch until trust is established, *because this gesture may be interpreted by the client as threatening.*

5. Use mirrors as well as drawings and pictures of the child to reinforce the child's learning of body parts and boundaries.

Outcome Criteria

1. Client is able to differentiate own body parts from those of others.
2. Client communicates ability to separate self from environment by discontinuing use of echolalia (repeating words heard) and echopraxia (imitating movements seen).

■ DISRUPTIVE BEHAVIOR DISORDERS

314.xx Attention-Deficit/Hyperactivity Disorder*

Defined

Attention-deficit/hyperactivity disorder (ADHD) is characterized by a persistent pattern of inattention and/or hyperactivity-impulsivity that is more frequent and severe than is typically observed in individuals at a comparable level of development (APA, 1994). The disorder is frequently not diagnosed until the child begins school because, prior to that time, childhood behavior is much more variable than that of older children. ADHD is 4 to 9 times more common in boys than in girls and may occur in as many as 3 to 5 percent of school-age children. The *DSM-IV* further categorizes the disorder into the following subtypes:

314.01 Combined Type
314.00 Predominantly Inattentive Type
314.01 Predominantly Hyperactive-Impulsive Type

The course can be chronic, persisting into adulthood.

Predisposing Factors

1. **Physiological**
   a. ***Genetics:*** A number of studies have indicated that hereditary factors may be implicated in the predisposition of ADHD. Siblings of hyperactive children are more likely than normal children to have the disorder.

---

*Reprinted with permission from the *Diagnostic and Statistical Manual of Mental Disorders, Fourth Edition*. Copyright 1994 American Psychiatric Association, 1994.

b. ***Biochemical:*** A deficit of the neurotransmitters dopamine and norepinephrine has been suggested as a causative factor.
c. ***Prenatal and Perinatal Factors:*** Some studies link maternal smoking and substance use with ADHD in offspring. Premature birth, fetal distress, precipitated or prolonged labor, and perinatal asphyxia have also been implicated.

2. **Psychosocial**
   a. ***Psychodynamic Theory:*** Mahler's (1975) theory suggests that the child with ADHD is fixed in the symbiotic phase of development and has not differentiated self from mother. Ego development is retarded, and impulsive behavior dictated by the id is manifested.
   b. ***Theory of Family Dynamics:*** Bowen (1978) proposes that when a dysfunctional spousal relationship exists, the focus of the disturbance is displaced onto the child, whose behavior in time begins to reflect the patterns of the dysfunctional system.

Symptomatology *(Subjective and Objective Data)*

The *DSM-IV* (APA, 1994) identifies the following signs and symptoms of ADHD:

1. **Inattention**
   a. Often fails to give close attention to details or makes careless mistakes in schoolwork, work, or other activities.
   b. Often has difficulty sustaining attention in tasks or play activities.
   c. Often does not seem to listen when spoken to directly.
   d. Often does not follow through on instructions and fails to finish schoolwork, chores, or duties in the workplace (not because of oppositional behavior or failure to understand instructions).
   e. Often has difficulty organizing tasks and activities.
   f. Often avoids, dislikes, or is reluctant to engage in tasks that require sustained mental effort (such as schoolwork or homework).
   g. Often loses things necessary for tasks or activities (e.g., toys, school assignments, pencils, books, or tools).
   h. Is often easily distracted by extraneous stimuli.
   i. Is often forgetful in daily activities.

2. **Hyperactivity**
   a. Often fidgets with hands or feet or squirms in seat.
   b. Often leaves seat in classroom or in other situations in which remaining seated is expected.
   c. Often runs about or climbs excessively in situations in which it is inappropriate (in adolescents or adults, may be limited to subjective feelings of restlessness).
   d. Often has difficulty playing or engaging in leisure activities quietly.
   e. Is often "on the go" or often acts as if "driven by a motor."
   f. Often talks excessively.
3. **Impulsivity**
   a. Often blurts out answers before questions have been completed.
   b. Often has difficulty awaiting turn.
   c. Often interrupts or intrudes on others (e.g., butts into conversations or games).

312.8 Conduct Disorder*

Defined

The *DSM-IV* describes the essential feature of this disorder as a repetitive and persistent pattern of conduct in which the basic rights of others or major age-appropriate societal norms or rules are violated. The conduct is more serious than the ordinary mischief and pranks of children and adolescents. The disorder is more common in boys than in girls, and the behaviors may continue into adulthood, often meeting the criteria for antisocial personality disorder. Conduct disorder is divided into two subtypes based on the age at onset:

1. **Childhood-Onset Type:** The onset of at least one characteristic of conduct disorder prior to age 10.
2. **Adolescent-Onset Type:** The absence of behaviors associated with conduct disorder prior to age 10.

Predisposing Factors

1. **Physiological**
   a. ***Birth Temperament:*** The term *temperament* refers to personality traits that become evident very early

---

*Reprinted with permission from the *Diagnostic and Statistical Manual of Mental Disorders, Fourth Edition.* Copyright 1994 American Psychiatric Association, 1994.

in life and may be present at birth. Evidence suggests an association between difficult temperament in childhood and behavioral problems later in life (Plomin, 1983).

2. **Psychosocial**
   a. ***Psychodynamic Theory:*** Mahler's (1975) theory suggests that this child is fixed in the separation-individuation phase of development. The child has failed to separate from mother and remains in the dependent position. Fears of abandonment nurture this dependency. The ego remains in an underdeveloped condition.
   b. ***Theory of Family Dynamics:*** The following factors related to family dynamics have been implicated as contributors in the predisposition to this disorder (Clunn, 1991; Popper and Steingard, 1994):
      - Parental rejection
      - Inconsistent management with harsh discipline
      - Early institutional living
      - Frequent shifting of parental figures
      - Large family size
      - Absent father
      - Parents with antisocial personality disorder and/or alcohol dependence
      - Association with a delinquent subgroup

Symptomatology *(Subjective and Objective Data)*

The *DSM-IV* has identified the following signs and symptoms of conduct disorder:

1. Often bullies, threatens, or intimidates others.
2. Often initiates physical fights.
3. Has used a weapon that can cause serious physical harm to others (e.g., a bat, brick, broken bottle, knife, gun).
4. Has been physically cruel to people.
5. Has been physically cruel to animals.
6. Has stolen while confronting a victim (e.g., mugging, purse snatching, extortion, armed robbery).
7. Has forced someone into sexual activity.
8. Has deliberately engaged in fire setting with the intention of causing serious damage.
9. Has deliberately destroyed others' property (other than by fire setting).
10. Has broken into someone else's house, building, or car.

11. Often lies to obtain goods or favors or to avoid obligations (i.e., "cons" others).
12. Has stolen items of nontrivial value without confronting a victim (e.g., shoplifting, but without breaking and entering; forgery).
13. Often stays out at night despite parental prohibitions, beginning before age 13 years.
14. Has run away from home overnight at least twice while living in parental or parental surrogate home (or once without returning for a lengthy period).
15. Is often truant from school, beginning before age 13 years.

313.81 Oppositional Defiant Disorder*

Defined

The *DSM-IV* defines this disorder as a pattern of negativistic, defiant, disobedient, and hostile behavior toward authority figures that occurs more frequently than is typically observed in individuals of comparable age and developmental level. The disorder typically begins by 8 years of age, and usually not later than early adolescence. The disorder is more prevalent in boys than in girls and is often a developmental antecedent to conduct disorder.

Predisposing Factors

1. **Physiological**
   a. Refer to this section under Conduct Disorder.
2. **Psychosocial**
   a. ***Theory of Family Dynamics:*** It is thought that some parents interpret average or increased levels of developmental oppositionalism as hostility and a deliberate effort on the part of the child to be in control. If power and control are issues for parents, or if they exercise authority for their own needs, a power struggle can be established between the parents and the child that sets the stage for the development of oppositional defiant disorder (Kaplan and Sadock, 1989).

---

*Reprinted with permission from the *Diagnostic and Statistical Manual of Mental Disorders, Fourth Edition.* Copyright 1994 American Psychiatric Association, 1994.

Symptomatology *(Subjective and Objective Data)*

The *DSM-IV* has identified the following signs and symptoms of oppositional defiant disorder:

1. Often loses temper.
2. Often argues with adults.
3. Often actively defies or refuses to comply with adult requests or rules.
4. Often deliberately annoys people.
5. Often blames others for his or her mistakes or misbehavior.
6. Is often touchy or easily annoyed by others.
7. Is often angry and resentful.
8. Is often spiteful or vindictive.

Common Nursing Diagnoses and Interventions for Disruptive Behavior Disorders

(Interventions are applicable to various health-care settings, such as inpatient and partial hospitalization, community outpatient clinic, home health, and private practice.)

RISKS FOR VIOLENCE: SELF-DIRECTED OR DIRECTED AT OTHERS

Definition: Behaviors in which an individual demonstrates that he/she can be physically, emotionally, and/or sexually harmful either to self or to others.

Related/Risk Factors ("related to")

[Retarded ego development]
[Unsatisfactory parent-child relationship]
[Neurological alteration related to premature birth, fetal distress, precipitated or prolonged labor]
[Dysfunctional family system]
[Disorganized or chaotic environments]
[Child abuse or neglect]
[Birth temperament]
[Fears of abandonment]
Body language—rigid posture, clenching of fists and jaw, hyperactivity, pacing, breathlessness, and threatening stances.
[History or threats of violence toward self or others or of destruction to the property of others]

Implusivity
History of cruelty to animals
Suicidal ideation, plan, available means

Goals/Objectives

Short-Term Goal

Client will seek out staff at any time if thoughts of harming self or others should occur.

Long-Term Goal

Client will not harm self or others.

Interventions with *Selected Rationales*

1. Observe client's behavior frequently. Do this through routine activities and interactions to avoid appearing watchful and suspicious. ***Clients at high risk for violence require close observation to prevent harm to self or others.***
2. Observe for suicidal behaviors: Verbal statements, such as "I'm going to kill myself" or "Very soon my mother won't have to worry herself about me any longer," or nonverbal behaviors, such as giving away cherished items, and mood swings. ***Most clients who attempt suicide have communicated their intent, either verbally or nonverbally.***
3. Determine suicidal intent and available means. Ask "Do you plan to kill yourself?" and "How do you plan to do it?" ***Direct, closed-ended questions are appropriate in this instance. The client who has a usable plan is at higher risk than one who does not.***
4. Obtain verbal or written contract from client agreeing not to harm self and agreeing to seek out staff in the event that such ideation occurs. ***Discussion of suicidal feelings with a trusted individual provides a degree of relief to the client. A contract gets the subject out in the open and places some of the responsibility for his or her safety with the client. An attitude of acceptance of the client as a worthwhile individual is conveyed.***
5. Assist client in recognizing when anger occurs and to accept those feelings as his or her own. Have client keep an "anger notebook," in which a record of anger experienced on a 24-hour basis is kept. Information regarding source of anger, behavioral response, and client's perception of the situation should also be noted. Discuss entries

with client, suggesting alternative behavioral responses for those identified as maladaptive.

6. Act as a role model for appropriate expression of angry feelings, and give positive reinforcement to client for attempting to conform. ***It is vital that the client express angry feelings, because suicide and other self-destructive behaviors are often viewed as a result of anger turned inward on the self.***
7. Remove all dangerous objects from client's environment. ***The client's physical safety is a nursing priority.***
8. Try to redirect violent behavior with physical outlets for the client's anxiety (e.g., punching bag, jogging, volleyball). ***Anxiety and tension can be relieved safely and with benefit to the client in this manner.***
9. Be available to stay with client as anxiety level and tensions begin to rise. ***The presence of a trusted individual provides a feeling of security.***
10. Staff should maintain and convey a calm attitude to client. ***Anxiety is contagious and can be communicated from staff to client and vice versa. A calm attitude conveys a sense of control and a feeling of security to the client.***
11. Have sufficient staff available to indicate a show of strength to client if it becomes necessary. ***This conveys to the client an evidence of control over the situation and provides some physical security for staff.***
12. Administer tranquilizing medications as ordered by physician, or obtain an order if necessary. Monitor medication for effectiveness and for adverse side effects. ***Antianxiety medications (e.g., diazepam, chlordiazepoxide, alprazolam) provide relief from the immobilizing effects of anxiety and facilitate client's cooperation with therapy.***
13. Mechanical restraints or isolation room may be required if less restrictive interventions are unsuccessful. ***It is the client's right to expect the use of techniques that ensure safety of the client and others by the least restrictive means.***

Outcome Criteria

1. Anxiety is maintained at a level at which client feels no need for aggression.
2. Client seeks out staff to discuss true feelings.
3. Client recognizes, verbalizes, and accepts possible consequences of own maladaptive behaviors.
4. Client does not harm self or others.

DEFENSIVE COPING

Definition: The state in which an individual repeatedly projects falsely positive self-evaluation based on a self-protective pattern that defends against underlying perceived threats to positive self-regard.

Possible Etiologies ("related to")

[Low self-esteem]
[Retarded ego development]
[Negative role models]
[Lack of positive feedback]
[Repeated negative feedback, resulting in feelings of diminished self-worth]
[Unsatisfactory parent-child relationship]
[Disorganized or chaotic environments]
[Child abuse or neglect]
[Dysfunctional family system]
[Neurological alteration related to premature birth, fetal distress, precipitated or prolonged labor]

Defining Characteristics ("evidenced by")

Denial of obvious problems or weaknesses
Projection of blame or responsibility
Rationalizes failures
Hypersensitive to criticism
Grandiosity
Superior attitude toward others
Difficulty establishing or maintaining relationships
Hostile laughter or ridicule of others
Difficulty in reality testing of perceptions
Lack of follow-through or participation in treatment or therapy

Goals/Objectives

Short-Term Goal

Client will verbalize personal responsibility for difficulties experienced in interpersonal relationships.

Long-Term Goal

Client will demonstrate ability to interact with others without becoming defensive, rationalizing behaviors, or expressing grandiose ideas.

Interventions with *Selected Rationales*

1. Recognize and support basic ego strengths. *Focusing on positive aspects of the personality may help to improve self-concept.*

2. Encourage client to recognize and verbalize feelings of inadequacy and need for acceptance from others, and how these feelings provoke defensive behaviors, such as blaming others for own behaviors. ***Recognition of the problem is the first step in the change process toward resolution.***
3. Provide immediate, matter-of-fact, nonthreatening feedback for unacceptable behaviors. ***Client may lack knowledge about how he or she is being perceived by others. Providing this information in a nonthreatening manner may help to eliminate these undesirable behaviors.***
4. Help client identify situations that provoke defensiveness and practice through role play more appropriate responses. ***Role playing provides confidence to deal with difficult situations when they actually occur.***
5. Provide immediate positive feedback for acceptable behaviors. ***Positive feedback enhances self-esteem and encourages repetition of desirable behaviors.***
6. Help client set realistic, concrete goals and determine appropriate actions to meet those goals. ***Success increases self-esteem.***
7. With client, evaluate the effectiveness of the new behaviors and discuss any modifications for improvement. ***Because of limited problem-solving ability, assistance may be required to reassess and develop new strategies in the event that certain of the new coping methods prove ineffective.***

Outcome Criteria

1. Client verbalizes and accepts responsibility for own behavior.
2. Client verbalizes correlation between feelings of inadequacy and the need to defend the ego through rationalization and grandiosity.
3. Client does not ridicule or criticize others.
4. Client interacts with others in group situations without taking a defensive stance.

IMPAIRED SOCIAL INTERACTION

Definition: The state in which an individual participates in an insufficient or excessive quantity or ineffective quality of social exchange.

Possible Etiologies ("related to")

Self-concept disturbance
[Retarded ego development]

[Neurological alterations related to premature birth, fetal distress, precipitated or prolonged labor]
[Dysfunctional family system]
[Disorganized or chaotic environments]
[Child abuse or neglect]
[Unsatisfactory parent-child relationship]
[Negative role models]

Defining Characteristics ("evidenced by")

Verbalized or observed discomfort in social situations
Verbalized or observed inability to receive or communicate a satisfying sense of belonging, caring, interest, or shared history
Observed use of unsuccessful social interaction behaviors
Dysfunctional interaction with peers, family, or others
[Behavior unaccepted for appropriate age by dominant cultural group]

Goals/Objectives

Short-Term Goal

Client will interact in age-appropriate manner with nurse in one-to-one relationship within 1 week.

Long-Term Goal

Client will be able to interact with staff and peers, by the time of discharge from treatment, with no indication of discomfort.

Interventions with *Selected Rationales*

1. Develop trusting relationship with client. Be honest; keep all promises; convey acceptance of person, separate from unacceptable behaviors ("It is not *you*, but *your behavior*, that is unacceptable." ***Acceptance of the client increases his or her feelings of self-worth.***
2. Offer to remain with client during initial interactions with others on the unit. ***Presence of a trusted individual provides a feeling of security.***
3. Provide constructive criticism and positive reinforcement for efforts. ***Positive feedback enhances self-esteem and encourages repetition of desirable behaviors.***
4. Confront client, and withdraw attention, when interactions with others are manipulative or exploitative. ***Attention to the unacceptable behavior may reinforce it.***
5. Act as role model for client through appropriate interactions with other clients and staff members.
6. Provide group situations for client. ***It is through these group interactions that client will learn socially ac-***

ceptable behavior, with positive and negative feedback from his or her peers.

Outcome Criteria

1. Client seeks out staff member for social, as well as therapeutic interaction.
2. Client has formed, and satisfactorily maintained, one interpersonal relationship with another client.
3. Client willingly and appropriately participates in group activities.
4. Client verbalizes reasons for inability to form close interpersonal relationships with others in the past.

INEFFECTIVE INDIVIDUAL COPING

Definition: Inability to form a valid appraisal of the stressors, inadequate choices of practiced responses, and/or inability to use available resources.

Possible Etiologies ("related to")

Situational crises
Maturational crises
Inadequate support systems
[Inadequate coping strategies]
[Negative role models]
[Neurological alteration related to premature birth, fetal distress, precipitated or prolonged labor]
[Retarded ego development]
[Low self-esteem]
[Dysfunctional family system]
[Disorganized or chaotic environments]
[Child abuse or neglect]

Defining Characteristics ("evidenced by")

Inability to meet [age-appropriate] role expectations
Inadequate problem solving
Poor concentration
[Manipulation of others in the environment for purposes of fulfilling own desires]
[Verbal hostility toward staff and peers]
[Hyperactivity, evidenced by excessive motor activity, easily distracted, short attention span]
[Unable to delay gratification]
[Oppositional and defiant responses to adult requests or rules]

Goals/Objectives

Short-Term Goal

Within 7 days, client will demonstrate ability and willingness to follow unit rules.

Long-Term Goal

By discharge from treatment, client will develop, and utilize, age-appropriate, socially acceptable coping skills.

Interventions with *Selected Rationales*

1. If client is hyperactive, make environment safe for continuous large muscle movement. Rearrange furniture and other objects to prevent injury. ***Client physical safety is a nursing priority.***
2. Provide large motor activities in which client may participate. Nurse may join in some of these activities ***to facilitate relationship development. Tension is released safely and with benefit to the client through physical activities.***
3. Provide frequent, nutritious snacks that client may "eat on the run," ***to ensure adequate calories to offset client's excessive use of energy.***
4. Set limits on manipulative behavior. ("I understand why you are saying these things [or doing these things] and I will not tolerate these behaviors from you.")
5. Identify for the client the consequences of manipulative behavior. All staff must follow through and be consistent. ***Client may try to play one staff member against another, so consistency is vital if intervention is to be successful. Negative consequences may work to decrease unacceptable behaviors.***
6. Do not debate, argue, rationalize, or bargain with the client. ***Ignoring these attempts may work to decrease manipulative behaviors.***
7. Caution should be taken to avoid reinforcing manipulative behaviors by providing desired attention.
8. Confront client's use of manipulative behaviors and explore their damaging effects on interpersonal relationships. ***Manipulative clients often deny responsibility for their behaviors.***
9. Encourage discussion of angry feelings. Help client identify the true object of the hostility. ***Dealing with the feelings honestly and directly will discourage displacement of the anger onto others.***
10. Explore with client alternative ways for handling frustration that would be most suited to his or her lifestyle. Provide support and positive feedback to client as new cop-

ing strategies are tried. Positive feedback encourages use of acceptable behaviors.

Outcome Criteria

1. Client is able to delay gratification, without resorting to manipulation of others.
2. Client is able to express anger in socially acceptable manner.
3. Client is able to verbalize alternative, socially acceptable, and lifestyle-appropriate coping skills he or she plans to use in response to frustration.

SELF-ESTEEM DISTURBANCE

Definition: **Negative self-evaluation and feelings about self or self-capabilities, which may be directly or indirectly expressed.**

Possible Etiologies ("related to")

[Retarded ego development]
[Negative role models]
[Lack of positive feedback]
[Repeated negative feedback, resulting in diminished self-worth]
[Unsatisfactory parent-child relationship]
[Disorganized or chaotic environments]
[Child abuse or neglect]
[Dysfunctional family system]

Defining Characteristics ("evidenced by")

[Lack of eye contact]
Self-negating verbalizations
Expressions of shame or guilt
Evaluates self as unable to deal with events
Rationalizes away or rejects positive feedback and exaggerates negative feedback about self
Hesitant to try new things or situations
Denial of problems obvious to others
Projection of blame or responsibility for problems
Rationalization of personal failures
Hypersensitivity to criticism
Grandiosity

Goals/Objectives

Short-Term Goal

Client will independently direct own care and ADLs within 1 week.

Long-Term Goal

By discharge from treatment, client will exhibit increased feelings of self-worth as evidenced by verbal expression of positive aspects about self, past accomplishments, and future prospects.

Interventions with *Selected Rationales*

1. Ensure that goals are realistic. It is important for client to achieve something, so plan for activities in which the possibility for success is likely. ***Success enhances self-esteem.***
2. Convey unconditional positive regard for client. ***Communication of your acceptance of him or her as a worthwhile human being increases self-esteem.***
3. Spend time with client, both on a one-to-one basis and in group activities. ***This conveys to client that you feel he or she is worth your time.***
4. Assist client in identifying positive aspects of self and in developing plans for changing the characteristics he or she views as negative.
5. Help client decrease use of denial as a defense mechanism. Given positive reinforcement for problem identification and development of more adaptive coping behaviors. ***Positive reinforcement enhances self-esteem and increases client's use of acceptable behaviors.***
6. Encourage and support client in confronting the fear of failure by attending therapy activities and undertaking new tasks. Offer recognition of successful endeavors and positive reinforcement for attempts made. ***Recognition and positive reinforcement enhance self-esteem.***

Outcome Criteria

1. Client verbalizes positive perception of self.
2. Client participates in new activities without exhibiting extreme fear of failure.

ANXIETY (MODERATE TO SEVERE)

Definition: A vague uneasy feeling of discomfort or dread accompanied by an autonomic response; the source is often nonspecific or unknown to the individual; a feeling of apprehension caused by anticipation of danger. It is an altering signal that warns of impending danger and enables the individual to take measures to deal with threat.

Possible Etiologies ("related to")

Situational and maturational crises
Threat to self-concept [perceived or real]
[Threat (or perceived threat) to physical integrity]
Unmet needs
[Fear of failure]
[Dysfunctional family system]
[Unsatisfactory parent-child relationship]
[Innately, easily agitated temperament since birth]

Defining Characteristics ("evidenced by")

Overexcited
Fearful
Feelings of inadequacy
Fear of unspecific consequences
Restlessness
Insomnia
Poor eye contact
Focus on self
[Continuous attention-seeking behaviors]
[Difficulty concentrating; selective inattention]
Increased respiratory and heart rates]

Goals/Objectives

Short-Term Goals

Client will be able to verbalize behaviors that become evident as anxiety starts to rise within 7 days.
Client will be able to verbalize strategies to interrupt escalation of anxiety within 7 days.

Long-Term Goal

Client, will be able to maintain anxiety below the moderate level, as evidenced by absence of disabling behaviors in response to stress, by discharge from treatment.

Interventions with *Selected Rationales*

1. Establish a trusting relationship with client. Be honest, consistent in responses, and available. Show genuine positive regard. ***Honesty, availablity, and acceptance promote trust in the nurse-client relationship.***
2. Provide activities geared toward reduction of tension and decreased anxiety (walking or jogging, volleyball, musical exercises, housekeeping chores, group games). ***Tension and anxiety are released safely and with benefit to the client through physical activities.***

3. Encourage client to identify true feelings and to acknowledge ownership of those feelings. ***Anxious clients often deny a relationship between emotional problems and their anxiety. Use of the defense mechanisms of projection and displacement is exaggerated.***
4. The nurse must maintain an atmosphere of calmness; ***anxiety is easily transmitted from one person to another.***
5. Offer support during times of elevated anxiety. Reassure client of physical and psychological safety. ***Client safety is a nursing priority.***
6. Use of touch is comforting to some clients. However, the nurse must be cautious with its use, ***because anxiety may foster suspicion in some individuals who might misinterpret touch as aggression.***
7. As anxiety diminishes, assist client in recognizing specific events that preceded its onset. Work on alternative responses to future occurrences. ***A plan of action provides the client with a feeling of security for more successfully handling the difficult situation should it recur.***
8. Assist client in recognizing signs of escalating anxiety, and explore ways client may intervene before behaviors become disabling.
9. Administer tranquilizing medication, as ordered. Assess for effectiveness, and instruct client regarding possible adverse side effects. ***Antianxiety medications (e.g., diazepam, chlordiazeproxide, alprazolam) provide relief from the immobilizing effects of anxiety and may facilitate client's cooperation with therapy.***

Outcome Criteria

1. Client is able to verbalize behaviors that become evident as anxiety starts to rise and takes actions appropriate to interrupt progression of the condition.
2. Client is able to maintain anxiety at a manageable level.

NONCOMPLIANCE

Definition: The extent to which a person's and/or caregiver's behavior coincides or fails to coincide with a health-promoting or therapeutic plan agreed upon by the person [or caregiver] and health-care professional.

Possible Etiologies ("related to")

[Biochemical alteration]

[Neurological alteration related to premature birth, fetal distress, precipitated or prolonged labor]
[Negative temperament]
[Dysfunctional family system]
[Negative role models]
[Retarded ego development]
[Low frustration tolerance and short attention span]
[Denial of problems]

Defining Characteristics ("evidenced by")

Behavior indicative of failure to adhere (to treatment regimen)
[Inability to sit still long enough to complete a task]
[Expression of opposition to requests for participation]
Refusal to follow directions or suggestions of treatment team

Goals/Objectives

Short-Term Goal

Client will participate in and cooperate during therapeutic activities.

Long-Term Goal

Client will complete assigned tasks willingly and independently or with a minimum of assistance.

Interventions with *Selected Rationales*

(For the client with inattention and hyperactivity:)

1. Provide an environment for task efforts that is as free of distractions as possible. ***Client is highly distractible and is unable to perform in the presence of even minimal stimulation.***
2. Provide assistance on a one-to-one basis, beginning with simple, concrete instructions. ***Client lacks the ability to assimilate information that is complicated or has abstract meaning.***
3. Ask client to repeat instructions to you ***to determine level of comprehension.***
4. Establish goals that allow client to complete a part of the task, rewarding completion of each step with a break for physical activity. ***Short-term goals are not so overwhelming to one with such a short attention span. The positive reinforcement (physical activity) increases self-esteem and provides incentive for client to pursue the task to completion.***
5. Gradually decrease the amount of assistance given to task performance, while assuring the client that assistance is still available if deemed necessary. ***This encourages the client***

to perform independently while providing a feeling of security with the presence of a trusted individual.

(For the client with oppositional tendencies:)

6. Set forth a structured plan of therapeutic activities. Start with minimum expectations and increase as client begins to manifest evidence of compliance. ***Structure provides security, and one or two activities may not seem as overwhelming as the whole schedule of activities presented at one time.***
7. Establish a system of rewards for compliance with therapy and consequences for noncompliance. Ensure that the rewards and consequences are concepts of value to the client. ***Positive and negative reinforcements can contribute to desired changes in behavior.***
8. Convey acceptance of the client separate from the undesirable behaviors being exhibited. ("It is not *you*, but your *behavior,* that is unacceptable.") ***Unconditional acceptance enhances self-worth and may contribute to a decrease in the need for passive-aggressive behavior toward others.***

Outcome Criteria

1. Client cooperates with staff in an effort to complete assigned tasks.
2. Client complies with treatment by participating in therapies without negativism.
3. Client takes direction from staff without becoming defensive.

307.23 TOURETTE'S DISORDER*

Defined

Tourette's disorder is characterized by the presence of multiple motor tics and one or more vocal tics that may appear simultaneously or at different periods during the illness (APA, 1994). Onset can be as early as age 2, but it occurs most commonly during childhood or early adolescence, with the median age being 7 years. The disorder is more common in boys than in girls. The duration of the disorder is usually lifelong, but the symptoms usually diminish during adolescence and adulthood.

---

*Reprinted with permission from the *Diagnostic and Statistical Manual of Mental Disorders, Fourth Edition.* Copyright 1994 American Psychiatric Association, 1994.

Predisposing Factors

1. **Physiological**
   a. ***Genetics:*** Family studies have shown that Tourette's disorder is more common in relatives of individuals with the disorder than in the general population. Autosomal dominant transmission may be involved (Kaplan and Sadock, 1998).
   b. ***Brain Alterations:*** Altered levels of neurotransmitters and dysfunction in the area of the basal ganglia have been implicated in the etiology of Tourette's disorder.
   c. ***Biochemical Factors:*** Abnormalities in levels of dopamine, serotonin, dynorphin, gamma-aminobutyric acid (GABA), acetylcholine, and norepinephrine have been associated with Tourette's disorder (Popper and Steingard, 1994).
2. **Psychosocial**
   a. It is believed that the genetic predisposition to Tourette's disorder may be reinforced by certain factors in the environment, such as increased prenatal complications, low birth weight, and emotional stress during pregnancy.

Symptomatology (Subjective and Objective Data)

The *DSM-IV* identifies the following signs and symptoms of Tourette's disorder.

1. The disorder may begin with a single motor tic, such as eye blinking, neck jerking, shoulder shrugging, facial grimacing, or coughing.
2. Complex motor tics may follow and include touching, squatting, hopping, skipping, deep knee bends, retracing steps, and twirling when walking.
3. Vocal tics include various words or sounds such as clicks, grunts, yelps, barks, sniffs, snorts, coughs, and in about 10% of cases a complex vocal tic involving the uttering of obscenities.
4. Vocal tics may include repeating certain words or phrases out of context, repeating one's own sounds or words (palilalia), or repeating what others say (echolalia).
5. The movements and vocalizations are experienced as compulsive and irresistible, but they can be suppressed for varying lengths of time.

6. Tics are exacerbated by stress and attenuated during periods in which the individual becomes totally absorbed by an activity.
7. Tics are markedly diminished during sleep.

Common Nursing Diagnoses and Interventions

(Interventions are applicable to various health-care settings, such as inpatient and partial hospitalization, community outpatient clinic, home health, and private practice.)

RISK FOR VIOLENCE: SELF-DIRECTED OR DIRECTED AT OTHERS

Definition: Behaviors in which an individual demonstrates that he/she can be physically, emotionally, and/or sexually harmful either to self or to others.

Related/Risk Factors ("related to")

[Low tolerance for frustration]
[Abnormalities in brain neurotransmitters]
Body language—rigid posture, clenching of fists and jaw, hyperactivity, pacing, breathlessness, and threatening stances
[History or threats of violence toward self or others or of destruction to the property of others]
Impulsivity
Suicidal ideation, plan, available means

Goals/Objectives

Short-Term Goal

Client will seek out staff/support person at any time if thoughts of harming self or others should occur.

Long-Term Goal

Client will not harm self or others.

Interventions with *Selected Rationales*

1. Observe client's behavior frequently through routine activities and interactions. Become aware of behaviors that indicate a rise in agitation. *Stress commonly increases tic behaviors. Recognition of behaviors that precede the onset of aggression may provide the opportunity to intervene before violence occurs.*

2. Monitor for self-destructive behavior and impulses. A staff member may need to stay with the client to prevent self-mutilation. ***Client safety is a nursing priority.***
3. Provide hand coverings and other restraints that prevent the client from self-multilative behaviors. ***Provide immediate external controls against self-aggressive behaviors.***
4. Redirect violent behavior with physical outlets for frustration. ***Excess energy is released through physical activities and a feeling of relaxation is induced.***
5. Administer medication as ordered by the physician. Several medications have been used to treat Tourette's disorder. The most common ones include the following:
   a. ***Haloperidol (Haldol):*** Haloperidol has been the drug of choice for Tourette's disorder. Children on this medication must be monitored for adverse effects associated with most antipsychotic medications (see Chap. 27). Because of the potential for adverse effects, haloperidol should be reserved for children with severe symptoms or with symptoms that interfere with their ability to function.
   b. ***Pimozide (Orap):*** The response rate and side effect profile of primozide are similar to haloperidol. It is used in the management of severe motor or vocal tics that have failed to respond to more conventional treatment. It is not recommended for children under age 12.
   c. ***Clonidine (Catapres):*** Clonidine is an antihypertensive medication, the efficacy of which in the treatment of Tourette's disorder has been mixed. Some physicians like it and use it as a drug of first choice because of its relative safety and few side effects.

Outcome Criteria

1. Anxiety is maintained at a level at which client feels no need for aggression.
2. Client seeks out staff or support person for expression of true feelings.
3. Client has not harmed self or others.

IMPAIRED SOCIAL INTERACTION

Definition: The state in which an individual participates in an insufficient or excessive quantity or ineffective quality of social exchange.

Possible Etiologies ("related to")

Self-concept disturbance

Low tolerance for frustration
Impulsiveness
Oppositional behavior
Aggressive behavior

Defining Characteristics ("evidenced by")

Verbalized or observed discomfort in social situations
Verbalized or observed inability to receive or communicate a satisfying sense of belonging, caring, interest, or shared history
Observed use of unsuccessful social interaction behaviors
Dysfunctional interaction with peers, family, or others

Goals/Objectives

Short-Term Goal

Client will develop a one-to-one relationship with a nurse or support person within 1 week.

Long-Term Goal

Client will be able to interact with staff and peers, using age-appropriate, acceptable behaviors.

Interventions with *Selected Rationales*

1. Develop a trusting relationship with the client. Convey acceptance of the person separate from the unacceptable behavior. ***Unconditional acceptance increases feelings of self-worth.***
2. Discuss with client which behaviors are and are not acceptable. Describe in matter-of-fact manner the consequences of unacceptable behavior. Follow through. ***Negative reinforcement can alter undesirable behaviors.***
3. Provide group situations for client. ***Appropriate social behavior is often learned from the positive and negative feedback of peers.***
4. Act as a role model for client through appropriate interactions with others. ***Role modeling of a respected individual is one of the strongest forms of learning.***

Outcome Criteria

1. Client seeks out staff or support person for social as well as for therapeutic interaction.
2. Client verbalizes reasons for inability to form close interpersonal relationships with others in the past.
3. Client interacts with others, using age-appropriate, acceptable behaviors.

SELF-ESTEEM DISTURBANCE

Definition: Negative self-evaluation and feelings about self or self-capabilities, which may be directly or indirectly expressed.

Possible Etiologies ("related to")

[Shame associated with tic behaviors]

Defining Characteristics ("evidenced by")

[Lack of eye contact]
Self-negating verbalizations
Expressions of shame or guilt
Hesitant to try new things or situations
[Manipulation of others]

Goals/Objectives

Short-Term Goal

Client will verbalize positive aspects about self not associated with tic behaviors.

Long-Term Goal

Client will exhibit increased feeling of self-worth as evidenced by verbal expression of positive aspects about self, past accomplishments, and future prospects.

Interventions with *Selected Rationales*

1. Convey unconditional acceptance and positive regard. *Communication of client as worthwhile human being may increase self-esteem.*
2. Set limits on manipulative behavior. Take caution not to reinforce manipulative behaviors by providing desired attention. Identify the consequences of manipulation. Administer consequences matter of factly when manipulation occurs. *Negative consequences may work to decrease unacceptable behaviors.*
3. Help client understand that he or she uses this behavior to try to increase own self-esteem. Interventions should reflect other actions to accomplish this goal. *When client feels better about self, the need to manipulate others will diminish.*
4. If client chooses to suppress tics in the presence of others, provide a specified "tic time," during which he or she "vents" tics, feelings, and behaviors (alone or with staff). *Allows for release of tics and assists in sense of control and management of symptoms (Rosner and Pollice, 1991).*

5. Ensure that client has regular one-to-one time with staff or support person. *Provides opportunity for educating about illness and teaching management tactics. Assists in exploring feelings around illness and incorporating illness into a healthy sense of self (Rosner and Pollice, 1991).*

Outcome Criteria

1. Client verbalizes positive perception of self.
2. Client willingly participates in new activities and situations.

■ 309.21 SEPARATION ANXIETY DISORDER*

Defined

The APA (1994) defines separation anxiety disorder as excessive anxiety concerning separation from the home or from those to whom the person is attached. Onset may occur as early as preschool age, rarely as late as adolescence, but always before age 18, and is more common in girls than in boys.

Predisposing Factors

1. **Physiological**
   a. ***Genetics:*** The results of studies indicate that a greater number of children with relatives who manifest anxiety problems develop anxiety disorders themselves than do children with no such family patterns.
   b. ***Temperament:*** Studies have shown that differences in temperamental characteristics at birth may be correlated to the acquisition of fear and anxiety disorders in childhood. This may denote an inherited vulnerability or predisposition toward developing these disorders.
2. **Psychosocial**
   a. ***Stressful Life Events:*** Studies indicate that children who are predisposed to anxiety disorders may be affected significantly by stressful life events.

---

*Reprinted with permission from the *Diagnostic and Statistical Manual of Mental Disorders, Fourth Edition*. Copyright 1994 American Psychiatric Association, 1994.

b. ***Family Influences:*** Several theories relate the development of separation anxiety to the following dynamics within the family:
   - An overattachment to the mother (primary caregiver)
   - Separation conflicts between parent and child
   - Enmeshment of members within a family
   - Overprotection of the child by the parents
   - Transfer of parents' fears and anxieties to the children through role modeling

Symptomatology (Subjective and Objective Data)

The *DSM-IV* identifies the following signs and symptoms of separation anxiety disorder:

1. Recurrent, excessive distress when separation from home or major attachment figures occurs or is anticipated
2. Persistent and excessive worry about losing, or about possible harm befalling, major attachment figures
3. Persistent and excessive worry that an untoward event will lead to separation from a major attachment figure
4. Persistent reluctance or refusal to go to school or elsewhere because of fear of separation
5. Persistent and excessive fear or reluctance to be alone or without major attachment figures at home or without significant adults in other settings
6. Persistent reluctance or refusal to go to sleep without being near a major attachment figure or to sleep away from home
7. Repeated nightmares involving the theme of separation
8. Repeated complaints of physical symptoms, such as headaches, stomach aches, nausea, or vomiting, when separation from major attachment figures occurs or is anticipated

Common Nursing Diagnoses and Interventions

(Interventions are applicable to various health-care settings, such as inpatient and partial hospitalization, community outpatient clinic, home health, and private practice.)

ANXIETY (SEVERE)

Definition: A vague uneasy feeling of discomfort or dread accompanied by an autonomic response; the source is often nonspecific or unknown to the individual; a feeling of apprehension caused by anticipation of danger. It is an altering signal that warns of impending danger and enables the individual to take measures to deal with threat.

Possible Etiologies ("related to")

Family history
Birth temperament
Overattachment to parent
Negative role modeling

Defining Characteristics ("evidenced by")

[Excessive distress when separated from attachment figure]
[Fear of anticipation of separation from attachment figure]
[Fear of being alone or without attachment figure]
[Reluctance or refusal to go to school or anywhere else without attachment figure]
[Nightmares about being separated from attachment figure]
[Somatic symptoms occurring as a result of fear of separation]

Goals/Objectives

Short-Term Goal

Client will discuss fears of separation with trusted individual.

Long-Term Goal

Client will maintain anxiety at no higher than moderate level in the face of events that formerly have precipitated panic.

Interventions with *Selected Rationales*

1. Establish an atmosphere of calmness, trust, and genuine positive regard. *Trust and unconditional acceptance are necessary for satisfactory nurse-client relationship. Calmness is important because anxiety is easily transmitted from one person to another.*
2. Assure client of his or her safety and security. *Symptoms of panic anxiety are very frightening.*
3. Explore the child's or adolescent's fears of separating from the parents. Explore with the parents possible fears they may have of separation from the child. *Some parents may*

have an underlying fear of separation from the child, of which they are unaware and which they are unconsciously transferring to the child.

4. Help parents and child initiate realistic goals (e.g., child to stay with sitter for 2 hours with minimal anxiety, or child to stay at friend's house without parents until 9:00 PM without experiencing panic anxiety). ***Parents may be so frustrated with the child's clinging and demanding behaviors that assistance with problem solving may be required.***
5. Give, and encourage parents to give, positive reinforcement for desired behaviors. ***Positive reinforcement encourages repetition of desirable behaviors.***

Outcome Criteria

1. Client and parents are able to discuss their fears regarding separation.
2. Client experiences no somatic symptoms from fear of separation.
3. Client maintains anxiety at moderate level when separation occurs or is anticipated.

INEFFECTIVE INDIVIDUAL COPING

Definition: The impairment of adaptive behaviors and abilities of a person in meeting life's demands and roles.

Possible Etiologies ("related to")

[Unresolved separation conflicts]
[Inadequate coping skills]

Defining Characteristics ("evidenced by")

[Somatic complaints in response to occurrence or anticipation of separation from attachment figure]

Goals/Objectives

Short-Term Goal

Client will verbalize correlation of somatic symptoms to fear of separation.

Long-Term Goal

Client will demonstrate use of more adaptive coping strategies (than physical symptoms) in response to stressful situations.

Interventions with *Selected Rationales*

1. Encourage child or adolescent to discuss specific situations in life that produce the most distress and describe his or her response to these situations. Include parents in the discussion. ***Client and family may be unaware of the correlation between stressful situations and the exacerbation of physical symptoms.***
2. Help the child or adolescent who is perfectionistic to recognize that self-expectations may be unrealistic. Connect times of unmet self-expectations to the exacerbation of physical symptoms. ***Recognition of maladaptive patterns is the first step in the change process.***
3. Encourage parents and child to identify more adaptive coping strategies that the child could use in the face of anxiety that feels overwhelming. Practice through role play. ***Practice facilitates the use of the desired behavior when the individual is actually faced with the stressful situation.***

Outcome Criteria

1. Client and family verbalize the correlation between separation anxiety and somatic symptoms.
2. Client verbalizes the correlation between unmet self-expectations and somatic symptoms.
3. Client responds to stressful situations without exhibiting physical symptoms.

IMPAIRED SOCIAL INTERACTION

Definition: The state in which an individual participates in an insufficient or excessive quantity or ineffective quality of social exchange.

Possible Etiologies ("related to")

[Reluctance to be away from attachment figure]

Defining Characteristics ("evidenced by")

[Symptoms of severe anxiety]
Verbalized or observed discomfort in social situations
Verbalized or observed inability to receive or communicate a satisfying sense of belonging, caring, interest, or shared history
Observed use of unsuccessful social interaction behaviors
Dysfunctional interaction with others

Goals/Objectives

Short-Term Goal

Client will spend time with staff or other support person, without presence of attachment figure, without excessive anxiety.

Long-Term Goal

Client will be able to spend time with others (without presence of attachment figure) without excessive anxiety.

Interventions with *Selected Rationales*

1. Develop a trusting relationship with client. ***This is the first step in helping the client learn to interact with others.***
2. Attend groups with the child and support efforts to interact with others. Give positive feedback. ***Presence of a trusted individual provides security during times of distress. Positive feedback encourages repetition.***
3. Convey to the child the acceptability of his or her not participating in group in the beginning. Gradually encourage small contributions until client is able to participate more fully. ***Small successes will gradually increase self-confidence and decrease self-consciousness, so that client will feel less anxious in the group situation.***
4. Help client set small personal goals (e.g., "Today I will speak to one person I don't know."). ***Simple, realistic goals provide opportunities for success that increase self-confidence and may encourage the client to attempt more difficult objectives in the future.***

Outcome Criteria

1. Client spends time with others using acceptable, age-appropriate behaviors.
2. Client is able to interact with others away from the attachment figure without excessive anxiety.

■ INTERNET REFERENCES

Additional information about Attention-Deficit/Hyperactivity Disorder may be located at the following Websites:

- http://www.chadd.org
- http://www.laurus.com

Additional information about Autism may be located at the following Websites:

- http://www.autism-society.org/autism.html
- http://www.laurus.com

Additional information about medications to treat Attention-Deficit/Hyperactivity Disorder may be located at the following Websites:

- http://www.fadavis.com
- http://www.laurus.com

CHAPTER 4

Delirium, Dementia, and Amnestic Disorders

■ BACKGROUND ASSESSMENT DATA

293.0 Delirium

Defined

The *DSM-IV* defines delirium as a disturbance of consciousness and a change in cognition that develop rapidly over a short period of time (APA, 1994). The symptoms of delirium usually begin quite abruptly, and the duration is usually brief (e.g., 1 week; rarely more than 1 month). The disorder subsides completely on recovery from the underlying determinant. If the underlying condition persists, the delirium may gradually shift to the syndrome of dementia or progress to coma. The individual then recovers, becomes chronically vegetative, or dies.

Predisposing Factors

The *DSM-IV* differentiates among the disorders of delirium by their etiology, although they share a common symptom presentation. Categories of delirium include the following:

1. **Delirium Due to a General Medical Condition:** Certain medical conditions, such as systematic infections, metabolic disorders, fluid and electrolyte imbalances, liver or kidney disease, encephalopathy, and head trauma, can cause the symptoms of delirium.

2. **Substance-Induced Delirium:** The symptoms of delirium can be induced by the exposure to a toxin or the ingestion of a medication, such as anticonvulsants, neuroleptics, anxiolytics, antidepressants, cardiovascular medications, antineoplastics, and hormones.
3. **Substance-Intoxication Delirium:** Delirium symptoms can occur in response to taking high doses of cannabis, cocaine, hallucinogens, alcohol, anxiolytics, or narcotics.
4. **Substance-Withdrawal Delirium:** Reduction or termination of long-term, high-dose use of certain substances, such as alcohol, sedatives, hypnotics, or anxiolytics, can result in withdrawal delirium symptoms.
5. **Delirium Due to Multiple Etiologies:** Symptoms of delirium may be related to more than one general medical condition or to the combined effects of a general medical condition and substance use.

Symptomatology *(Subjective and Objective Data)*

The following symptoms have been identified with the syndrome of delirium:

1. Altered consciousness ranging from hypervigilance to stupor or semicoma.
2. Extreme distractibility with difficulty focusing attention.
3. Disorientation to time and place.
4. Impaired reasoning ability and goal-directed behavior.
5. Disturbance in the sleep-wake cycle.
6. Emotional instability as manifested by fear, anxiety, depression, irritability, anger, euphoria, or apathy.
7. Misperceptions of the environment, including illusions and hallucinations.
8. Autonomic manifestations, such as tachycardia, sweating, flushed face, dilated pupils, and elevated blood pressure.
9. Incoherent speech.
10. Impairment of recent memory.

290.xx Dementia

Defined

Dementia is defined as a syndrome of acquired, persistent intellectual impairment with compromised function in multiple spheres of mental activity, such as memory, language, visuospatial skills, emotion or personality, and cognition (Wise and Gray, 1994). The disease usually has a slow, insidious onset and is chronic, progressive, and irreversible.

Predisposing Factors

The *DSM-IV* identifies the following etiologic categories for the syndrome of dementia:

1. **Dementia of the Alzheimer's Type:** The exact cause of Alzheimer's disease is unknown, but several theories have been proposed, such as reduction in brain acetylcholine, accumulation of aluminum in the brain, immune system alterations, head trauma, and genetic factors. Pathological changes in the brain include atrophy, enlarged ventricles, and the presence of numerous neurofibrillary plaques and tangles. Definitive diagnosis is by biopsy or autopsy examination of brain tissue, although refinement of diagnostic criteria now enables clinicians to use specific clinical features to identify the disease at an accuracy rate approaching 85 percent.
2. **Vascular Dementia:** This type of dementia is caused by significant cerebrovascular disease. The client suffers the equivalent of small strokes caused by arterial hypertension or cerebral emboli or thrombi, which destroy many areas of the brain. The onset of symptoms is more abrupt than in Alzheimer's disease and runs a highly variable course, progressing in steps rather than as a gradual deterioration.
3. **Dementia Due to HIV Disease:** The immune dysfunction associated with human immunodeficiency virus (HIV) disease can lead to brain infections by other organisms. HIV also appears to cause dementia directly.
4. **Dementia Due to Head Trauma:** The syndrome of symptoms associated with dementia can be brought on by a traumatic brain injury.
5. **Dementia Due to Parkinson's Disease:** Parkinson's disease is caused by a loss of nerve cells in the substantia nigra of the basal ganglia. The symptoms of dementia associated with Parkinson's disease closely resemble those of Alzheimer's disease.
6. **Dementia Due to Huntington's Disease:** This disease is transmitted as a mendelian dominant gene,

and damage occurs in the areas of the basal ganglia and the cerebral cortex. A profound dementia occurs within 5 to 10 years of onset.

7. **Dementia Due to Pick's Disease:** Pathology occurs from atrophy in the frontal and temporal lobes of the brain. Symptoms are strikingly similar to those of Alzheimer's disease, and Pick's disease is often misdiagnosed as Alzheimer's.
8. **Dementia Due to Creutzfeldt-Jakob Disease:** This form of dementia is caused by a transmissible virus. The clinical presentation is typical of the syndrome of dementia, and the course is extremely rapid, with progressive deterioration and death within 1 year.
9. **Dementia Due to Other General Medical Conditions:** These include endocrine, hepatic, renal, cardiopulmonary, or neurological conditions, brain lesions, or systemic infections.
10. **Substance-Induced Persisting Dementia:** This type of dementia is related to the persisting effects of substances such as alcohol, inhalants, sedatives, hypnotics, anxiolytics, other medications, and environmental toxins. The term "persisting" is used to indicate that the dementia persists long after the effects of substance intoxication or substance withdrawal have subsided.

***Symptomatology** (Subjective and Objective Data)*

The following symptoms have been identified with the syndrome of dementia:

1. Memory impairment (impaired ability to learn new information or to recall previously learned information).
2. Impairment in abstract thinking, judgment, and impulse control.
3. Impairment in language ability, such as difficulty naming objects. In some instances, the individual may not speak at all (aphasia).
4. Personality changes are common.
5. Impaired ability to execute motor activities despite intact motor abilities (apraxia).
6. Disorientation.
7. Wandering.
8. Delusions are common (particularly delusions of persecution).

294.0: Amnestic Disorders

Defined

Amnestic disorders are characterized by an inability to learn new information (short-term memory deficit) despite normal attention, and an inability to recall previously learned information (long-term memory deficit). No other cognitive deficits exist.

Predisposing Factors

The *DSM-IV* identifies the following categories as etiologies for the syndrome of symptoms known as amnestic disorders:

1. **Amnestic Disorder Due to a General Medical Condition:** The symptoms may be associated with head trauma, cerebrovascular disease, cerebral neoplastic disease, cerebral anoxia, herpes simplex encephalitis, poorly controlled insulin-dependent diabetes, and surgical intervention to the brain (APA, 1994; Wise and Gray, 1994). Transient amnestic syndromes can also occur from epileptic seizures, electroconvulsive therapy, severe migraine, and drug overdose (Wise and Gray, 1994).
2. **Substance-Induced Persisting Amnestic Disorder:** This type of amnestic disorder is related to the persisting effects of substances such as alcohol, sedatives, hypnotics, anxiolytics, other medications, and environmental toxins. The term "persisting" is used to indicate that the symptoms persist long after the effects of substance intoxication or substance withdrawal have subsided.

Symptomatology *(Subjective and Objective Data)*

The following symptoms have been identified with amnestic disorder:

1. Disorientation to place and time may occur with profound amnesia.
2. There is an inability to recall events from the recent past and events from the remote past. (Events from the very remote past are often more easily recalled than recently occurring ones.)
3. The individual is prone to confabulation; that is, the individual may create imaginary events to fill in the memory gaps.
4. Apathy, lack of initiative, and emotional blandness are common.

Common Nursing Diagnoses and Interventions for Delirium, Dementia, and Amnestic Disorders

(Interventions are applicable to various health-care settings, such as inpatient and partial hospitalization, community outpatient clinic, home health, and private practice.)

RISK FOR TRAUMA

Definition: [The client has] accentuated risk of accidental tissue injury (e.g., wound, burn, fracture).

Related/Risk Factors ("related to")

[Chronic alteration in structure or function of brain tissue, secondary to the aging process, multiple infarcts, HIV disease, head trauma, chronic substance abuse, or progressively dysfunctional physical condition resulting in the following symptoms:
- Disorientation; confusion
- Weakness
- Muscular incoordination
- Seizures
- Memory impairment
- Poor vision
- Extreme psychomotor agitation observed in the late stages of delirium]

[Frequent shuffling of feet and stumbling]
[Falls, caused by muscular incoordination or seizures]
[Bumping into furniture]
[Exposing self to frigid conditions with insufficient protective clothing]
[Cutting self when using sharp instruments]
[History of attempting to light burner or oven and leaving gas on in house]
[Smoking and leaving burning cigarettes in various places; smoking in bed; falling asleep on couch or chair with lit cigarette in hand]
[Purposeless, thrashing movements; hyperactivity that is out of touch with the environment]

Goals/Objectives

Short-Term Goal

Client will call for assistance when ambulating or carrying out other activities.

Long-Term Goal

Client will not experience physical injury.

Interventions with *Selected Rationales*

1. Assess client's level of disorientation and confusion to determine specific requirements for safety. ***Knowledge of client's level of functioning is necessary to formulate appropriate plan of care.***
2. Institute appropriate safety measures, such as the following:
   a. Place furniture in room in an arrangement that best accommodates client's disabilities.
   b. Observe client behaviors frequently; assign staff on one-to-one basis if condition warrants; accompany and assist client when ambulating; use wheelchair for transporting long distances.
   c. Store items that client uses frequently within easy access.
   d. Remove potentially harmful articles from client's room: cigarettes, matches, lighters, sharp objects.
   e. Remain with client while he or she smokes.
   f. Pad side rails and headboard of client with seizure disorder. Institute seizure precautions as described in procedure manual of individual institution.

   Client safety is a nursing priority.
3. Frequently orient client to reality and surroundings. ***Disorientation may endanger client safety if he or she unknowingly wanders away from safe environment.***
4. Use tranquilizing medications and soft restraints, as prescribed by physician, for client's protection during periods of excessive hyperactivity. ***Use restraints judiciously, because they can increase agitation. They may be required, however, to provide for client safety.***
5. Teach prospective caregivers methods that have been successful in preventing client injury. ***These caregivers will be responsible for client's safety after discharge from the hospital. Sharing successful interventions may be helpful.***

Outcome Criteria

1. Client is able to accomplish daily activities within the environment without experiencing injury.
2. Prospective caregivers are able to verbalize means of providing safe environment for client.

RISK FOR VIOLENCE: SELF-DIRECTED OR DIRECTED AT OTHERS

Definition: Behaviors in which an individual demonstrates that he/she can be physically, emotionally, and/or sexually harmful either to self or to others.

Related/Risk Factors ("related to")

[Chronic alteration in structure or function of brain tissue, secondary to the aging process, multiple infarcts, HIV disease, head trauma, chronic substance abuse, or progressively dysfunctional physical condition resulting in the following symptoms:
Delusional thinking
Suspiciousness of others
Hallucinations
Illusions
Disorientation or confusion
Impairment of impulse control]
[Inaccurate perception of the environment]
Body language—rigid posture, clenching of fists and jaw, hyperactivity, pacing, breathlessness, and threatening stances.
Suicidal ideation, plan, available means
Cognitive impairment
[Depressed mood]

Goals/Objectives

Short-Term Goal

Client will maintain agitation at manageable level so as not to become violent.

Long-Term Goal

Client will not harm self or others.

Interventions with *Selected Rationales*

1. Assess client's level of anxiety and behaviors that indicate the anxiety is increasing. ***Recognizing these behaviors, the nurse may be able to intervene before violence occurs.***
2. Maintain low level of stimuli in client's environment (low lighting, few people, simple decor, low noise level). ***Anxiety increases in a highly stimulating environment.***
3. Remove all potentially dangerous objects from client's environment. ***In a disoriented, confused state, the client may use these objects to harm self or others.***

4. Have sufficient staff available to execute a physical confrontation, if necessary. ***Assistance may be required from others to provide for physical safety of client or primary nurse or both.***
5. Maintain a calm manner with client. Attempt to prevent frightening the client unnecessarily. Provide continual reassurance and support. ***Anxiety is contagious and can be transferred to the client.***
6. Interrupt periods of unreality and reorient. ***Client safety is jeopardized during periods of disorientation. Correcting misinterpretations of reality enhances client's feelings of self-worth and personal dignity.***
7. Use tranquilizing medications and soft restraints, as prescribed by physician, ***for protection of client and others during periods of elevated anxiety. Use restraints judiciously, because agitation is sometimes increased; they may be required, however, to ensure client safety.***
8. Sit with client and provide one-to-one observation if assessed to be actively suicidal. ***Client safety is a nursing priority.***
9. Teach relaxation exercise ***to intervene in times of increasing anxiety.***
10. Teach prospective caregivers to recognize client behaviors that indicate anxiety is increasing and ways to intervene before violence occurs.

Outcome Criteria

1. Prospective caregivers are able to verbalize behaviors that indicate an increasing anxiety level and ways they may assist client to manage the anxiety before violence occurs.
2. Client is able to control impulse to perform acts of violence against self or others, with assistance from caregivers.

ALTERED THOUGHT PROCESSES

Definition: A state in which an individual experiences a disruption in cognitive operations and activities.

Possible Etiologies ("related to")

[Alteration in structure/function of brain tissue, secondary to the following conditions:
- Advanced age
- Vascular disease
- Hypertension

- Cerebral hypoxia
- Long-term abuse of mood- or behavior-altering substances
- Exposure to environmental toxins
- Various other physical disorders that predispose to cerebral abnormalities (see Predisposing Factors)]

Defining Characteristics ("evidenced by")

[Delusional thinking]
Inaccurate interpretation of environment
Memory deficit or problems [and confabulation]
Altered attention span; distractibility
[Disorientation to time, place, person, circumstances, and events]
[Impaired ability to make decisions, problem-solve, reason, abstract or conceptualize, calculate]
Inappropriate or non–reality-based thinking

Goals/Objectives

Short-Term Goal

Client will accept explanations of inaccurate interpretations within the environment within 5 days.

Long-Term Goal

With assistance from caregiver, client will be able to interrupt non–reality-based thinking.

Interventions with *Selected Rationales*

1. Frequently orient client to reality and surroundings. Allow client to have familiar objects around him or her. Use other items, such as clock, calendar, and daily schedules, to assist in maintaining reality orientation. ***Client safety is jeopardized during periods of disorientation. Maintaining reality orientation enhances client's sense of self-worth and personal dignity.***
2. Teach prospective caregivers how to orient client to time, person, place, and circumstances, as required. ***These caregivers will be responsible for client safety after discharge from the hospital. Sharing successful interventions may be helpful.***
3. Give positive feedback when thinking and behavior are appropriate or when client verbalizes that certain expressed ideas are not based in reality. ***Positive feedback increases self-esteem and enhances desire to repeat appropriate behaviors.***
4. Use simple explanations and face-to-face interaction when communicating with client. Do not shout message into client's ear. ***Speaking slowly and in a face-to-face posi-***

tion is most effective when communicating with an elderly individual experiencing a hearing loss. Visual cues facilitate understanding. Shouting causes distortion of high-pitched sounds and in some instances creates a feeling of discomfort for the client.

5. Express reasonable doubt if client relays suspicious beliefs in response to delusional thinking. Discuss with client the potential personal negative effects of continued suspiciousness of others. Reinforce accurate perception of people and situations. ***Expressions of doubt by a trusted individual may foster similar uncertainties about delusion on the part of the client.***
6. Do not permit rumination of false ideas. When this begins, talk to client about real people and real events. ***Reality orientation increases client's sense of self-worth and personal dignity.***
7. Close observation of client's behavior is indicated if delusional thinking reveals an intention for violence. ***Client safety is a nursing priority.***

Outcome Criteria

1. With assistance from caregiver, client is able to distinguish between reality-based and non–reality-based thinking.
2. Prospective caregivers are able to verbalize ways in which to orient client to reality, as needed.

SELF-CARE DEFICIT

Definition: A state in which the individual experiences an impaired ability to perform or complete [activities of daily living (ADLs)] independently.

Possible Etiologies ("related to")

[Disorientation]
[Confusion]
[Memory deficits]

Defining Characteristics ("evidenced by")

[Inability to fulfill ADLs]

Goals/Objectives

Short-Term Goal

Client will participate in ADLs with assistance from caregiver.

Long-Term Goal

Client will accomplish ADLs to the best of his or her ability. Unfulfilled needs will be met by caregiver.

Interventions with *Selected Rationales*

1. Provide a simple, structured environment ***to minimize confusion:***
   a. Identify self-care deficits and provide assistance as required.
   b. Allow plenty of time for client to perform tasks.
   c. Provide guidance and support for independent actions by talking the client through the task one step at a time.
   d. Provide a structured schedule of activities that does not change from day to day.
   e. ADLs should follow home routine as closely as possible.
   f. Provide for consistency in assignment of daily caregivers.
2. In planning for discharge:
   a. Perform ongoing assessment of client's ability to fulfill nutritional needs, ensure personal safety, follow medication regimen, and communicate need for assistance with those activities that he or she cannot accomplish independently. ***Client safety and security are nursing priorities.***
   b. Assess prospective caregivers' ability to anticipate and fulfill client's unmet needs. Provide information to assist caregivers with this responsibility. Ensure that caregivers are aware of available community support systems from whom they can seek assistance when required. ***This will facilitate transition to discharge from treatment center.***
   c. National support organizations can provide information:

      National Parkinson Foundation Inc.
      1501 NW 9th Ave.
      Miami, FL 33136
      1-800-327-4545

      Alzheimer's Association
      919 N. Michigan Ave., Suite 1000
      Chicago, IL 60611
      1-800-272-3900

      The Centers for Disease Control and Prevention (CDC)
      AIDS Hotline
      1-800-342-AIDS
      (24 hours/day, 7 days/week)

Outcome Criteria

1. Client willingly participates in ADLs.
2. Client accomplishes ADLs to the best of his or her ability.
3. Client's unfulfilled needs are met by caregivers.

SENSORY-PERCEPTUAL ALTERATIONS (SPECIFY)

Definition: A state in which an individual experiences a change in the amount or patterning of incoming stimuli [either internally or externally initiated] accompanied by a diminished, exaggerated, distorted, or impaired response to such stimuli.

Possible Etiologies ("related to")

[Alteration in structure/function of brain tissue, secondary to the following conditions:

- Advanced age
- Vascular disease
- Hypertension
- Cerebral hypoxia
- Abuse of mood- or behavior-altering substances
- Exposure to environmental toxins
- Various other physical disorders that predispose to cerebral abnormalities (see Predisposing Factors)]

Defining Characteristics ("evidenced by")

[Disorientation to time, place, person, or circumstances]
[Inability to concentrate]
[Visual and auditory distortions]
Inappropriate responses
[Talking and laughing to self]
[Suspiciousness]
Hallucinations

Goals/Objectives

Short-Term Goal

With assistance from caregiver, client will maintain orientation to time, place, person, and circumstances for specified period of time.

Long-Term Goal

Client will demonstrate accurate perception of the environment by responding appropriately to stimuli indigenous to the surroundings.

Interventions with *Selected Rationales*

1. Decrease the amount of stimuli in the client's environment (e.g., low noise level, few people, simple decor). *This decreases the possibility of forming inaccurate sensory perceptions.*
2. Do not reinforce the hallucination. Let client know that you do not share the perception. Maintain reality through reorientation and focus on real situations and people. *Reality orientation decreases false sensory perceptions and enhances client's sense of self-worth and personal dignity.*
3. Provide reassurance of safety if client responds with fear to inaccurate sensory perception. *Client safety and security is a nursing priority.*
4. Correct client's description of inaccurate perception, and describe the situation as it exists in reality. *Explanation of, and participation in, real situations and real activities interferes with the ability to respond to hallucinations.*
5. Allow for care to be given by same personnel on a regular basis, if possible, *to provide a feeling of security and stability in the client's environment.*
6. Teach prospective caregivers how to recognize signs and symptoms of client's inaccurate sensory perceptions. Explain techniques they may use to restore reality to the situation.

Outcome Criteria

1. With assistance from caregiver, client is able to recognize when perceptions within the environment are inaccurate.
2. Prospective caregivers are able to verbalize ways in which to correct inaccurate perceptions and restore reality to the situation.

SELF-ESTEEM DISTURBANCE

Definition: Negative self-evaluation or feelings about self or self capabilities, which may be directly or indirectly expressed.

Possible Etiologies ("related to")

[Loss of independent functioning]
[Loss of capacity for remembering]
[Loss of capability for effective verbal communication]

Defining Characteristics ("evidenced by")

[Withdraws into social isolation]
[Lack of eye contact]
[Excessive crying alternating with expressions of anger]
[Refusal to participate in therapies]
[Refusal to participate in own self-care activities]
[Becomes increasingly dependent on others to perform ADLs]
Expressions of shame or guilt

Goals/Objectives

Short-Term Goal

Client will voluntarily spend time with staff and peers in dayroom activities within 1 week.

Long-Term Goal

By discharge, client will exhibit increased feelings of self-worth as evidenced by voluntary participation in own self-care and interaction with others.

Interventions with *Selected Rationales*

1. Encourage client to express honest feelings in relation to loss of prior level of functioning. Acknowledge pain of loss. Support client through process of grieving. ***Client may be fixed in anger stage of grieving process, which is turned inward on the self, resulting in diminished self-esteem.***
2. Devise methods of assisting client with memory deficit. Examples follow:
   a. Name sign on door identifying client's room.
   b. Identifying sign on outside of dining room door.
   c. Identifying sign on outside of restroom door.
   d. Large clock, with oversized numbers and hands, appropriately placed.
   e. Large calendar, indicating one day at a time, with month, day, and year identified in bold print.
   f. Printed, structured daily schedule, with one copy for client and one posted on unit wall.
   g. "News board" on unit wall where current national and local events may be posted.

   These aids may assist client to function more independently, thereby increasing self-esteem.
3. Encourage client's attempts to communicate. If verbalizations are not understandable, express to client what you think he or she intended to say. It may be necessary to reorient client frequently. ***The ability to communicate effectively with others may enhance self-esteem.***
4. Encourage reminiscence and discussion of life review. Also

discuss present-day events. Sharing picture albums, if possible, is especially good. ***Reminiscence and life review help the client resume progression through the grief process associated with disappointing life events and increase self-esteem as successes are reviewed.***

5. Encourage participation in group activities. Caregiver may need to accompany client at first, until he or she feels secure that the group members will be accepting, regardless of limitations in verbal communication. ***Positive feedback from group members will increase self-esteem.***
6. Offer support and empathy when client expresses embarrassment at inability to remember people, events, and places. Focus on accomplishments ***to lift self-esteem.***
7. Encourage client to be as independent as possible in self-care activities. Provide written schedule of tasks to be performed. Intervene in areas in which client requires assistance. ***The ability to perform independently preserves self-esteem.***

Outcome Criteria

1. Client initiates own self-care according to written schedule and willingly accepts assistance as needed.
2. Client interacts with others in group activities, maintaining anxiety at minimal level in response to difficulties with verbal communication.

CAREGIVER ROLE STRAIN

Definition: A caregiver's felt or exhibited difficulty in performing the family caregiver role.

Possible Etiologies ("related to")

[Severity of the care receiver's illness]
[Duration of the care receiver's illness]
Lack of respite and recreation for the caregiver
Caregiver's competing role commitments
Inadequate physical environment for providing care
Family or caregiver isolation
Complexity and amount of caregiving tasks

Defining Characteristics ("evidenced by")

Apprehension about possible institutionalization of care receiver
Apprehension about future regarding care receiver's health and caregiver's ability to provide care

Difficulty performing required activities
Inability to complete caregiving tasks
Apprehension about care receiver's care when caregiver is ill or deceased

Goals/Objectives

Short-Term Goal

Caregivers will verbalize understanding of ways to facilitate the caregiver role.

Long-Term Goal

Caregivers will demonstrate effective problem-solving skills and develop adaptive coping mechanisms to regain equilibrium.

Interventions with *Selected Rationales*

1. Assess caregivers' ability to anticipate and fulfill client's unmet needs. Provide information to assist caregivers with this responsibility. ***Caregivers may be unaware of what client will realistically be able to accomplish. They may be unaware of the progressive nature of the illness.***
2. Ensure that caregivers are aware of available community support systems from which they can seek assistance when required. Examples include adult day-care centers, housekeeping and homemaker services, respite-care services, or perhaps a local chapter of the Alzheimer's Disease and Related Disorders Association (ADRDA). This organization sponsors a nationwide 24-hour hotline to provide information and link families who need assistance with nearby chapters and affiliates. The hotline number is 1-800-272-3900. ***Caregivers require relief from the pressures and strain of providing 24-hour care for their loved one. Studies have shown that elder abuse arises out of caregiving situations that place overwhelming stress on the caregivers.***
3. Encourage caregivers to express feelings, particularly anger. ***Release of these emotions can serve to prevent psychopathology, such as depression or psychophysiological disorders from occurring.***
4. Encourage participation in support groups composed of members with similar life situations. ***Hearing others who are experiencing the same problems discuss ways in which they have coped may help caregiver adopt more adaptive strategies. Individuals who are experiencing similar life situations provide empathy and support for each other.***

Outcome Criteria

1. Caregivers are able to problem-solve effectively regarding care of elderly client.
2. Caregivers demonstrate adaptive coping strategies for dealing with stress of caregiver role.
3. Caregivers openly express feelings.
4. Caregivers express desire to join support group of other caregivers.

■ INTERNET REFERENCES

Additional information about Alzheimer's Disease may be located at the following Websites:

- http://www.alz.org
- http://www.alzheimers.org/adear
- http://www.brain.nwu.edu/

Information on caregiving can be located at the following Website:

- http://www.aarp.org

Additional information about medications to treat Alzheimer's Disease may be located at the following Websites:

- http://www.fadavis.com
- http://www.laurus.com

CHAPTER 5

Substance-Related Disorders

■ BACKGROUND ASSESSMENT DATA

The substance-related disorders are composed of two groups: the substance-use disorders (dependence and abuse) and the substance-induced disorders (intoxication and withdrawal). Other substance-induced disorders (delirium, dementia, amnesia, psychosis, mood disorder, anxiety disorder, sexual dysfunction, and sleep disorders) are included in the chapters with which they share symptomatology (e.g., substance-induced mood disorders are included in Chap. 7; substance-induced sexual dysfunction is included in Chap. 11, etc.).

■ SUBSTANCE-USE DISORDERS

Substance Abuse*

Defined

The *DSM-IV* (APA, 1994) defines substance abuse as a maladaptive pattern of substance use manifested by recurrent and significant adverse consequences related to repeated use of the substance. Criteria include the following:

1. Recurrent substance use resulting in a failure to fulfill major role obligations at work, school, or home.
2. Recurrent substance use in situations in which it is physically hazardous.

---

*Reprinted with permission from the *Diagnostic and Statistical Manual of Mental Disorders, Fourth Edition*. Copyright 1994 American Psychiatric Association, 1994.

3. Recurrent substance-related legal problems.
4. Continued substance use despite having persistent or recurrent social or interpersonal problems caused or exacerbated by the effects of the substance.

Substance Dependence*

Defined

The *DSM-IV* defines substance dependence by the following criteria:

1. Evidence of tolerance, as identified by either of the following:
   a. A need for increased amounts of the substance to achieve intoxication or the desired effect.
   b. Diminished effect with continued use of the same amount of the substance.
2. Evidence of withdrawal symptoms, as manifested by either of the following:
   a. The characteristic withdrawal syndrome for the substance.
   b. The same (or closely related) substance is taken to relieve or avoid withdrawal symptoms.
3. The substance is often taken in larger amounts or over a longer period than was intended.
4. There is a persistent desire or unsuccessful effort to cut down or control substance use.
5. A great deal of time is spent in activities necessary to obtain, use, or recover from the effects of the substance.

■ SUBSTANCE-INDUCED DISORDERS

Substance Intoxication*

Defined

The *DSM-IV* defines substance intoxication by the following criteria:

1. The development of a reversible substance-specific syndrome caused by recent ingestion of (or exposure to) a substance.
2. Clinically significant maladaptive behavior or psycho-

*Reprinted with permission from the *Diagnostic and Statistical Manual of Mental Disorders, Fourth Edition.* Copyright 1994 American Psychiatric Association, 1994.

logical changes that are caused by the effect of the substance on the central nervous system (CNS) and develop during or shortly after use of the substance.

Substance Withdrawal*

Defined

The *DSM-IV* defines substance withdrawal by the following criteria:

1. The development of a substance-specific syndrome caused by the cessation of (or reduction in) heavy and prolonged substance use.
2. The substance-specific syndrome causes clinically significant distress or impairment in social, occupational, or other important areas of functioning.

■ CLASSIFICATION OF SUBSTANCES

Alcohol

303.90	Alcohol Dependence
305.00	Alcohol Abuse
303.00	Alcohol Intoxication
291.8	Alcohol Withdrawal

Even though alcohol is a depressant, it will be considered separately because of the complex effects and widespread nature of its use. Low to moderate consumption produces a feeling of well-being and reduced inhibitions. At higher concentrations, motor and intellectual functioning are impaired, mood becomes very labile, and behaviors characteristic of depression, euphoria, and aggression are exhibited. The only medical use for alcohol (with the exception of its inclusion in a number of pharmacological concentrates) is as an antidote for methanol consumption.

Examples: Beer, wine, bourbon, scotch, gin, vodka, rum, tequila, liqueurs.

Common substances containing alcohol and used by some dependent individuals to satisfy their need include liquid cough medications, liquid cold preparations, mouthwashes, isopropyl rubbing alcohol, nail polish removers, colognes, and aftershave and preshave preparations.

---

*Reprinted with permission from the *Diagnostic and Statistical Manual of Mental Disorders, Fourth Edition.* Copyright 1994 American Psychiatric Association, 1994.

Opioids

304.00	Opioid Dependence
305.50	Opioid Abuse
292.89	Opioid Intoxication
292.0	Opioid Withdrawal

Opioids have a medical use as analgesics, antitussives, and antidiarrheals. They produce the effects of analgesia and euphoria by stimulating the opiate receptors in the brain and thereby mimicking the naturally occurring endorphins.

Examples: Opium, morphine, codeine, heroin, hydromorphone, meperidine, methadone.

Common Street Names: Horse, junk, H (heroin); black stuff, poppy, big O (opium); M, morph (morphine); dollies (methadone); terp (terpin hydrate or cough syrup with codeine).

CNS Depressants

304.10	Sedative, Hypnotic, or Anxiolytic Dependence
305.40	Sedative, Hypnotic, or Anxiolytic Abuse
292.89	Sedative, Hypnotic, or Anxiolytic Intoxication
292.0	Sedative, Hypnotic, or Anxiolytic Withdrawal

CNS depressants have a medical use as antianxiety agents, sedatives, hypnotics, anticonvulsants, and anesthetics. They depress the action of the CNS, resulting in an overall calming, relaxing effect on the individual. At higher dosages they can induce sleep.

Examples: Benzodiazepines, barbiturates, chloral hydrate, ethchlorvynol, meprobamate.

Common Street Names: Peter, Mickey (chloral hydrate); green and whites, roaches (Librium); blues (Valium, 10 mg); yellows (Valium, 5 mg); red birds, red devils (secobarbital); blue birds (Amytal capsules); yellow birds (Nembutal); downers (barbiturates; tranquilizers).

CNS Stimulants

304.40	Amphetamine Dependence
305.70	Amphetamine Abuse
292.89	Amphetamine Intoxication
292.0	Amphetamine Withdrawal
305.90	Caffeine Intoxication
304.20	Cocaine Dependence

305.60 Cocaine Abuse
292.89 Cocaine Intoxication
292.0 Cocaine Withdrawal
305.10 Nicotine Dependence
292.0 Nicotine Withdrawal

CNS stimulants have a medical use in the management of hyperkinesia, narcolepsy, and weight control. They stimulate the action of the CNS, resulting in increased alertness, excitation, euphoria, increased pulse rate and blood pressure, insomnia, and loss of appetite.

Examples: Amphetamines, methylphenidate (Ritalin), phendimetrazine, cocaine, hydrochloride cocaine, caffeine, tobacco.

Common Street Names: Bennies, wake-ups, uppers, speed (amphetamines); coke, snow, gold dust, girl (cocaine); crack, rock (hydrochloride cocaine); speedball (mixture of heroin and cocaine).

Hallucinogens

304.50 Hallucinogen Dependence
305.30 Hallucinogen Abuse
292.89 Hallucinogen Intoxication
304.90 Phencyclidine Dependence
305.90 Phencyclidine Abuse
292.89 Phencyclidine Intoxication

Hallucinogens act as sympathomimetic agents, producing effects resembling those resulting from stimulation of the sympathetic nervous system (e.g., excitation, increased energy, distortion of the senses). Therapeutic medical uses for lysergic acid diethylamide (LSD) have been proposed in the treatment of chronic alcoholism and in the reduction of intractable pain, such as terminal malignant disease and phantom limb sensations.

Examples: LSD, mescaline, phencyclidine (PCP).

Common Street Names: Acid, cube, big D, California sunshine (LSD); angel dust, hog, peace pill, crystal (PCP); cactus, mescal, mesc (mescaline).

Cannabinols

304.30 Cannabis Dependence
305.20 Cannabis Abuse
292.89 Cannabis Intoxication

Cannabinols depress higher centers in the brain and consequently release lower centers from inhibitory influence. They produce an anxiety-free state of relaxation characterized by a feeling of extreme well-being. Large doses of the drug can produce hallucinations. Marijuana has been used therapeutically in the relief of nausea and vomiting associated with antineoplastic chemotherapy.

Examples: Marijuana, hashish.

Common Street Names: Joints, reefers, pot, grass, Mary Jane (marijuana); hash (hashish).

A profile summary of these psychoactive substances is presented in Table 5–1.

Predisposing Factors

1. **Physiological**
   a. ***Genetics:*** An apparent genetic link is involved in the development of substance-related disorders. This is especially evident with alcoholism, less so with other substances. About half of the children of alcoholics become alcoholic, suggesting a possible heredity factor. The statistics are inconclusive regarding abuse of other substances, although children of people who themselves have substance-related disorders are at higher risk for developing these disorders.
   b. ***Biochemical:*** A second physiological hypothesis relates to the possibility that alcohol may produce morphinelike substances in the brain that are responsible for alcohol addiction. This occurs when the products of alcohol metabolism react with biologically active amines.
2. **Psychosocial**
   a. ***Psychodynamic Theory:*** This theory suggests that individuals who abuse substances have underdeveloped egos because of a failure in completing tasks of separation-individuation. The person retains a highly dependent nature, with characteristics of poor impulse control, low frustration tolerance, and low self-esteem. The superego is weak, resulting in absence of guilt feelings for their behavior (Freud, 1959).
   b. ***Theory of Family Dynamics:*** This theory relates a predisposition to substance-related disorders to the dysfunctional family system. There is often one parent who is absent or who is an overpowering tyrant, and one who is weak and ineffectual. Substance abuse may be evident as the primary method of relieving stress. The child has negative

TABLE 5–1 **Psychoactive Substances: A Profile Summary**

Class of Drugs	Symptoms of Use	Therapeutic Uses	Symptoms of Overdose	Trade Names	Common Names
CNS depressants: Alcohol	Relaxation, loss of inhibitions, lack of concentration, drowsiness, slurred speech, sleep	Antidote for methanol consumption; ingredient in many pharmacological concentrates.	Nausea, vomiting; shallow respirations; cold, clammy skin; weak, rapid pulse; coma; possible death	Ethyl alcohol, beer, gin, rum, vodka, bourbon, whiskey, liqueurs, wine, brandy, sherry, champagne	Booze, alcohol, liquor, drinks, cocktails, highballs, nightcaps, moonshine, white lightening
Other (barbiturates and non-barbiturates)	Same as Alcohol	Relief from anxiety and insomnia; as anticonvulsants and anesthetics.	Anxiety, fever, agitation, hallucinations, disorientation, tremors, delirium, convulsions, possible death	Seconal, Nembutal, Amytal Valium, Librium Chloral hydrate Equanil, Miltown	Red birds, yellow birds, blue birds Blues/yellows, green & whites Mickies Downers
CNS Stimulants: Amphetamines and related drugs	Hyperactivity, agitation, euphoria, insomnia, loss of appetite	Management of narcolepsy, hyperkinesia, and weight control.	Cardiac arrhythmias, headache, convulsions, hypertension, rapid heart rate, coma,	Dexedrine, Didrex, Tenuate, Ritalin, Plegine, Cylert,	Uppers, pep pills, wake-ups, bennies, eye-openers, speed, black beauties,

Table continued on following page

TABLE 5–1 **Psychoactive Substances: A Profile Summary (*Continued*)**

Class of Drugs	Symptoms of Use	Therapeutic Uses	Symptoms of Overdose	Trade Names	Common Names
			possible death	Sanorex	sweet A's
Cocaine	Euphoria, hyperactivity, restlessness, talkativeness, increased pulse, dilated pupils	Topical anesthetic.	Hallucinations, convulsions, pulmonary edema, respiratory failure, coma, cardiac arrest, possible death	Cocaine hydrochloride	Coke, flake, snow, dust, happy dust, gold dust, girl, cecil, C, toot, blow, crack
Opioids	Euphoria, lethargy, drowsiness, lack of motivation	As analgesics; methadone in substitution therapy; heroin has no therapeutic use.	Shallow breathing, slowed pulse, clammy skin, pulmonary edema, respiratory arrest, convulsions, coma, possible death	Heroin	Snow, Stuff, H, Harry, Horse
				Morphine	M, Morph, Miss Emma
				Codeine	Schoolboy
				Dilaudid	Lords
				Demerol	Doctors
				Methadone	Dollies
				Percodan	Perkies
				Talwin	T's
				Opium	Big O, black stuff

Hallucinogens	Visual hallucinations, disorientation, confusion, paranoid delusions, euphoria, anxiety, panic, increased pulse	LSD has been proposed in the treatment of chronic alcoholism and in the reduction of intractable pain.	Agitation, extreme hyperactivity, violence, hallucinations, psychosis, convulsions, possible death	LSD PCP Mescaline DMT STP	Acid, cube, big D Angel dust, hog, peace pill Mesc Businessman's trip Serenity and peace
Cannabinols	Relaxation, talkativeness, lowered inhibitions, euphoria, mood swings	Marijuana has been used for relief of nausea and vomiting associated with antineoplastic chemotherapy and to reduce eye pressure in glaucoma patients.	Fatigue, paranoia, delusions, hallucinations, possible psychosis	Cannabis Hashish	Marijuana, pot, grass, joint, Mary Jane, MJ Hash, rope, Sweet Lucy

Source: From Townsend, 2000, pp. 376–377, with permission.

role models and learns to respond to stressful situations in like manner (Leigh, 1985).

■ COMMON PATTERNS OF USE IN SUBSTANCE-RELATED DISORDERS

Symptomatology (Subjective and Objective Data)

Alcohol Abuse/Dependence

1. Begins with social drinking that provides feeling of relaxation and well-being. Soon requires more and more to produce the same effects.
2. Drinks in secret; hides bottles of alcohol; drinks first thing in the morning (to "steady my nerves") and at any other opportunity that arises during the day.
3. As the disease progresses, the individual may drink in binges. During a binge, drinking continues until the individual is too intoxicated or too sick to consume any more. Behavior borders on the psychotic, with the individual wavering in and out of reality.
4. Begins to have blackouts. Periods of amnesia occur (in the absence of intoxication or loss of consciousness), during which the individual is unable to remember periods of time or events that have occurred.
5. Chronic use results in multisystem physiological impairments that include (but are not limited to) the following:
   a. ***Peripheral Neuropathy:*** Numbness, tingling, pain in extremities (caused by thiamine deficiency).
   b. ***Wernicke-Korsakoff Syndrome:*** Mental confusion, agitation, diplopia (caused by thiamine deficiency). Rapid deterioration to coma and death will occur without immediate thiamine replacement.
   c. ***Alcoholic Cardiomyopathy:*** Enlargement of the heart caused by an accumulation of excess lipids in myocardial cells. Symptoms of tachycardia, dyspnea, and arrhythmias may be evident.
   d. ***Esophagitis:*** Inflammation of, and pain in, the esophagus.
   e. ***Esophageal Varices:*** Distended veins in the esophagus, with risk of rupture and subsequent hemorrhage.
   f. ***Gastritis:*** Inflammation of lining of stomach caused by irritation from the alcohol, resulting in

pain, nausea, vomiting, and possibility of bleeding because of erosion of blood vessels.

g. ***Pancreatitis:*** Inflammation of the pancreas, resulting in pain, nausea and vomiting, and abdominal distention. With progressive destruction to the gland, symptoms of diabetes mellitus could occur.
h. ***Alcoholic Hepatitis:*** Inflammation of the liver, resulting in enlargement, jaundice, right upper quadrant pain, and fever.
i. ***Cirrhosis of the Liver:*** Fibrous and degenerative changes occurring in response to chronic accumulation of large amounts of fatty acids in the liver. In cirrhosis, symptoms of alcoholic hepatitis progress to include the following:
   - **Portal Hypertension:** Elevation of blood pressure through the portal circulation resulting from defective blood flow through the cirrhotic liver.
   - **Ascites:** An accumulation of serous fluid in the peritoneal cavity.
   - **Hepatic Encephalopathy:** Liver disorder caused by inability of the liver to convert ammonia to urea (the body's natural method of discarding excess ammonia); as serum ammonia levels rise, confusion occurs, accompanied by restlessness, slurred speech, fever, and, without intervention, an eventual progression to coma and death.

Alcohol Intoxication

1. Symptoms of alcohol intoxication include disinhibition of sexual or aggressive impulses, mood lability, impaired judgment, impaired social or occupational functioning, slurred speech, incoordination, unsteady gait, nystagmus, and flushed face.
2. Intoxication usually occurs at blood alcohol levels between 100 and 200 mg/dL.

Alcohol Withdrawal

1. Occurs within 4 to 12 hours of cessation of, or reduction in, heavy and prolonged (several days or longer) alcohol use.
2. Symptoms include coarse tremor of hands, tongue, or eyelids; nausea or vomiting; malaise or weakness; tachycardia; sweating, elevated blood pressure; anxi-

ety; depressed mood or irritability; transient hallucinations or illusions; headache; and insomnia.

3. Without aggressive intervention, the individual may progress to *alcohol withdrawal delirium* about the second or third day following cessation of, or reduction in, prolonged, heavy alcohol use. Symptoms include those described under the syndrome of delirium (see Chap. 4).

Amphetamine (or Amphetamine-like) Dependence/Abuse

1. The use of amphetamines is often initiated for their appetite-suppressant effect in an attempt to lose or control weight.
2. Amphetamines are also taken for the initial feeling of well-being and confidence.
3. They are typically taken orally, intravenously, or by nasal inhalation.
4. Chronic daily (or almost daily) use usually results in an increase in dosage over time to produce the desired effect.
5. Episodic use often takes the form of binges, followed by an intense and unpleasant "crash" in which the individual experiences anxiety, irritability, and feelings of fatigue and depression.
6. Continued use appears to be related to a "craving" for the substance, rather than to prevention or alleviation of withdrawal symptoms.

Amphetamine (or Amphetamine-like) Intoxication

1. Amphetamine intoxication usually begins with a "high" feeling, followed by the development of symptoms such as euphoria with enhanced vigor, gregariousness, hyperactivity, restlessness, hypervigilance, interpersonal sensitivity, talkativeness, anxiety, tension, alertness, grandiosity, stereotypical and repetitive behavior, anger, fighting, and impaired judgment (APA, 1994).
2. Physical signs and symptoms that occur with amphetamine intoxication include tachycardia or bradycardia, pupillary dilation, elevated or lowered blood pressure, perspiration or chills, nausea or vomiting, psychomotor retardation or agitation, muscular weakness, respiratory depression, chest pain or cardiac ar-

rhythmias, confusion, seizures, dyskinesias, dystonias, or coma (APA, 1994).

Amphetamine (or Amphetamine-like) Withdrawal

1. Amphetamine withdrawal symptoms occur after cessation of (or reduction in) amphetamine (or a related substance) use that has been heavy and prolonged.
2. Symptoms of amphetamine withdrawal develop within a few hours to several days and include fatigue; vivid, unpleasant dreams; insomnia or hypersomnia; increased appetite; and psychomotor retardation or agitation.

Cannabis Dependence/Abuse

1. Cannabis preparations are almost always smoked but may also be taken orally.
2. It is commonly regarded incorrectly to be a substance without potential for dependence.
3. Tolerance to the substance may result in increased frequency of its use.
4. Abuse is evidenced by participation in hazardous activities while motor coordination is impaired from cannabis use.

Cannabis Intoxication

1. Cannabis intoxication is characterized by impaired motor coordination, euphoria, anxiety, sensation of slowed time, impaired judgment, and social withdrawal that developed during or shortly after cannabis use (APA, 1994).
2. Physical symptoms of cannabis intoxication include conjunctival injection, increased appetite, dry mouth, and tachycardia.
3. The impairment of motor skills lasts for 8 to 12 hours.

Cocaine Dependence/Abuse

1. Various forms are smoked, inhaled, injected, or taken orally.
2. Chronic daily (or almost daily) use usually results in an increase in dosage over time to produce the desired effect.
3. Episodic use often takes the form of binges, followed by an intense and unpleasant "crash" in which the in-

dividual experiences anxiety, irritability, and feelings of fatigue and depression.

4. The drug user often abuses, or is dependent on, a CNS depressant to relieve the residual effects of cocaine.
5. Cocaine abuse and dependence lead to tolerance of the substance and subsequent use of increasing doses.
6. Continued use appears to be related to a "craving" for the substance, rather than to prevention or alleviation of withdrawal symptoms.

Cocaine Intoxication

1. Symptoms of cocaine intoxication develop during, or shortly after, use of cocaine.
2. Symptoms of cocaine intoxication include euphoria or affective blunting, changes in sociability, hypervigilance, interpersonal sensitivity, anxiety, tension, anger, stereotyped behaviors, impaired judgment, and impaired social or occupational functioning.
3. Physical symptoms of cocaine intoxication include tachycardia or bradycardia, pupillary dilation, elevated or lowered blood pressure, perspiration or chills, nausea or vomiting, psychomotor agitation or retardation, muscle weakness, respiratory depression, chest pain, or cardiac arrhythmias, confusion, seizures, dyskinesias, dystonias, or coma.

Cocaine Withdrawal

1. Symptoms of withdrawal occur after cessation of, or reduction in, cocaine use that has been heavy and prolonged.
2. Symptoms of cocaine withdrawal include dysphoric mood; fatigue; vivid, unpleasant dreams; insomnia or hypersomnia; increased appetite; psychomotor retardation or agitation.

Hallucinogen Dependence/Abuse

1. Hallucinogenic substances are taken orally.
2. Because the cognitive and perceptual impairment may last for up to 12 hours, use is generally episodic, because the individual must organize time during the daily schedule for its use.
3. Frequent use results in tolerance to the effects of the substance.

4. Dependence is rare, and most people are able to resume their previous lifestyle, following a period of hallucinogen use, without much difficulty.
5. Flashbacks may occur following cessation of hallucinogen use. These episodes consist of visual or auditory misperceptions usually lasting only a few seconds, but sometimes lasting up to several hours.
6. Hallucinogens are highly unpredictable in the effects they may induce each time they are used.

Hallucinogen Intoxication

1. Symptoms of intoxication develop during or shortly after hallucinogen use.
2. Symptoms include marked anxiety or depression, ideas of reference, fear of losing one's mind, paranoid ideation, impaired judgment, and impaired social or occupational functioning.
3. Other symptoms include subjective intensification of perceptions, depersonalization, derealization, illusions, hallucinations, and synesthesias.

Inhalant Dependence/Abuse

1. Effects are induced by inhaling the vapors of volatile substances through the nose or mouth.
2. Examples of substances include glue, gasoline, paint, paint thinners, various cleaning chemicals, typewriter correction fluid.
3. Use of inhalants often begins in childhood, and considerable family dysfunction is characteristic.
4. Use may be daily or episodic, and chronic use may continue into adulthood.
5. Tolerance has been reported among individuals with heavy use, but a withdrawal syndrome from these substances has not been well documented.

Inhalant Intoxication

1. Symptoms of intoxication develop during, or shortly after, use of, or exposure to, volatile inhalants.
2. Symptoms of inhalant intoxication include belligerence, assaultiveness, apathy, impaired judgment, and impaired social or occupational functioning.
3. Physical symptoms of inhalant intoxication include dizziness, nystagmus, incoordination, slurred speech,

unsteady gait, lethargy, depressed reflexes, psychomotor retardation, tremor, generalized muscle weakness, blurred vision or diplopia, stupor or coma, and euphoria.

Nicotine Dependence

1. The effects of nicotine are induced through inhaling the smoke of cigarettes, cigars, or pipe tobacco, and orally through the use of snuff or chewing tobacco.
2. Continued use results in a "craving" for the substance.
3. Nicotine is commonly used to relieve or to avoid withdrawal symptoms that occur when the individual has been in a situation in which use is restricted.
4. Continued use despite knowledge of medical problems related to smoking is a particularly important health problem.

Nicotine Withdrawal

1. Symptoms of withdrawal develop within 24 hours after abrupt cessation of (or reduction in) nicotine use.
2. Symptoms of nicotine withdrawal include dysphoric or depressed mood, insomnia, irritability, frustration, anger, anxiety, difficulty concentrating, restlessness, decreased heart rate, and increased appetite.

Opioid Dependence/Abuse

1. Various forms are taken by mouth, by intravenous injection, by nasal inhalation, and by smoking.
2. Dependence occurs after recreational use of the substance "on the street" or after prescribed use of the substance for relief of pain or cough.
3. Chronic use leads to remarkably high levels of tolerance.
4. Once abuse or dependence is established, substance procurement often comes to dominate the person's life.
5. Cessation or decreased consumption results in a "craving" for the substance and produces a specific syndrome of withdrawal.

Opioid Intoxication

1. Symptoms of intoxication develop during or shortly after opioid use.

2. Symptoms of opioid intoxication include euphoria (initially) followed by apathy, dysphoria, psychomotor agitation or retardation, impaired judgment, and impaired social or occupational functioning.
3. Physical symptoms of opioid intoxication include pupillary constriction, drowsiness or coma, slurred speech, and impairment in attention or memory.

Opioid Withdrawal

1. Symptoms of opioid withdrawal occur after cessation of (or reduction in) heavy and prolonged opioid use. Symptoms of withdrawal can also occur after administration of an opioid antagonist after a period of opioid use.
2. Symptoms of opioid withdrawal can occur within minutes to several days following use (or antagonist) and include dysphoric mood, nausea or vomiting, muscle aches, lacrimation or rhinorrhea, pupillary dilation, piloerection, sweating, abdominal cramping, diarrhea, yawning, fever, and insomnia.

Phencyclidine (PCP) Dependence/Abuse

1. Phencyclidine is taken by mouth, by intravenous injection, or by smoking or inhaling.
2. Use can be on a chronic daily basis but more often is taken episodically in binges that can last several days.
3. Abuse or dependence can occur after only a short period of occasional use.
4. Unclear if tolerance or withdrawal symptoms develop with use of PCP.

Phencyclidine Intoxication

1. Symptoms of intoxication develop during or shortly after PCP use.
2. Symptoms of PCP intoxication include belligerence, assaultiveness, impulsiveness, unpredictability, psychomotor agitation, impaired judgment, and impaired social or occupational functioning.
3. Physical symptoms occur within an hour or less of PCP use and include vertical or horizontal nystagmus, hypertension or tachycardia, numbness or diminished responsiveness to pain, ataxia, dysarthria, muscle rigidity, seizures or coma, and hyperacusis.

Sedative, Hypnotic, or Anxiolytic Dependence/Abuse

1. Effects are produced through oral intake of these substances.
2. Dependence can occur following recreational use of the substance "on the street" or after prescribed use of the substance for relief of anxiety or insomnia.
3. Chronic use leads to remarkably high levels of tolerance.
4. Once dependence develops, there is evidence of strong substance-seeking behaviors (obtaining prescriptions from several physicians or resorting to illegal sources to maintain adequate supplies of the substance).
5. Abrupt cessation of these substances can result in life-threatening withdrawal symptoms.

Sedative, Hypnotic, or Anxiolytic Intoxication

1. Symptoms of intoxication develop during or shortly after intake of sedatives, hypnotics, or anxiolytics.
2. Symptoms of intoxication include inappropriate sexual or aggressive behavior, mood lability, impaired judgment, and impaired social or occupational functioning.
3. Physical symptoms of sedative, hypnotic, or anxiolytic intoxication include slurred speech, incoordination, unsteady gait, nystagmus, impairment in attention or memory, stupor, or coma.

Sedative, Hypnotic, or Anxiolytic Withdrawal

1. Withdrawal symptoms occur after cessation of (or reduction in) heavy and prolonged use of sedatives, hypnotics, or anxiolytics.
2. Symptoms of withdrawal occur within several hours to a few days after abrupt cessation or reduction in use of the drug.
3. Symptoms of withdrawal include autonomic hyperactivity (e.g., sweating or pulse rate > 100); increased hand tremor; insomnia; nausea or vomiting; transient visual, tactile, or auditory hallucinations or illusions; psychomotor agitation; anxiety; or grand mal seizures.

A summary of symptoms associated with the syndromes of intoxication and withdrawal is presented in Table 5–2.

TABLE 5–2 **Summary of Symptoms Associated with the Syndromes of Intoxication and Withdrawal**

Class of Drugs	Intoxication	Withdrawal	Comments
Alcohol	Aggressiveness, impaired judgment, impaired attention, irritability, euphoria, depression, emotional lability, slurred speech, incoordination, unsteady gait, nystagmus, flushed face	Tremors, nausea/vomiting, malaise, weakness, tachycardia, sweating, elevated blood pressure, anxiety, depressed mood, irritability, hallucinations, headache, insomnia, seizures	Alcohol withdrawal begins within 4-6 hr after last drink. May progress to delirium tremens on 2nd or 3rd day. Use of Librium or Serax is common for substitution therapy.
Amphetamines and related substances	Fighting, grandiosity, hyper-vigilance, psychomotor agitation, impaired judgment, tachycardia, pupillary dilation, elevated blood pressure, perspiration or chills, nausea and vomiting	Anxiety, depressed mood, irritability, craving for the substance, fatigue, insomnia or hypersomnia, psychomotor agitation, paranoid and suicidal ideation	Withdrawal symptoms usually peak within 2-4 days, although depression and irritability may persist for months. Antidepressants may be used.
Caffeine	Restlessness, nervousness, excitement, insomnia, flushed face, diuresis, gastrointestinal complaints, muscle twitching, rambling flow of thought and speech, cardiac arrhythmia, periods of inexhaustibility, psychomotor agitation	Headache	Caffeine is contained in coffee, tea, colas, cocoa, chocolate, some over-the-counter analgesics, "cold" preparations, and stimulants.

Table continued on following page

TABLE 5–2 **Summary of Symptoms Associated with the Syndromes of Intoxication and Withdrawal (*Continued*)**

Class of Drugs	Intoxication	Withdrawal	Comments
Cannabis	Euphoria, anxiety, suspiciousness, sensation of slowed time, impaired judgment, social withdrawal, tachycardia, conjunctival redness, increased appetite, hallucinations	Restlessness, irritability, insomnia, loss of appetite	Intoxication occurs immediately and lasts about 3 hr. Oral ingestion is more slowly absorbed and has longer-lasting effects.
Cocaine	Euphoria, fighting, grandiosity, hypervigilence, psychomotor agitation, impaired judgment, tachycardia, elevated blood pressure, pupillary dilation, perspiration or chills, nausea/vomiting, hallucinations, delirium	Depression, anxiety, irritability, fatigue, insomnia or hypersomnia, psychomotor agitation, paranoid or suicidal ideation, apathy, social withdrawal	Large doses of the drug can result in convulsions or death from cardiac arrhythmias or respiratory paralysis.
Inhalants	Belligerence, assaultiveness, apathy, impaired judgment, dizziness, nystagmus, slurred speech, unsteady gait, lethargy, depressed reflexes, tremor, blurred vision, stupor or coma, euphoria, irritation	No withdrawal symptoms well documented	Intoxication occurs within 5 min of inhalation. Symptoms last 60-90 min. Large doses can result in death from CNS depression or cardiac arrhythmia.

	around eyes, throat, and nose		
Nicotine		Craving for the drug, irritability, anger, frustration, anxiety, difficulty concentrating, restlessness, decreased heart rate, increased appetite, weight gain, tremor, headaches, insomnia	Symptoms begin within 24 hr of last drug use and decrease in intensity over days, weeks, or sometimes longer.
Opioids	Euphoria, lethargy, somnolence, apathy, dysphoria, impaired judgment, pupillary constriction, drowsiness, slurred speech, constipation, nausea, decreased respiratory rate and blood pressure	Craving for the drug, nausea/vomiting, muscle aches, lacrimation or rhinorrhea, pupillary dilation, piloerection or sweating, diarrhea, yawning, fever, insomnia	Withdrawal symptoms appear within 6-8 hr after last dose, reach a peak in the 2nd or 3rd day, and disappear in 7-10 days.
Phencyclidine and related substances	Belligerence, assaultiveness, impulsiveness, psychomotor agitation, impaired judgment, nystagmus, increased heart rate and blood pressure, diminished pain response, ataxia, dysarthria, muscle rigidity, seizures, hyperacusis, delirium	Unclear whether withdrawal symptoms occur	Delirium can occur within 24 hr after use of phencyclidine or may occur up to a week following recovery from an overdose of the drug.

Table continued on following page

TABLE 5–2 **Summary of Symptoms Associated with Syndromes of Intoxication and Withdrawal *Continued*)**

Class of Drugs	Intoxication	Withdrawal	Comments
Sedatives, hypnotics, anxiolytics	Disinhibition of sexual or aggressive impulses, mood lability, impaired judgment, slurred speech, incoordination, unsteady gait, impairment in attention or memory, disorientation, confusion	Nausea/vomiting, malaise, weakness, tachycardia, sweating, anxiety, irritability, orthostatic hypotension, tremor, insomnia, seizures	Withdrawal may progress to delirium, usually within 1 wk of last use. Long-acting barbiturates or benzodiazepines may be used in withdrawal substitution therapy.

Source: From Townsend, 2000, pp. 378–379, with permission.

Common Nursing Diagnoses and Interventions

(Interventions are applicable to various health-care settings, such as inpatient and partial hospitalization, community outpatient clinic, home health, and private practice.)

RISK FOR INJURY

Definition: A state in which the individual is at risk of injury as a result of [internal or external] environmental conditions interacting with the individual's adaptive and defensive resources.

Related/Risk Factors ("related to")

[Substance intoxication]
[Substance withdrawal]
[Disorientation]
[Seizures]
[Hallucinations]
[Psychomotor agitation]
[Unstable vital signs]
[Delirium]
[Flashbacks]
[Panic level of anxiety]

Goals/Objectives

Short-Term Goal

Client's condition will stabilize within 72 hours.

Long-Term Goal

Client will not experience physical injury.

Interventions with *Selected Rationales*

1. Assess client's level of disorientation to determine specific requirements for safety. ***Knowledge of client's level of functioning is necessary to formulate appropriate plan of care.***
2. Obtain a drug history, if possible, to determine
   a. Type of substance(s) used.
   b. Time of last ingestion and amount consumed.
   c. Length and frequency of consumption.
   d. Amount consumed on a daily basis.
3. Obtain urine sample for laboratory analysis of substance content. ***Subjective history is often not accurate.***

Knowledge regarding substance ingestion is important for accurate assessment of client condition.

4. Place client in quiet, private room. ***Excessive stimuli increase client agitation.***
5. Institute necessary safety precautions:
   a. Observe client behaviors frequently; assign staff on one-to-one basis if condition is warranted; accompany and assist client when ambulating; use wheelchair for transporting long distances.
   b. Be sure that side rails are up when client is in bed.
   c. Pad headboard and side rails of bed with thick towels to protect client in case of seizure.
   d. Use mechanical restraints as necessary to protect client if excessive hyperactivity accompanies the disorientation.

   Client safety is a nursing priority.
6. Ensure that smoking materials and other potentially harmful objects are stored outside client's access. ***Client may harm self or others in disoriented, confused state.***
7. Frequently orient client to reality and surroundings. ***Disorientation may endanger client safety if he or she unknowingly wanders away from safe environment.***
8. Monitor vital signs every 15 minutes initially and less frequently as acute symptoms subside. ***Vital signs provide the most reliable information regarding client condition and need for medication during acute detoxification period.***
9. Follow medication regimen, as ordered by physician. Common medical intervention for detoxification from the following substances includes:
   a. ***Alcohol:*** Chlordiazepoxide (Librium) is given orally every 4 to 8 hours in decreasing doses until withdrawal is complete. In clients with liver disease, accumulation of the longer-acting agents, such as chlordiazepoxide (Librium), may be problematic, and the use of the shorter-acting benzodiazepine oxazepam (Serax) is more appropriate. Some physicians may order anticonvulsant medication to be used prophylactically; however, this is not a universal intervention. Multivitamin therapy, in combination with daily thiamine (either by mouth or by injection), is common protocol.
   b. ***Narcotics:*** Narcotic antagonists, such as naloxone (Narcan), nalorphine (Nalline), or levallorphan (Lorfan), are administered intravenously for narcotic overdose. Withdrawal is managed with rest and nutritional therapy. Substitution therapy may be instituted to decrease withdrawal symptoms using propoxyphene (Darvon) for

weaker effects or methadone (Dolophine) for longer effects.

c. ***Depressants:*** Substitution therapy may be instituted to decrease withdrawal symptoms using a long-acting barbiturate, such as phenobarbital (Luminal). Some physicians prescribe oxazepam (Serax) as needed for objective symptoms, gradually decreasing the dosage until the drug is discontinued.
d. ***Stimulants:*** Treatment of overdose is geared toward stabilization of vital signs. Intravenous antihypertensives may be used, along with intravenous diazepam (Valium) to control seizures. Chlordiazepoxide may be administered orally for the first few days while the client is "crashing."
e. ***Hallucinogens and Cannabinols:*** Medications are normally not prescribed for withdrawal from these substances. However, in the event of overdose, diazepam (Valium) or chlordiazepoxide (Librium) may be given as needed to decrease agitation.

Outcome Criteria

1. Client is no longer exhibiting any signs or symptoms of substance intoxication or withdrawal.
2. Client shows no evidence of physical injury obtained during substance intoxication or withdrawal.

INEFFECTIVE DENIAL

Definition: The state of a conscious or unconscious attempt to disavow the knowledge or meaning of an event to reduce anxiety or fear to the detriment of health.

Possible Etiologies ("related to")

[Weak, underdeveloped ego]
[Underlying fears and anxieties]
[Low self-esteem]
[Fixation in early level of development]

Defining Characteristics ("evidenced by")

[Denies substance abuse or dependence]
[Denies that substance use creates problems in his or her life]
[Continues to use substance, knowing it contributes to impairment in functioning or exacerbation of physical symptoms]
[Uses substance(s) in physically hazardous situations]
[Use of rationalization and projection to explain maladaptive behaviors]
Unable to admit impact of disease on life pattern

Goals/Objectives

Short-Term Goal

Client will divert attention away from external issues and focus on behavioral outcomes associated with substance use.

Long-Term Goal

Client will verbalize acceptance of responsibility for own behavior and acknowledge association between substance use and personal problems.

Interventions with *Selected Rationales*

1. Begin by working to develop a trusting nurse-client relationship. Be honest. Keep all promises. ***Trust is the basis of a therapeutic relationship.***
2. Convey an attitude of acceptance to the client. Ensure that he or she understands "It is not *you* but your *behavior* that is unacceptable." ***An attitude of acceptance promotes feelings of dignity and self-worth.***
3. Provide information to correct misconceptions about substance abuse. Client may rationalize his or her behavior with statements such as, "I'm not an alcoholic. I can stop drinking any time I want. Besides, I only drink beer." or "I only smoke pot to relax before class. So what? I know lots of people who do. Besides, you can't get hooked on pot." ***Many myths abound regarding use of specific substances. Factual information presented in a matter-of-fact, nonjudgmental way explaining what behaviors constitute substance-related disorders may help the client focus on his or her own behaviors as an illness that requires help.***
4. Identify recent maladaptive behaviors or situations that have occurred in the client's life, and discuss how use of substances may have been a contributing factor. ***The first step in decreasing use of denial is for client to see the relationship between substance use and personal problems.***
5. Use confrontation with caring. Do not allow client to fantasize about his or her lifestyle. (Examples: "It is my understanding that the last time you drank alcohol, you . . ." or "The lab report shows that you were under the influence of alcohol when you had the accident that injured three people.") ***Confrontation interferes with client's ability to use denial; a caring attitude preserves self-esteem and avoids putting the client on the defensive.***
6. Do not accept the use of rationalization or projection as client attempts to make excuses for, or blame his or her behavior on, other people or situations. ***Rationalization and***

projection prolong the stage of denial that problems exist in the client's life because of substance use.

7. Encourage participation in group activities. ***Peer feedback is often more accepted than feedback from authority figures. Peer pressure can be a strong factor, as well as the association with individuals who are experiencing or who have experienced similar problems.***
8. Offer immediate positive recognition of client's expressions of insight gained regarding illness and acceptance of responsibility for own behavior. ***Positive reinforcement enhances self-esteem and encourages repetition of desirable behaviors.***

Outcome Criteria

1. Client verbalizes understanding of the relationship between personal problems and the use of substances.
2. Client verbalizes acceptance of responsibility for own behavior.
3. Client verbalizes understanding of substance dependence and abuse as an illness requiring ongoing support and treatment.

INEFFECTIVE INDIVIDUAL COPING

Definition: Inability to form a valid appraisal of the stressors, inadequate choices of practiced responses, and/or inability to use available resources.

Possible Etiologies ("related to")

[Inadequate support systems]
[Inadequate coping skills]
[Underdeveloped ego]
[Possible hereditary factor]
[Dysfunctional family system]
[Negative role modeling]
[Personal vulnerability]

Defining Characteristics ("evidenced by")

[Low self-esteem]
[Chronic anxiety]
[Chronic depression]
Inability to meet role expectations
[Alteration in societal participation]
Inability to meet basic needs
[Inappropriate use of defense mechanisms]

[Low frustration tolerance]
[Need for immediate gratification]
[Manipulative behavior]
Abuse of chemical agents

Goals/Objectives

Short-Term Goal

Client will express true feelings associated with use of substances as a method of coping with stress.

Long-Term Goal

Client will be able to verbalize adaptive coping mechanisms to use, instead of substance abuse, in response to stress.

Interventions with *Selected Rationales*

1. Establish trusting relationship with client (be honest; keep appointments; be available to spend time). ***The therapeutic nurse-client relationship is built on trust.***
2. Set limits on manipulative behavior. Be sure that the client knows what is acceptable, what is not, and the consequences for violating the limits set. Ensure that all staff maintain consistency with this intervention. ***Client is unable to establish own limits, so you must do so for him or her. Unless administration of consequences for violation of limits is consistent, manipulative behavior will not be eliminated.***
3. Encourage client to verbalize feelings, fears, anxieties. Answer any questions he or she may have regarding the disorder. ***Verbalization of feelings in a nonthreatening environment may help client come to terms with long-unresolved issues.***
4. Explain the effects of substance abuse on the body. Emphasize that prognosis is closely related to abstinence. ***Many clients lack knowledge regarding the deleterious effects of substance abuse on the body.***
5. Explore with client the options available to assist with stressful situations rather than resorting to substance abuse (e.g., contacting various members of Alcoholics Anonymous or Narcotics Anonymous; physical exercise; relaxation techniques; meditation). ***Client may have persistently resorted to chemical abuse, and thus may possess little or no knowledge of adaptive responses to stress.***
6. Provide positive reinforcement for evidence of gratification delayed appropriately. ***Positive reinforcement enhances self-esteem and encourages client to repeat acceptable behaviors.***

7. Encourage client to be as independent as possible in own self-care. Provide positive feedback for independent decision making and effective use of problem-solving skills.

Outcome Criteria

1. Client is able to verbalize adaptive coping strategies for use as alternatives to substance use in response to stress.
2. Client is able to verbalize the names of support people from whom he or she may seek help when the desire for substance use is intense.

ALTERED NUTRITION: LESS THAN BODY REQUIREMENTS

Definition: The state in which an individual experiences an intake of nutrients insufficient to meet metabolic needs.

Possible Etiologies ("related to")

[Drinking alcohol instead of eating nourishing food]
[Eating only "junk food"]
[Eating nothing (or very little) while on a "binge"]
[No money for food (having spent what is available on substances)]
[Problems with malabsorption caused by chronic alcohol abuse]

Defining Characteristics ("evidenced by")

Loss of weight
Pale conjunctiva and mucous membranes
Poor muscle tone
[Poor skin turgor]
[Edema of extremities]
[Electrolyte imbalances]
[Cheilosis (cracks at corners of mouth)]
[Scaley dermatitis]
[Weakness]
[Neuropathies]
[Anemias]
[Ascites]

Goals/Objectives

Short-Term Goals

Client will gain 2lb during next 7 days.
Client's electrolytes will be restored to normal within 1 week.

Long-Term Goal

Client will exhibit no signs or symptoms of malnutrition by discharge. (This would not be a realistic goal for a chronic alcoholic in the end stages of the disease. For such a client, it would be more appropriate to establish short-term goals, as realistic step objectives, to use in the evaluation of care given.)

Interventions with *Selected Rationales*

1. In collaboration with dietitian, determine number of calories required to provide adequate nutrition and realistic (according to body structure and height) weight gain.
2. Strict documentation of intake, output, and calorie count. ***This information is necessary to make an accurate nutritional assessment and maintain client safety.***
3. Weigh daily. ***Weight loss or gain is important assessment information.***
4. Determine client's likes and dislikes and collaborate with dietitian to provide favorite foods. ***Client is more likely to eat foods that he or she particularly enjoys.***
5. Ensure that client receives small, frequent feedings, including a bedtime snack, rather than three larger meals. ***Large amounts of food may be objectionable, or even intolerable, to the client.***
6. Administer vitamin and mineral supplements, as ordered by physician, ***to improve nutritional state.***
7. If appropriate, ask family members or significant others to bring in special foods that client particularly enjoys.
8. Monitor laboratory work, and report significant changes to physician.
9. Explain the importance of adequate nutrition. ***Client may have inadequate or inaccurate knowledge regarding the contribution of good nutrition to overall wellness.***

Outcome Criteria

1. Client has achieved and maintained at least 90 percent of normal body weight.
2. Vital signs, blood pressure, and laboratory serum studies are within normal limits.
3. Client is able to verbalize importance of adequate nutrition.

SELF-ESTEEM DISTURBANCE

Definition: Negative self-evaluation and feelings about self or self-capabilities, which may be directly or indirectly expressed.

Possible Etiologies ("related to")

[Retarded ego development]
[Dysfunctional family system]
[Lack of positive feedback]
[Perceived failures]

Defining Characteristics ("evidenced by")

[Difficulty accepting positive reinforcement]
[Failure to take responsibility for self-care]
[Self-destructive behavior (substance abuse)]
[Lack of eye contact]
[Withdraws into social isolation]
[Highly critical and judgmental of self and others]
[Sense of worthlessness]
[Fear of failure]
[Unable to recognize own accomplishments]
[Setting self up for failure by establishing unrealistic goals]
[Unsatisfactory interpersonal relationships]
[Negative or pessimistic outlook]
Denial of problems obvious to others
Projection of blame or responsibility for problems
Rationalizing personal failures
Hypersensitivity to slight criticism
Grandiosity

Goals/Objectives

Short-Term Goal

Client will accept responsibility for personal failures and verbalize the role substances played in those failures.

Long-Term Goal

By discharge, client will exhibit increased feelings of self-worth as evidenced by verbal expression of positive aspects about self, past accomplishments, and future prospects.

Interventions with *Selected Rationales*

1. Be accepting of client and his or her negativism. ***An attitude of acceptance enhances feelings of self-worth.***
2. Spend time with client ***to convey acceptance and contribute toward feelings of self-worth.***
3. Help client to recognize and focus on strengths and accomplishments. Discuss past (real or perceived) failures, but minimize amount of attention devoted to them beyond client's need to accept responsibility for them. ***Client must accept responsibility for own behavior before change in behavior can occur. Minimizing attention***

to past failures may help to eliminate negative ruminations and increase client's sense of self-worth.

4. Encourage participation in group activities *from which client may receive positive feedback and support from peers.*
5. Help client identify areas he or she would like to change about self and assist with problem solving toward this effort. *Low self-worth may interfere with client's perception of own problem-solving ability. Assistance may be required.*
6. Assure that client is not becoming increasingly dependent and that he or she is accepting responsibility for own behaviors. *Client must be able to function independently if he or she is to be successful within the less structured community environment.*
7. Ensure that therapy groups offer client simple methods of achievement. Offer recognition and positive feedback for actual accomplishments. *Successes and recognition increase self-esteem.*
8. Provide instruction in assertiveness techniques: the ability to recognize the difference among passive, assertive, and aggressive behaviors; the importance of respecting the human rights of others while protecting one's own basic human rights. *Self-esteem is enhanced by the ability to interact with others in an assertive manner.*
9. Teach effective communication techniques, such as the use of "I" messages and placing emphasis on ways to avoid making judgmental statements.

Outcome Criteria

1. Client is able to verbalize positive aspects about self.
2. Client is able to communicate assertively with others.
3. Client expresses an optimistic outlook for the future.

KNOWLEDGE DEFICIT (Effects of Substance Abuse on the Body)

Definition: Absence or deficiency of cognitive information related to [the effects of substance abuse on the body and its interference with achievement and maintenance of optimal wellness].

Possible Etiologies ("related to")

Lack of interest in learning
[Low self-esteem]

[Denial of need for information]
[Denial of risks involved with substance abuse]
Unfamiliarity with information resources

Defining Characteristics ("evidenced by")

[Abuse of substances]
[Statement of lack of knowledge]
[Statement of misconception]
[Request for information]
Verbalization of the problem

Goals/Objectives

Short-Term Goal

Client will be able to verbalize effects of [substance used] on the body following implementation of teaching plan.

Long-Term Goal

Client will verbalize the importance of abstaining from use of [substance] to maintain optimal wellness.

Interventions with *Selected Rationales*

1. Assess client's level of knowledge regarding effects of [substance] on body. ***Baseline assessment of knowledge is required to develop appropriate teaching plan for client.***
2. Assess client's level of anxiety and readiness to learn. ***Learning does not take place beyond moderate level of anxiety.***
3. Determine method of learning most appropriate for client (e.g., discussion, question and answer, use of audio or visual aids, oral or written method). ***Level of education and development are important considerations as to methodology selected.***
4. Develop teaching plan, including measurable objectives for the learner. ***Measurable objectives provide criteria on which to base evaluation of the teaching experience.***
5. Include significant others, if possible. ***Lifestyle changes often affect all family members.***
6. Implement teaching plan at a time that facilitates, and in a place that is conducive to, optimal learning (e.g., in the evening when family members visit, in an empty, quiet classroom or group therapy room). ***Learning is enhanced by an environment with few distractions.***
7. Begin with simple concepts and progress to the more complex. ***Retention is increased if presented introductory material is easy to understand.***

8. Include information on physical effects of [substance], its capacity for physiological and psychological dependence, its effects on family functioning, its effects on a fetus (and the importance of contraceptive use until abstinence has been achieved), and the importance of regular participation in an appropriate treatment program.
9. Provide activities for client and significant others in which to actively participate during the learning exercise. ***Active participation increases retention.***
10. Ask client and significant others to demonstrate knowledge gained by verbalizing presented information. ***Verbalization of knowledge gained is a measurable method of evaluating the teaching experience.***
11. Provide positive feedback for participation, as well as for accurate demonstration of knowledge gained. ***Positive feedback enhances self-esteem and encourages repetition of acceptable behaviors.***
12. Evaluate teaching plan. Identify strengths and weaknesses, as well as any changes that may enhance the effectiveness of the plan.

Outcome Criteria

1. Client is able to verbalize effects of [substance] on the body.
2. Client verbalizes understanding of risks involved in use of [substance].
3. Client is able to verbalize community resources for obtaining knowledge and support with substance-related problems.

■ INTERNET REFERENCES

Additional information on Addictions may be located at the following Websites:

- http://www.recovery-works.com
- http://www.ncbi.nlm.nih.gov
- http://www.liebertpub.com
- http://www.drugs.indiana.edu

Additional information on self-help organizations may be located at the following Websites:

- http://www.ca.org (Cocaine Anonymous)
- http://www.alcoholics-anonymous.org (AA)
- http://www.delphi.com (Narcotics Anonymous)

Additional information about medications for treatment of Alcohol and Drug Dependence may be located at the following Websites:

- http://www.fadavis.com
- http://www.laurus.com

CHAPTER 6

*Schizophrenia and Other Psychotic Disorders**

■ BACKGROUND ASSESSMENT DATA

The syndrome of symptoms associated with schizophrenia and other psychotic disorders reveals alterations in content and organization of thoughts, perception of sensory input, affect or emotional tone, sense of identity, volition, psychomotor behavior, and ability to establish satisfactory interpersonal relationships.

Categories

295.30 Paranoid Schizophrenia

Paranoid schizophrenia is characterized by extreme suspiciousness of others and by delusions and hallucinations of a persecutory or grandiose nature. The individual is often tense and guarded and may be argumentative, hostile, and aggressive.

295.10 Disorganized Schizophrenia

In disorganized schizophrenia, behavior is typically regressive and primitive. Affect is inappropriate, with common characteristics being silliness, incongruous giggling, facial grimaces, and extreme social withdrawal. Communication is consistently incoherent.

---

*Reprinted with permission from the *Diagnostic and Statistical Manual of Mental Disorders, Fourth Edition.* Copyright 1994 American Psychiatric Association, 1994.

295.20 Catatonic Schizophrenia

Catatonic schizophrenia manifests itself in the form of *stupor* (marked psychomotor retardation, mutism, waxy flexibility [posturing], negativism, and rigidity) or *excitement* (extreme psychomotor agitation, leading to exhaustion or the possibility of hurting self or others if not curtailed).

295.90 Undifferentiated Schizophrenia

Undifferentiated schizophrenia is characterized by disorganized behaviors and psychotic symptoms (e.g., delusions, hallucinations, incoherence, and grossly disorganized behavior) that may appear in more than one category.

295.60 Residual Schizophrenia

Behavior in residual schizophrenia is eccentric, but psychotic symptoms, if present at all, are not prominent. Social withdrawal and inappropriate affect are characteristic. The patient has a history of at least one episode of schizophrenia in which psychotic symptoms were prominent.

295.70 Schizoaffective Disorder

Schizoaffective disorder refers to behaviors characteristic of schizophrenia, in addition to those indicative of disorders of mood, such as depression or mania.

298.8 Brief Psychotic Disorder

The essential features of brief psychotic disorder include a sudden onset of psychotic symptoms in response to a severe psychosocial stressor. The symptoms last at least 1 day but less than 1 month with a virtual return to the premorbid level of functioning. The diagnosis is further specified by whether it follows a severe identifiable stressor or whether the onset occurs within 4 weeks postpartum.

295.40 Schizophreniform Disorder

The essential features of schizophreniform disorder are identical to those of schizophrenia, with the exception that the duration is at least 1 month but less than 6 months. The diagnosis is termed "provisional" if a diagnosis must be made prior to recovery.

297.1 Delusional Disorder

Delusional disorder is characterized by the presence of one or more nonbizarre delusions that persist for at least 1 month. Hallucinatory activity is not prominent. Apart from the delusions, behavior is not bizarre. The following types are based on the predominant delusional theme. (APA, 1994):

1. **Persecutory Type:** Delusions that one is being malevolently treated in some way.
2. **Jealous Type:** Delusions that one's sexual partner is unfaithful.
3. **Erotomanic Type:** Delusions that another person of higher status is in love with him or her.
4. **Somatic Type:** Delusions that the person has some physical defect, disorder, or disease.
5. **Grandiose Type:** Delusions of inflated worth, power, knowledge, special identity, or special relationship to a deity or famous person.

297.3 Shared Psychotic Disorder (Folie à Deux)

In shared psychotic disorder, a delusional system develops in the context of a close relationship with another person who already has a psychotic disorder with prominent delusions.

293.xx Psychotic Disorder Due to a General Medical Condition

The *DSM-IV* identifies the essential features of this disorder as prominent hallucinations and delusions that can be directly attributed to a general medical condition. Examples of general medical conditions that may cause psychotic symptoms include neurological conditions (e.g., neoplasms, Huntington's disease, CNS infections); endocrine conditions (e.g., hyperthyroidism, hypothyroidism, hypoadrenocorticism); metabolic conditions (e.g., hypoxia, hypercarbia, hypoglycemia); autoimmune disorders (e.g., systemic lupus erythematosus); and others (e.g., fluid or electrolyte imbalances, hepatic or renal diseases).

Substance-Induced Psychotic Disorder (Refer to Substance-Related Disorders for substance-specific codes)

The essential features of this disorder are the presence of prominent hallucinations and delusions that are judged to be directly attributable to the physiological effects of a substance (i.e., a drug of abuse, a medication, or toxin exposure) (APA, 1994).

Predisposing Factors

1. **Physiological**
   a. ***Genetics:*** Studies (Black and Andreasen, 1994; Kaplan and Sadock, 1998) have indicated that certain genetic factors may be involved in the development of a psychotic disorder. Results have shown that individuals are at higher risk for the disorder if there is a familial pattern of involvement (parents, siblings, other relatives).
   b. ***Histological Changes:*** Scheibel (1991) has suggested that schizophrenic disorders may in fact be a birth defect, occurring in the hippocampus region of the brain, and related to an influenza virus encountered by the mother during the second trimester of pregnancy. The studies have shown a "disordering" of the pyramidal cells in the brains of schizophrenics, but the cells in the brains of nonschizophrenic individuals appeared to be arranged in an orderly fashion. Further research is required to determine the possible link between this birth defect and the development of schizophrenia.
   c. ***The Dopamine Hypothesis:*** A biochemical theory suggests the involvement of elevated levels of the neurotransmitter dopamine, which is thought to produce the symptoms of overactivity and fragmentation of associations that are commonly observed in psychoses (Hollandsworth, 1990).
2. **Psychosocial**
   Early conceptualizations of schizophrenia focused on family relationship factors as major influences in the development of the illness. This probably occurred in light of the conspicuous absence of information related to a biological connection.

   In the past decade researchers have doubted these theories and are now focusing their studies more in terms of schizophrenia as a brain disorder. Can family interaction patterns cause schizophrenia? Cutting (1985) states: "These purely psychological causes are *theoretically* possible, even if difficult to prove in practice."

Kaplan and Sadock (1998) state: "Clinicians should consider the psychosocial factors affecting schizophrenia. Although, historically, theorists have attributed the development of schizophrenia to psychosocial factors, contemporary clinicians can benefit from using the relevant theories and guidelines of these past observations and hypotheses." (p. 465)

The following psychosocial theories are presented for enlightenment and discussion.

a. ***Family Systems Theory:*** Bowen (1978) describes the development of schizophrenia as it evolves out of a dysfunctional family system. Conflict between spouses drives one parent to attach to the child. This overinvestment in the child redirects the focus of anxiety in the family, and a more stable condition results. A symbiotic relationship develops between parent and child; the child remains totally dependent on the parent into adulthood and is unable to respond to the demands of adult functioning.
b. ***Interpersonal Theory:*** Sullivan (1953) relates that the psychotic person is the product of a parent-child relationship fraught with intense anxiety. The child receives confusing and conflicting messages from the parent and is unable to establish trust. High levels of anxiety are maintained, and the child's concept of self is one of ambiguity. Psychosis offers relief from anxiety and security from intimate relatedness.
c. ***Psychodynamic Theory:*** Birchwood and coworkers (1989) assert that psychosis is the result of a weak ego, development of which has been inhibited by a cold, overprotective, and domineering mother. *Double-bind communication* may also be a factor in this theory of causation. Double-bind communication occurs when a verbal statement is made accompanied by a nonverbal expression that is incongruent. These incompatible communications may also interfere with ego development, thereby causing the individual to generate false ideas and exhibit extreme mistrust of all communications. Because of weak ego development, the adolescent or young adult is unable to deal with the demands of adult living and retreats into a form of thinking from early childhood.

Symptomatology (Subjective/Objective Data)

1. **Autism:** There is a focus inward. The individual may create his or her own world. Words and events may take on special meaning to the psychotic person, meaning of a highly symbolic nature that only the individual can understand.
2. **Emotional Ambivalence:** Powerful emotions of love, hate, and fear produce much conflict within the individual. Each tends to balance the other until an emotional neutralization occurs, and the individual experiences apathy or indifference.
3. **Inappropriate Affect:** The affect is blunted or flat, and often inappropriate (e.g., person laughs when told of the death of a parent).
4. **Associative Looseness:** This term describes the very disorganized thoughts and verbalizations of the psychotic person. Ideas shift from one unrelated subject to another. When the condition is severe, speech may be incoherent.
5. **Echolalia:** The psychotic person often repeats words he or she hears.
6. **Echopraxia:** The psychotic person often repeats movements he or she sees in others. (Echolalia and echopraxia are products of the person's very weak ego boundaries.)
7. **Neologisms:** Words that are invented by the psychotic person that are meaningless to others but have symbolic meaning to the individual.
8. **Concrete Thinking:** The psychotic person has difficulty thinking on the abstract level and may use literal translations concerning aspects of the environment.
9. **Clang Associations:** The individual uses rhyming words in a nonsensical pattern.
10. **Word Salad:** The psychotic person may put together a random jumble of words without any logical connection.
11. **Mutism:** Psychotic individuals may refuse or be unable to speak.
12. **Circumstantiality:** Circumstantiality refers to a psychotic person's delay in reaching the point of a communication because of unnecessary and tedious details.
13. **Tangentiality:** Tangentiality differs from circumstantiality in that the person never really gets to the point of the communication. Unrelated topics are introduced, and the original discussion is lost.
14. **Perseveration:** The individual who exhibits perse-

veration persistently repeats the same word or idea in response to different questions.

15. **Delusions:** False ideas or beliefs. Types of delusions include the following:
    a. ***Grandeur:*** The person has an exaggerated feeling of importance or power.
    b. ***Persecution:*** The person feels threatened and believes others intend harm or persecution toward him or her in some way.
    c. ***Reference:*** All events within the environment are referred by the psychotic person to himself or herself.
    d. ***Control or Influence:*** The individual believes certain objects or people have control over his or her behavior.
16. **Hallucinations:** Hallucinations are false sensory perceptions that may involve any of the five senses. Auditory and visual hallucinations are most common, although olfactory, tactile, and gustatory hallucinations can occur.
17. **Regression:** A primary ego defense mechanism used in psychoses. Childlike mannerisms and comfort techniques are employed. Socially inappropriate behavior may be evident.
18. **Religiosity:** The psychotic person becomes preoccupied with religious ideas, a defense mechanism thought to be used in an attempt to provide stability and structure to disorganized thoughts and behaviors.

Common Nursing Diagnoses and Interventions

(Interventions are applicable to various health-care settings, such as inpatient and partial hospitalization, community outpatient clinic, home health, and private practice.)

RISK FOR VIOLENCE: SELF-DIRECTED OR DIRECTED AT OTHERS

Definition: Behaviors in which an individual demonstrates that he/she can be physically, emotionally, and/or sexually harmful either to self or to others.

Related/Risk Factors ("related to")

[Lack of trust (suspiciousness of others)]
[Panic level of anxiety]

[Catatonic excitement]
[Negative role modeling]
[Rage reactions]
[Command hallucinations]
[Delusional thinking]
Body language—rigid posture, clenching of fists and jaw, hyperactivity, pacing, breathlessness, and threatening stances
[History or threats of violence toward self or others or of destruction to the property of others]
Impulsivity
Suicidal ideation, plan, available means
[Perception of the environment as threatening]
[Receiving auditory or visual "suggestions" of a threatening nature]

Goals/Objectives

Short-Term Goal

Within [a specified time], client will recognize signs of increasing anxiety and agitation and report to staff for assistance with intervention.

Long-Term Goal

Client will not harm self or others.

Interventions with *Selected Rationales*

1. Maintain low level of stimuli in client's environment (low lighting, few people, simple decor, low noise level). ***Anxiety level rises in a stimulating environment. A suspicious, agitated client may perceive individuals as threatening.***
2. Observe client's behavior frequently (every 15 minutes). Do this in a manner of carrying out routine activities, ***so as to avoid creating suspiciousness in the individual. Close observation is necessary so that intervention can occur if required to ensure client (and others') safety.***
3. Remove all dangerous objects from client's environment, ***so that in his or her agitated, confused state, client may not use them to harm self or others.***
4. Try to redirect the violent behavior with physical outlets for the client's anxiety (e.g., punching bag). ***Physical exercise is a safe and effective way of relieving pent-up tension.***
5. Staff should maintain and convey a calm attitude toward client. ***Anxiety is contagious and can be transmitted from staff to client.***
6. Have sufficient staff available to indicate a show of strength to client if it becomes necessary. ***This shows the***

client evidence of control over the situation and provides some physical security for staff.

7. Administer tranquilizing medications as ordered by physician. Monitor medication for its effectiveness and for any adverse side effects. ***The avenue of the "least restrictive alternative" must be selected when planning interventions for a psychiatric client.***
8. If client is not calmed by "talking down" or by medication, use of mechanical restraints may be necessary. Be sure to have sufficient staff available to assist. Follow protocol established by the institution. Most states require that the physician re-evaluate and issue a new order for restraints every 3 hours, except between midnight and 8:00 AM. If the client has previously refused medication, administer after restraints have been applied. Most states consider this intervention appropriate in emergency situations or in the event that a client would likely harm self or others.
9. Observe the client in restraints every 15 minutes (or according to institutional policy). Ensure that circulation to extremities is not compromised (check temperature, color, pulses). Assist client with needs related to nutrition, hydration, and elimination. Position client so that comfort is facilitated and aspiration can be prevented. ***Client safety is a nursing priority.***
10. As agitation decreases, assess client's readiness for restraint removal or reduction. Remove one restraint at a time, while assessing client's response. ***This minimizes risk of injury to client and staff.***

Outcome Criteria

1. Anxiety is maintained at a level at which client feels no need for aggression.
2. Client demonstrates trust of others in his or her environment.
3. Client maintains reality orientation.

SOCIAL ISOLATION

Definition: Condition of aloneness experienced by the individual and perceived as imposed by others and as a negative or threatened state.

Possible Etiologies ("related to")

[Lack of trust]
[Panic level of anxiety]

[Regression to earlier level of development]
[Delusional thinking]
[Past experiences of difficulty in interactions with others]
[Weak ego development]
[Repressed fears]

Defining Characteristics ("evidenced by")

[Staying alone in room]
Uncommunicative, withdrawn, no eye contact, [mutism, autism]
Sad, dull affect
[Lying on bed in fetal position with back to door]
Inappropriate or immature interests and activities for developmental age or stage
Preoccupation with own thoughts; repetitive, meaningless actions
[Approaching staff for interaction, then refusing to respond to staff's acknowledgment]
Expression of feelings of rejection or of aloneness imposed by others

Goals/Objectives

Short-Term Goal

Client will willingly attend therapy activities accompanied by trusted staff member within 1 week.

Long-Term Goal

Client will voluntarily spend time with other clients and staff members in group activities on the unit by discharge.

Interventions with *Selected Rationales*

1. Convey an accepting attitude by making brief, frequent contacts. ***An accepting attitude increases feelings of self-worth and facilitates trust.***
2. Show unconditional positive regard. ***This conveys your belief in the client as a worthwhile human being.***
3. Be with the client to offer support during group activities that may be frightening or difficult for him or her. ***The presence of a trusted individual provides emotional security for the client.***
4. Be honest and keep all promises. ***Honesty and dependability promote a trusting relationship.***
5. Orient client to time, person, and place, as necessary.
6. Be cautious with touch. Allow client extra space and an avenue for exit if he or she becomes too anxious. ***A suspicious client may perceive touch as a threatening gesture.***

7. Administer tranquilizing medications as ordered by physician. Monitor for effectiveness and for adverse side effects. ***Antipsychotic medications help to reduce psychotic symptoms in some individuals, thereby facilitating interactions with others.***
8. Discuss with client the signs of increasing anxiety and techniques to interrupt the response (e.g., relaxation exercises, thought stopping). ***Maladaptive behaviors such as withdrawal and suspiciousness are manifested during times of increased anxiety.***
9. Give recognition and positive reinforcement for client's voluntary interactions with others. ***Positive reinforcement enhances self-esteem and encourages repetition of acceptable behaviors.***

Outcome Criteria

1. Client demonstrates willingness and desire to socialize with others.
2. Client voluntarily attends group activities.
3. Client approaches others in appropriate manner for one-to-one interaction.

INEFFECTIVE INDIVIDUAL COPING

Definition: Inability to form a valid appraisal of the stressors, inadequate choices of practiced responses, and/or inability to use available resources.

Possible Etiologies ("related to")

[Inability to trust]
[Panic level of anxiety]
[Personal vulnerability]
[Low self-esteem]
[Inadequate support systems]
[Negative role model]
[Repressed fears]
[Underdeveloped ego]
[Possible hereditary factor]
[Dysfunctional family system]

Defining Characteristics ("evidenced by")

[Suspiciousness of others, resulting in:
- Alteration in societal participation
- Inability to meet basic needs
- Inappropriate use of defense mechanisms]

Goals/Objectives

Short-Term Goal

Client will develop trust in at least one staff member within 1 week.

Long-Term Goal

Client will demonstrate use of more adaptive coping skills as evidenced by appropriateness of interactions and willingness to participate in the therapeutic community.

Interventions with *Selected Rationales*

1. Encourage same staff to work with client as much as possible ***in order to promote development of trusting relationship.***
2. Avoid physical contact. ***Suspicious clients may perceive touch as a threatening gesture.***
3. Avoid laughing, whispering, or talking quietly where client can see but not hear what is being said. ***Suspicious clients often believe others are discussing them, and secretive behaviors reinforce the paranoid feelings.***
4. Be honest and keep all promises. ***Honesty and dependability promote a trusting relationship.***
5. A creative approach may have to be used to encourage food intake (e.g., canned food and own can opener or family-style meals). ***Suspicious clients may believe they are being poisoned and refuse to eat food from the individually prepared tray.***
6. Mouth checks may be necessary following medication administration ***to verify whether client is swallowing the tablets or capsules. Suspicious clients may believe they are being poisoned with their medication and attempt to discard the pills.***
7. Activities should never include anything competitive. Activities that encourage a one-to-one relationship with the nurse or therapist are best. ***Competitive activities are very threatening to suspicious clients.***
8. Encourage client to verbalize true feelings. The nurse should avoid becoming defensive when angry feelings are directed at him or her. ***Verbalization of feelings in a nonthreatening environment may help client come to terms with long-unresolved issues.***
9. An assertive, matter-of-fact, yet genuine approach will be least threatening to the suspicious person. ***The suspicious client does not have the capacity to relate to an overly friendly, overly cheerful attitude.***

Outcome Criteria

1. Client is able to appraise situations realistically and refrain from projecting own feelings onto the environment.
2. Client is able to recognize and clarify possible misinterpretations of the behaviors and verbalizations of others.
3. Client eats food from tray and takes medications without evidence of mistrust.
4. Client appropriately interacts and cooperates with staff and peers in therapeutic community setting.

SENSORY-PERCEPTUAL ALTERATION: AUDITORY/VISUAL

Definition: A state in which an individual experiences a change in the amount or patterning of oncoming stimuli [either internally or externally initiated] accompanied by a diminished, exaggerated, distorted, or impaired response to such stimuli.

Possible Etiologies ("related to")

[Panic level of anxiety]
[Withdrawal into the self]
[Stress sufficiently severe to threaten an already weak ego]

Defining Characteristics ("evidenced by")

[Talking and laughing to self]
[Listening pose (tilting head to one side as if listening)]
[Stops talking in middle of sentence to listen]
[Disorientation]
[Poor concentration]
[Rapid mood swings]
[Disordered thought sequencing]
Inappropriate responses

Goals/Objectives

Short-Term Goal

Client will discuss content of hallucinations with nurse or therapist within 1 week.

Long-Term Goal

Client will be able to define and test reality, eliminating the occurrence of hallucinations.
(This goal may not be realistic for the individual with chronic

illness who has experienced auditory hallucinations for many years.) A more realistic goal may be:

Client will verbalize understanding that the voices are a result of his or her illness and demonstrate ways to interrupt the hallucination.

Interventions with *Selected Rationales*

1. Observe client for signs of hallucinations (listening pose, laughing or talking to self, stopping in midsentence). ***Early intervention may prevent aggressive responses to command hallucinations.***
2. Avoid touching the client before warning him or her that you are about to do so. ***Client may perceive touch as threatening and respond in an aggressive manner.***
3. An attitude of acceptance will encourage the client to share the content of the hallucination with you. ***This is important to prevent possible injury to the client or others from command hallucinations.***
4. Do not reinforce the hallucination. Use "the voices" instead of words like "they," which imply validation. Let client know that you do not share the perception. Say, "Even though I realize that the voices are real to you, I do not hear any voices speaking." ***The nurse must be honest with the client so that he or she may realize that the hallucinations are not real.***
5. Try to connect the times of the hallucinations to times of increased anxiety. Help the client to understand this connection. ***If client can learn to interrupt escalating anxiety, hallucinations may be prevented.***
6. Try to distract the client away from the hallucination. ***Involvement in interpersonal activities and explanation of the actual situation will help bring the client back to reality.***
7. For some clients, auditory hallucinations persist after the acute psychotic episode has subsided. Listening to the radio or watching television helps distract some clients from attention to the voices. Others have benefited from an intervention called ***voice dismissal.*** With this technique, the client is taught to say loudly, "Go away!" or "Leave me alone!", thereby exerting some conscious control over the behavior.

Outcome Criteria

1. Client is able to recognize that hallucinations occur at times of extreme anxiety.
2. Client is able to recognize signs of increasing anxiety and employ techniques to interrupt the response.

ALTERED THOUGHT PROCESSES

Definition: A state in which an individual experiences a disruption in cognitive operations and activities.

Possible Etiologies ("related to")

[Inability to trust]
[Panic level of anxiety]
[Repressed fears]
[Stress sufficiently severe to threaten an already weak ago]
[Possible hereditary factor]

Defining Characteristics ("evidenced by")

[Delusional thinking (false ideas)]
[Inability to concentrate]
Hypervigilance
[Altered attention span]—distractibility
Inaccurate interpretation of the environment
[Impaired ability to make decisions, problem-solve, reason, abstract or conceptualize, calculate]
[Inappropriate social behavior (reflecting inaccurate thinking)]
Inappropriate non–reality-based thinking

Goals/Objectives

Short-Term Goal

By the end of 2 weeks, client will recognize and verbalize that false ideas occur at times of increased anxiety.

Long-Term Goal

Depending on chronicity of disease process, choose the most realistic long-term goal for the client:

1. By discharge from treatment, client will experience (verbalize evidence of) no delusional thoughts.
2. By discharge from treatment, client will be able to differentiate between delusional thinking and reality.

Interventions with *Selected Rationales*

1. Convey your acceptance of client's need for the false belief, while letting him or her know that you do not share the belief. ***It is important to communicate to the client that you do not accept the delusion as reality.***
2. Do not argue or deny the belief. Use *reasonable doubt* as a therapeutic technique: "I find that hard to believe." ***Arguing with the client or denying the belief serves no useful purpose, because delusional ideas are not elim-***

inated by this approach, and the development of a trusting relationship may be impeded.

3. Help client try to connect the false beliefs to times of increased anxiety. Discuss techniques that could be used to control anxiety (e.g., deep-breathing exercises, other relaxation exercises, thought-stopping techniques). ***If the client can learn to interrupt escalating anxiety, delusional thinking may be prevented.***
4. Reinforce and focus on reality. Discourage long ruminations about the irrational thinking. Talk about real events and real people. ***Discussions that focus on the false ideas are purposeless and useless, and may even aggravate the psychosis.***
5. Assist and support client in his or her attempt to verbalize feelings of anxiety, fear, or insecurity. ***Verbalization of feelings in a nonthreatening environment may help client come to terms with long-unresolved issues.***

Outcome Criteria

1. Verbalizations reflect thinking processes oriented in reality.
2. Client is able to maintain ADLs to his or her maximal ability.
3. Client is able to refrain from responding to delusional thoughts, should they occur.

IMPAIRED VERBAL COMMUNICATION

Definition: The state in which an individual experiences a decreased, delayed, or absent ability to receive, process, transmit, and use a system of symbols.

Possible Etiologies ("related to")

[Inability to trust]
[Panic level of anxiety]
[Regression to earlier level of development]
[Withdrawal into the self]
[Disordered, unrealistic thinking]

Defining Characteristics ("evidenced by")

[Loose association of ideas]
[Use of words that are symbolic to the individual (neologisms)]
[Use of words in a meaningless, disconnected manner (word salad)]
[Use of words that rhyme in a nonsensical fashion (clang association)]
[Repetition of words that are heard (echolalia)]
[Does not speak (mutism)]

[Verbalizations reflect concrete thinking (ability to think in abstract terms)]
[Poor eye contact (either no eye contact or continuous staring into the other person's eyes)]

Goals/Objectives

Short-Term Goal

Client will demonstrate ability to remain on one topic, using appropriate, intermittent eye contact for 5 minutes with nurse or therapist.

Long-Term Goal

By discharge from treatment, client will demonstrate ability to carry on a verbal communication in a socially acceptable manner with staff and peers.

Interventions with *Selected Rationales*

1. Use the techniques of *consensual validation* and *seeking clarification* to decode communication patterns. (Examples: "Is it that you mean . . . ?" or "I don't understand what you mean by that. Would you please explain it to me?" ***These techniques reveal to the client how he or she is being perceived by others, while the responsibility for not understanding is accepted by the nurse.***
2. Maintain consistency of staff assignment over time, ***to facilitate trust and the ability to understand client's actions and communication.***
3. In a nonthreatening manner, explain to client how his or her behavior and verbalizations are viewed by, and may alienate, others.
4. If client is unable or unwilling to speak (mutism), use of the technique of *verbalizing the implied* is therapeutic. (Example: "That must have been very difficult for you when . . .") ***This may help to convey empathy, develop trust, and eventually encourage client to discuss painful issues.***
5. Anticipate and fulfill client's needs until satisfactory communication patterns return. ***Client comfort and safety are nursing priorities.***

Outcome Criteria

1. Client is able to communicate in a manner that is understood by others.
2. Client's nonverbal messages are congruent with verbalizations.
3. Client is able to recognize that disorganized thinking and impaired verbal communication occur at times of increased anxiety, and intervene to interrupt the process.

SELF-CARE DEFICIT (Identify Specific Area)

Definition: A state in which the individual experiences an impaired ability to perform or complete [activities of daily living].

Possible Etiologies ("related to")

[Withdrawal into the self]
[Regression to an earlier level of development]
[Panic level of anxiety]
Perceptual or cognitive impairment
[Inability to trust]

Defining Characteristics ("evidenced by")

[Difficulty bringing or] inability to bring food from receptacle to mouth.
Inability [or refusal] to wash body or body parts.
[Impaired ability or lack of interest in selecting appropriate clothing to wear, dressing, grooming, or maintaining appearance at a satisfactory level]
[Inability or unwillingness to carry out toileting procedures without assistance]

Goals/Objectives

Short-Term Goal

Client will verbalize a desire to perform ADLs by end of 1 week.

Long-Term Goal

Client will be able to perform ADLs in an independent manner and demonstrate a willingness to do so by discharge from treatment.

Interventions with *Selected Rationales*

1. Encourage client to perform normal ADLs to his or her level of ability. *Successful performance of independent activities enhances self-esteem.*
2. Encourage independence, but intervene when client is unable to perform. *Client comfort and safety are nursing priorities.*
3. Offer recognition and positive reinforcement for independent accomplishments. (Examples: "Mrs. J., I see you have put on a clean dress and combed your hair.") *Positive re-*

inforcement enhances self-esteem and encourages repetition of desirable behaviors.

4. Show client, on concrete level, how to perform activities with which he or she is having difficulty. (Example: If client is not eating, place spoon in his or her hand, scoop some food into it, and say, "Now, eat a bite of mashed potatoes (or other food)." ***Because concrete thinking prevails, explanations must be provided at the client's concrete level of comprehension.***
5. Keep strict records of food and fluid intakes. ***This information is necessary to acquire an accurate nutritional assessment.***
6. Offer nutritious snacks and fluids between meals. ***Client may be unable to tolerate large amounts of food at mealtimes and may therefore require additional nourishment at other times during the day to receive adequate nutrition.***
7. If client is not eating because of suspiciousness and fears of being poisoned, provide canned foods and allow client to open them. Or, if possible, suggest that food be served family-style, ***so that client may see everyone eating from the same servings.***
8. If client is soiling self, establish routine schedule for toileting needs. Assist client to bathroom on hourly or bi-hourly schedule, as need is determined, until he or she is able to fulfill this need without assistance.

Outcome Criteria

1. Client feeds self without assistance.
2. Client selects appropriate clothing, dresses and grooms self daily without assistance.
3. Client maintains optimal level of personal hygiene by bathing daily and carrying out essential toileting procedures without assistance.

SLEEP PATTERN DISTURBANCE

Definition: Time-limited disruption of sleep (natural, periodic suspension of consciousness) amount and quality.

Possible Etiologies ("related to")

[Panic level of anxiety]
[Repressed fears]

[Hallucinations]
[Delusional thinking]

Defining Characteristics ("evidenced by")

[Difficulty falling asleep]
[Awakening very early in the morning]
[Pacing; others signs of increasing irritability caused by lack of sleep]
[Frequent yawning, nodding off to sleep]

Goals/Objectives

Short-Term Goal

Within first week of treatment, client will fall asleep within 30 minutes of retiring and sleep 5 hours without awakening, with use of sedative if needed.

Long-Term Goal

By discharge from treatment, client will be able to fall asleep within 30 minutes of retiring and sleep 6 to 8 hours without a sleeping aid.

Interventions with *Selected Rationales*

1. Keep strict records of sleeping patterns. ***Accurate baseline data are important in planning care to assist client with this problem.***
2. Discourage sleep during the day ***to promote more restful sleep at night.***
3. Administer antipsychotic medication at bedtime ***so client does not become drowsy during the day.***
4. Assist with measures that promote sleep, such as warm, nonstimulating drinks, light snacks, warm baths, and back rubs.
5. Performing relaxation exercises to soft music may be helpful prior to sleep.
6. Limit intake of caffeinated drinks such as tea, coffee, and colas. ***Caffeine is a CNS stimulant and may interfere with the client's achievement of rest and sleep.***

Outcome Criteria

1. Client is able to fall asleep within 30 minutes after retiring.
2. Client sleeps at least 6 consecutive hours without awakening.
3. Client does not require a sedative to fall asleep.

■ INTERNET REFERENCES

Additional information about Schizophrenia may be located at the following Websites:

- http://www.schizophrenia.com
- http://www.nimh.nih.gov
- http://schizophrenia.nami.org
- http://mentalhealth.com

Support and information for patients with Schizophrenia and their families may be located at the following Websites:

- http://www.mhhub.com/psychosis.html
- http://www.health-center.com/english/brain/schiz/fact.htm

Additional information about medications to treat Schizophrenia may be located at the following Websites:

- http://www.mentalhealth.com/menu.htm/
- http://www.mediconsult.com
- http://www.fadavis.com
- http://www.laurus.com

CHAPTER 7

*Mood Disorders**

BACKGROUND ASSESSMENT DATA

Mood is defined as an individual's sustained emotional tone, which significantly influences behavior, personality, and perception. A disturbance in mood is the predominant feature of the mood disorders (APA, 1994). Mood disorders are classified as depressive or bipolar.

Depressive Disorders

296.xx Major Depressive Disorder

Major depressive disorder is described as a disturbance of mood involving depression or loss of interest or pleasure in the usual activities and pastimes. There is evidence of interference in social and occupational functioning for at least 2 weeks. There is no history of manic behavior and the symptoms cannot be attributed to use of substances or a general medical condition. The following specifiers may be used to further describe the depressive episode:

1. **Single Episode or Recurrent:** This specifier identifies whether the individual has experienced prior episodes of depression.
2. **Mild, Moderate, or Severe:** These categories are identified by the number and severity of symptoms.
3. **With Psychotic Features:** Impairment of reality testing, such as the presence of hallucinations or delusions, is evident.
4. **With Melancholic Features:** This is a typically severe

---

*Reprinted with permission from the *Diagnostic and Statistical Manual of Mental Disorders, Fourth Edition*. Copyright 1994 American Psychiatric Association, 1994.

form of major depressive episode. Symptoms are exaggerated. There is a loss of interest in all activities. Depression is regularly worse in the morning. There is a history of major depressive episodes that have responded well to somatic antidepressant therapy.

5. **Chronic:** This classification applies when the current episode of depressed mood has been evident continuously for at least the past 2 years.
6. **With Seasonal Pattern:** This diagnosis indicates the presence of depressive symptoms during the fall or winter months. This diagnosis is made when the number of seasonal depressive episodes substantially outnumbers the nonseasonal depressive episodes that have occurred over the individual's lifetime (APA, 1994). This disorder has previously been identified in the literature as seasonal affective disorder (SAD).
7. **With Postpartum Onset:** This specifier is used when symptoms of major depression occur within 4 weeks postpartum.

300.4 Dysthymic Disorder

A mood disturbance with characteristics similar to, if somewhat milder than, those ascribed to major depressive disorder. There is no evidence of psychotic symptoms.

Bipolar Disorders

These disorders are characterized by mood swings from profound depression to extreme euphoria (mania), with intervening periods of normalcy.

During an episode of *mania*, the mood is elevated, expansive, or irritable. Motor activity is excessive and frenzied. Psychotic features may be present. A somewhat milder form is called *hypomania*. It is usually not severe enough to require hospitalization, and it does not include psychotic features.

The diagnostic picture for *bipolar depression* is identical to that described for major depressive disorder, with one addition. The client must have a history of one or more manic episodes.

When the symptom presentation includes rapidly alternating moods (sadness, irritability, euphoria) accompanied by symptoms associated with both depression and mania, the individual is given a diagnosis of *bipolar disorder, mixed*.

296.xx Bipolar I Disorder

Bipolar I disorder is the diagnosis given to an individual who is experiencing, or has experienced, a full syndrome of manic or mixed symptoms. The client may also have experienced episodes of depression.

296.89 Bipolar II Disorder

Bipolar II disorder is characterized by recurrent bouts of major depression with the episodic occurrence of hypomania. This individual has never experienced a full syndrome of manic or mixed symptoms.

301.13 Cyclothymic Disorder

The essential feature is a chronic mood disturbance of at least 2 years' duration, involving numerous periods of depression and hypomania, but not of sufficient severity and duration to meet the criteria for either bipolar I or II disorder. There is an absence of psychotic features.

293.83 Mood Disorder Due to General Medical Condition

This disorder is characterized by a prominent and persistent disturbance in mood (either depression or mania) that is judged to be the direct result of the physiological effects of a general medical condition (APA, 1994).

Substance-Induced Mood Disorder (Refer to Substance-Related Disorders for substance-specific codes)

The disturbance of mood (depression or mania) associated with this disorder is considered to be the direct result of the physiological effects of a substance (e.g., use or abuse of a drug or a medication, or toxin exposure).

■ MAJOR DEPRESSIVE DISORDER; DYSTHYMIC DISORDER

Predisposing Factors

1. **Physiological**

a. ***Genetic:*** Numerous studies have been conducted that support the involvement of heredity in depressive illness. The disorder is 1.5 to 3 times more common among first-degree relatives of individuals with the disorder than among the general population.
b. ***Biochemical:*** A biochemical theory implicates the biogenic amines norepinephrine, dopamine, and serotonin. The levels of these chemicals have been found to be deficient in individuals with depressive illness (Janowsky et al., 1988).
c. ***Neuroendocrine Disturbances:*** Elevated levels of serum cortisol and decreased levels of thyroid-stimulating hormone have been associated with depressed mood in some individuals.
d. ***Medication Side Effects:*** A number of drugs can produce a depressive syndrome as a side effect. Common ones include anxiolytics, antipsychotics, and sedative-hypnotics. Antihypertensive medications such as propranolol and reserpine have been known to produce depressive symptoms.
e. ***Other Physiological Conditions:*** Depressive symptoms may occur in the presence of electrolyte disturbances, nutritional deficiencies, and with certain physical disorders, such as cardiovascular accident, systematic lupus erythematosus, hepatitis, and diabetes mellitus.

2. **Psychosocial**

a. ***Psychoanalytical:*** This theory (Klein, 1948) implicates an unsatisfactory, early mother-infant relationship as a predisposition to depressive illness. The infant's needs go unfulfilled, a condition that is viewed as a loss. The grief response goes unresolved, and rage and hostility are turned inward on the self. The ego remains weak, while the superego expands and becomes punitive.
b. ***Cognitive:*** These theorists (Beck et al., 1979) believe that depressive illness occurs as a result of impaired cognition. Disturbed thought processes foster a negative evaluation of self by the individual. The perceptions are of inadequacy and worthlessness. Outlook for the future is one of pessimism and hopelessness.

c. ***Learning Theory:*** This theory (Seligman, 1974) proposes that depressive illness is predisposed by the individual's belief that there is a lack of control over his or her life situations. It is thought that this belief arises out of experiences that result in failure (either perceived or real). Following numerous failures, the individual feels helpless to succeed at any endeavor and therefore gives up trying. This "learned helplessness" is viewed as a predisposition to depressive illness.

d. ***Object Loss Theory:*** This theory (Bowlby, 1973) suggests that depressive illness occurs if the person is separated from, or abandoned by, a significant other during the first 6 months of life. The bonding process is interrupted, and the child withdraws from people and the environment.

Symptomatology (Subjective and Objective Data)

1. The affect of a depressed person is one of sadness, dejection, helplessness, and hopelessness. The outlook is gloomy and pessimistic. A feeling of worthlessness prevails.
2. Thoughts are slowed and concentration is difficult. Obsessive ideas and rumination of negative thoughts are common. In severe depression (major depressive disorder or bipolar depression), psychotic features such as hallucinations and delusions may be evident, reflecting misinterpretations of the environment.
3. Physically, there is evidence of weakness and fatigue—very little energy to carry on ADLs. The individual may express an exaggerated concern over bodily functioning, seemingly experiencing heightened sensitivity to somatic sensations.

   Some individuals may be inclined toward excessive eating and drinking, while others may experience anorexia and weight loss.

   In response to a general slowdown of the body, digestion is often sluggish, constipation is common, and urinary retention is possible.

   Sleep disturbances are common, either insomnia or hypersomnia. At the less severe level (dysthymic disorder), individuals tend to feel their best early in the morning, then continually feel worse as the day progresses. The opposite is true of persons experiencing severe depression. The exact cause of this phenomenon is unknown, but it is thought to be related to the circadian rhythm of the hormones and their effects on the body.

4. A general slowdown of motor activity commonly accompanies depression (psychomotor retardation). Energy level is depleted, movements are lethargic, and performance of daily activities is extremely difficult. Regression is common, evidenced by withdrawal into the self and retreat to the fetal position.

   Severely depressed persons may manifest psychomotor activity through symptoms of agitation. These are constant, rapid, purposeless movements, out of touch with the environment.
5. Verbalizations are limited. When depressed persons do speak, the content may be either ruminations regarding their own life regrets or, in psychotic clients, a reflection of their delusional thinking.
6. Social participation is diminished. The depressed client has an inclination toward egocentrism and narcissism—an intense focus on the self. This discourages others from pursuing a relationship with the individual, which increases his or her feelings of worthlessness and penchant for isolation.

Common Nursing Diagnoses and Interventions for Depression

(Interventions are applicable to various health-care settings, such as inpatient and partial hospitalization, community outpatient clinic, home health, and private practice.)

RISK FOR SUICIDE

Definition: Risk for self-inflicted life-threatening injury.

Related/Risk Factors ("related to")

[Depressed mood]
[Feelings of worthlessness]
[Anger turned inward]
[Punitive superego and irrational feelings of guilt]
[Numerous failures (learned helplessness)]

[Feelings of abandonment by significant other]
[Hopelessness]
[Misinterpretations of reality]
[Making direct or indirect statements indicating a desire to commit suicide]
[History of previous suicide attempts]
[Has suicide plan and means to carry it out]
[Putting business affairs in order; writing a will; giving away prized possessions]
[Hallucinations]
[Delusional thinking]
[Statements regarding hopelessness for improvement of life situation]
Suicidal ideation, plan, available means

Goals/Objectives

Short-Term Goals

1. Client will seek out staff when feeling urge to harm self.
2. Client will make short-term verbal (or written) contract with nurse not to harm self.

Long-Term Goal

Client will not harm self.

Interventions with *Selected Rationales*

1. Ask client directly: "Have you thought about killing yourself? If so, what do you plan to do? Do you have the means to carry out this plan? ***This risk of suicide is greatly increased if the client has developed a plan and particularly if means exist for the client to execute the plan.***
2. Create a safe environment for the client. Remove all potentially harmful objects from client's access (sharp objects, straps, belts, ties, glass items). ***Client safety is a nursing priority.***
3. Formulate a short-term verbal contract with the client that he or she will not harm self during specific time period. When that contract expires, make another, and so forth. ***Discussion of suicidal feelings with a trusted individual provides a degree of relief to the client. A contract gets the subject out in the open and places some of the responsibility for the client's safety with the client. An attitude of acceptance of the client as a worthwhile individual is conveyed.***
4. Secure promise from client that he or she will seek out a staff member or support person if thoughts of suicide emerge. ***Suicidal clients are often very ambivalent***

about their feelings. Discussion of feelings with a trusted individual may provide assistance before the client experiences a crisis situation.

5. Encourage verbalizations of honest feelings. Through exploration and discussion, help client to identify symbols of hope in his or her life.
6. Encourage client to express angry feelings within appropriate limits. Provide safe method of hostility release. Help client to identify true source of anger and to work on adaptive coping skills for use outside the hospital. ***Depression and suicidal behaviors may be viewed as anger turned inward on the self. If this anger can be verbalized in a nonthreatening environment, the client may be able to resolve these feelings, regardless of the discomfort involved.***
7. Identify community resources that client may use as support system and from whom he or she may request help if feeling suicidal. ***Having a concrete plan for seeking assistance during a crisis may discourage or prevent self-destructive behaviors.***
8. Orient client to reality, as required. Point out sensory misperceptions or misinterpretations of the environment. Take care not to belittle client's fears or indicate disapproval of verbal expressions.
9. Most important, spend time with client. ***This provides a feeling of safety and security, while also conveying the message, "I want to spent time with you because I think you are a worthwhile person."***

Outcome Criteria

1. Client verbalizes no thoughts of suicide.
2. Client commits no acts of self-violence.
3. Client is able to verbalize names of resources outside the hospital from whom he or she may request help if feeling suicidal.

DYSFUNCTIONAL GRIEVING

Definition: Extended, unsuccessful use of intellectual and emotional responses by which individuals (families, communities) attempt to work through the process of modifying self-concept based upon the perception of [actual or] potential loss.

Possible Etiologies ("related to")

[Real or perceived loss of any concept of value to the individual]

[Bereavement overload (cumulative grief from multiple unresolved losses)]
[Thwarted grieving response to a loss]
[Absence of anticipatory grieving]
[Feelings of guilt generated by ambivalent relationship with lost concept]

Defining Characteristics ("evidenced by")

Idealization of lost [concept]
Denial of loss
[Excessive anger, expressed inappropriately]
[Obsessions with past experiences]
[Ruminations of guilt feelings, excessive and exaggerated out of proportion to the situation]
Developmental regression
Difficulty in expressing loss
Repetitive use of ineffectual behaviors associated with attempts to reinvest in relationships
Reliving of past experiences with little or no reduction of intensity of the grief
Prolonged interference with life functioning, with onset or exacerbation of somatic or psychosomatic responses
Labile affect
Alterations in eating habits, sleep patterns, dream patterns, activity level, libido

Goals/Objectives

Short-Term Goal

Client will express anger toward lost concept.

Long-Term Goal

Client will be able to verbalize behaviors associated with the normal stages of grief. Client will be able to recognize own position in grief process as he or she progresses at own pace toward resolution.

Interventions with *Selected Rationales*

1. Determine stage of grief in which client is fixed. Identify behaviors associated with this stage. *Accurate baseline assessment data are necessary to effectively plan care for the grieving client.*
2. Develop trusting relationship with client. Show empathy and caring. Be honest and keep all promises. *Trust is the basis for a therapeutic relationship.*
3. Convey an accepting attitude and enable the client to express feelings openly. *An accepting attitude conveys to*

the client that you believe he or she is a worthwhile person. Trust is enhanced.

4. Encourage client to express anger. Do not become defensive if initial expression of anger is displaced on nurse or therapist. Assist client to explore angry feelings so that they may be directed toward the intended object or person. ***Verbalization of feelings in a nonthreatening environment may help client come to terms with unresolved issues.***
5. Assist client in discharging pent-up anger through participation in large motor activities (e.g., brisk walks, jogging, physical exercises, volleyball, punching bag, exercise bike). ***Physical exercise provides a safe and effective method for discharging pent-up tension.***
6. Teach the normal stages of grief and behaviors associated with each stage. Help client to understand that feelings such as guilt and anger toward the lost concept are appropriate and acceptable during the grief process. ***Knowledge of acceptability of the feelings associated with normal grieving may help to relieve some of the guilt that these responses generate.***
7. Encourage client to review relationship with the lost concept. With support and sensitivity, point out reality of the situation in areas in which misrepresentations are expressed. ***Client must give up an idealized perception and be able to accept both positive and negative aspects about the lost concept before the grief process is complete.***
8. Communicate to client that crying is acceptable. Use of touch is therapeutic and appropriate with most clients. Knowledge of cultural influences specific to the client is important before using this technique.
9. Assist client in problem solving as he or she attempts to determine methods for more adaptive coping with the experienced loss. Provide positive feedback for strategies identified and decisions made. ***Positive feedback increases self-esteem and encourages repetition of desirable behaviors.***
10. Encourage client to reach out for spiritual support during this time in whatever form is desirable to him or her. Assess spiritual needs of client and assist as necessary in the fulfillment of those needs.

Outcome Criteria

1. Client is able to verbalize normal stages of the grief process and behaviors associated with each stage.

2. Client is able to identify own position within the grief process and express honest feelings related to the lost concept.
3. Client is no longer manifesting exaggerated emotions and behaviors related to dysfunctional grieving and is able to carry out ADLs independently.

SELF-ESTEEM DISTURBANCE

Definition: Negative self-evaluation and feelings about self or self-capabilities, which may be directly or indirectly expressed.

Possible Etiologies ("related to")

[Lack of positive feedback]
[Feelings of abandonment by significant other]
[Numerous failures (learned helplessness)]
[Underdeveloped ego and punitive superego]
[Impaired cognition fostering negative view of self]

Defining Characteristics ("evidenced by")

[Difficulty accepting positive reinforcement]
[Withdrawal into social isolation]
[Being highly critical and judgmental of self and others]
[Expressions of worthlessness]
[Fear of failure]
[Inability to recognize own accomplishments]
[Setting self up for failure by establishing unrealistic goals]
[Unsatisfactory interpersonal relationships]
[Negative, pessimistic outlook]
Hypersensitive to slight or criticism
Grandiosity

Goals/Objectives

Short-Term Goals

1. Within reasonable time period, client will discuss fear of failure with nurse.
2. Within reasonable time period, client will verbalize things he or she likes about self.

Long-Term Goals

1. By discharge from treatment, client will exhibit increased feelings of self-worth as evidenced by verbal expression of positive aspects about self, past accomplishments, and future prospects.

2. By discharge from treatment, client will exhibit increased feelings of self-worth by setting realistic goals and trying to reach them, thereby demonstrating a decrease in fear of failure.

Interventions with *Selected Rationales*

1. Be accepting of client and his or her negativism. ***An attitude of acceptance enhances feelings of self-worth.***
2. Spend time with client ***to convey acceptance and contribute toward feelings of self-worth.***
3. Help client to recognize and focus on strengths and accomplishments. Minimize attention given to past (real or perceived) failures. ***Lack of attention may help to eliminate negative ruminations.***
4. Encourage participation in group activities from ***which client may receive positive feedback and support from peers.***
5. Help client identify areas he or she would like to change about self, and assist with problem solving toward this effort. ***Low self-worth may interfere with client's perception of own problem-solving ability. Assistance may be required.***
6. Ensure that client is not becoming increasingly dependent and that he or she is accepting responsibility for own behaviors. ***Client must be able to function independently if he or she is to be successful within the less structured community environment.***
7. Ensure that therapy groups offer client simple methods of achievement. Offer recognition and positive feedback for actual accomplishments. ***Successes and recognition increase self-esteem.***
8. Teach assertiveness techniques: the ability to recognize the differences among passive, assertive, and aggressive behaviors, and the importance of respecting the human rights of others while protecting one's own basic human rights. ***Self-esteem is enhanced by the ability to interact with others in an assertive manner.***
9. Teach effective communication techniques, such as the use of "I" messages. Emphasize ways to avoid making judgmental statements.
10. Assist client in performing aspects of self-care when required. Offer positive feedback for tasks performed independently. ***Positive feedback enhances self-esteem and encourages repetition of desirable behaviors.***

Outcome Criteria

1. Client is able to verbalize positive aspects about self.

2. Client is able to communicate assertively with others.
3. Client expresses some optimism and hope for the future.
4. Client sets realistic goals for self and demonstrates willing attempt to reach them.

SOCIAL ISOLATION/IMPAIRED SOCIAL INTERACTION

Definition: Social isolation is the condition of aloneness experienced by the individual and perceived as imposed by others and as a negative or threatened state; impaired social interaction is the state in which an individual participates in an insufficient or excessive quantity or ineffective quality of social exchange.

Possible Etiologies ("related to")

[Developmental regression]
[Egocentric behaviors (which offend others and discourage relationships)]
Altered thought processes [delusional thinking]
[Fear of rejection or failure of the interaction]
[Impaired cognition fostering negative view of self]
[Unresolved grief]
Absence of available significant others or peers

Defining Characteristics ("evidenced by")

Sad, dull affect
Being uncommunicative, withdrawn; lacking eye contact
Preoccupation with own thoughts; performance of repetitive, meaningless actions
Seeking to be alone
[Assuming fetal position]
Expression of feelings of aloneness or rejection
Verbalization or observation of discomfort in social situations
Dysfunctional interaction with peers, family, and others

Goals/Objectives

Short-Term Goal

Client will develop trusting relationship with nurse or counselor within reasonable period of time

Long-Term Goals

1. Client will voluntarily spend time with other clients and nurse or therapist in group activities by discharge from treatment.

2. Client will refrain from using egocentric behaviors that offend others and discourage relationships by discharge from treatment.

Interventions with *Selected Rationales*

1. Spend time with client. This may mean just sitting in silence for a while. ***Your presence may help improve client's perception of self as a worthwhile person.***
2. Develop a therapeutic nurse-client relationship through frequent, brief contacts and an accepting attitude. Show unconditional positive regard. ***Your presence, acceptance, and conveyance of positive regard enhance the client's feelings of self-worth.***
3. After client feels comfortable in a one-to-one relationship, encourage attendance in group activities. May need to attend with client the first few times to offer support. Accept client's decision to remove self from group situation if anxiety becomes too great. ***The presence of a trusted individual provides emotional security for the client.***
4. Verbally acknowledge client's absence from any group activities. ***Knowledge that his or her absence was noticed may reinforce the client's feelings of self-worth.***
5. Teach assertiveness techniques. Interactions with others may be discouraged by client's use of passive or aggressive behaviors. ***Knowledge of the use of assertive techniques could improve client's relationships with others.***
6. Provide direct feedback about client's interactions with others. Do this in a nonjudgmental manner. Help client learn how to respond more appropriately in interactions with others. Teach client skills that may be used to approach others in a more socially acceptable manner. Practice these skills through role play. ***Client may not realize how he or she is being perceived by others. Direct feedback from a trusted individual may help to alter these behaviors in a positive manner. Having practiced these skills in role play facilitates their use in real situations.***
7. The depressed client must have lots of structure in his or her life because of the impairment in decision-making and problem-solving ability. Devise a plan of therapeutic activities and provide client with a written time schedule. ***Remember:*** The client who is moderately depressed feels best early in the day, whereas later in the day is a better time for the severely depressed individual to participate in activities.
8. Provide positive reinforcement for client's voluntary interactions with others. ***Positive reinforcement enhances***

self-esteem and encourages repetition of desirable behaviors.

Outcome Criteria

1. Client demonstrates willingness and desire to socialize with others.
2. Client voluntarily attends group activities.
3. Client approaches others in appropriate manner for one-to-one interaction.

POWERLESSNESS

Definition: The perception of the individual that his or her own action will not significantly affect an outcome; a perceived lack of control over a current situation or immediate happening.

Possible Etiologies ("related to")

Lifestyle of helplessness
Health-care environment
[Dysfunctional grieving process]
[Lack of positive feedback]
[Consistent negative feedback]

Defining Characteristics ("evidenced by")

Verbal expressions of having no control or influence over situation, outcome, or self-care
Nonparticipation in care or decision making when opportunities are provided
Expression of doubt regarding role performance
Reluctance to express true feelings, fearing alienation from caregivers
Apathy
Dependence on others that may result in irritability, resentment, anger, and guilt
Passivity

Goals/Objectives

Short-Term Goal

Client will participate in decision making regarding own care within 5 days.

Long-Term Goal

Client will be able to effectively problem-solve ways to take control of his or her life situation by discharge from treatment, thereby decreasing feelings of powerlessness.

Interventions with *Selected Rationales*

1. Encourage client to take as much responsibility as possible for own self-care practices. ***Providing client with choices will increase his or her feelings of control.*** Examples:
   a. Include client in setting the goals of care he or she wishes to achieve.
   b. Allow client to establish own schedule for self-care activities.
   c. Provide client with privacy as need is determined.
   d. Provide positive feedback for decisions made. Respect client's right to make those decisions independently, and refrain from attempting to influence him or her toward those that may seem more logical.
2. Assist client to set realistic goals. ***Unrealistic goals set the client up for failure and reinforce feelings of powerlessness.***
3. Help client identify areas of life situation that he or she can control. ***Client's emotional condition interferes with his or her ability to solve problems. Assistance is required to perceive the benefits and consequences of available alternatives accurately.***
4. Help client identify areas of life situation that are not within his or her ability to control. Encourage verbalization of feelings related to this inability ***in an effort to deal with unresolved issues and accept what cannot be changed.***
5. Identify ways in which client can achieve. Encourage participation in these activities, and provide positive reinforcement for participation, as well as for achievement. ***Positive reinforcement enhances self-esteem and encourages repetition of desirable behaviors.***

Outcome Criteria

1. Client verbalizes choices made in a plan to maintain control over his or her life situation.
2. Client verbalizes honest feelings about life situations over which he or she has no control.
3. Client is able to verbalize system for problem solving as required for adequate role performance.

ALTERED THOUGHT PROCESSES

Definition: A state in which an individual experiences a disruption in cognitive operations and activities.

Possible Etiologies ("related to")

[Withdrawal into the self]

[Underdeveloped ego; punitive superego]
[Impaired cognition fostering negative perception of self and the environment]

Defining Characteristics ("evidenced by")

Inaccurate interpretation of environment
[Delusional thinking]
Hypovigilance
[Altered attention span]—distractibility
Egocentricity
[Impaired ability to make decisions, problem-solve, reason]
[Negative ruminations]

Goals/Objectives

Short-Term Goal

Client will recognize and verbalize when interpretations of the environment are inaccurate within 1 week.

Long-Term Goal

Client will experience no delusional or distorted thinking by discharge from treatment

Interventions with *Selected Rationales*

1. Convey your acceptance of client's need for the false belief, while letting him or her know that you do not share the delusion. ***A positive response would convey to the client that you accept the delusion as reality.***
2. Do not argue or deny the belief. Use *reasonable doubt* as a therapeutic technique: "I find that hard to believe." ***Arguing with the client or denying the belief serves no useful purpose, as delusional ideas are not eliminated by this approach, and the development of a trusting relationship may be impeded.***
3. Use the techniques of *consensual validation* and *seeking clarification* when communication reflects alteration in thinking. (Examples: "Is it that you mean . . . ?" or "I don't understand what you mean by that. Would you please explain?") ***These techniques reveal to the client how he or she is being perceived by others, while the responsibility for not understanding is accepted by the nurse.***
4. Reinforce and focus on reality. Talk about real events and real people. Use real situations and events to divert client away from long, purposeless, repetitive verbalizations of false ideas.
5. Give positive reinforcement as client is able to differentiate between reality-based and non–reality-based thinking.

Positive reinforcement enhances self-esteem and encourages repetition of desirable behaviors.

6. Teach client to intervene, using thought-stopping techniques, when irrational or negative thoughts prevail. ***Thought stopping*** involves using the command "Stop!" or a loud noise (such as hard clapping) to interrupt unwanted thoughts. ***This noise or command distracts the individual from the undesirable thinking that often precedes undesirable emotions or behaviors.***
7. Use touch cautiously, particularly if thoughts reveal ideas of persecution. ***Clients who are suspicious may perceive touch as threatening and may respond with aggression.***

Outcome Criteria

1. Client's thinking processes reflect accurate interpretation of the environment.
2. Client is able to recognize negative or irrational thoughts and intervene to "stop" their progression.

ALTERED NUTRITION, LESS THAN BODY REQUIREMENTS

Definition: The state in which an individual experiences an intake of nutrients insufficient to meet metabolic needs.

Possible Etiologies ("related to")

Inability to ingest food because of:

[Depressed mood]
[Loss of appetite]
[Energy level too low to meet own nutritional needs]
[Regression to lower level of development]
[Ideas of self-destruction]
Lack of interest in food

Defining Characteristics ("evidenced by")

Loss of weight
Pale conjunctiva and mucous membranes
Poor muscle tone
[Amenorrhea]
[Poor skin turgor]
[Edema of extremities]
[Electrolyte imbalances]
[Weakness]
[Constipation]
[Anemias]

Goals/Objectives

Short-Term Goal

Client will gain 2 lb per week for the next 3 weeks.

Long-Term Goal

Client will exhibit no signs or symptoms of malnutrition by discharge from treatment (e.g., electrolytes and blood counts will be within normal limits; a steady weight gain will be demonstrated; constipation will be corrected; client will exhibit increased energy in participation of activities).

Interventions with *Selected Rationales*

1. In collaboration with dietitian, determine number of calories required to provide adequate nutrition and realistic (according to body structure and height) weight gain.
2. To prevent constipation, ensure that diet includes foods high in fiber content. Encourage client to increase fluid consumption and physical exercise to promote normal bowel functioning. ***Depressed clients are particularly vulnerable to constipation because of psychomotor retardation. Constipation is also a common side effect of many antidepressant medications.***
3. Keep strict documentation of intake, output, and calorie count. ***This information is necessary to make an accurate nutritional assessment and maintain client safety.***
4. Weigh client daily. ***Weight loss or gain is important assessment information.***
5. Determine client's likes and dislikes and collaborate with dietitian to provide favorite foods. ***Client is more likely to eat foods that he or she particularly enjoys.***
6. Ensure that client receives small, frequent feedings, including a bedtime snack, rather than three larger meals. ***Large amounts of food may be objectionable, or even intolerable, to the client.***
7. Administer vitamin and mineral supplements and stool softeners or bulk extenders, as ordered by physician.
8. If appropriate, ask family members or significant others to bring in special foods that client particularly enjoys.
9. Stay with client during meals ***to assist as needed and to offer support and encouragement.***
10. Monitor laboratory values, and report significant changes to physician. ***Laboratory values provide objective data regarding nutritional status.***
11. Explain the importance of adequate nutrition and fluid intake. ***Client may have inadequate or inaccurate***

knowledge regarding the contribution of good nutrition to overall wellness.

Outcome Criteria

1. Client has shown a slow, progressive weight gain during hospitalization.
2. Vital signs, blood pressure, and laboratory serum studies are within normal limits.
3. Client is able to verbalize importance of adequate nutrition and fluid intake.

SLEEP PATTERN DISTURBANCE

Definition: Time-limited disruption of sleep (natural, periodic suspension of consciousness) amount and quality.

Possible Etiologies ("related to")

Depression
[Repressed fears]
[Feelings of hopelessness]
Anxiety
[Hallucinations]
[Delusional thinking]

Defining Characteristics ("evidenced by")

Verbal complaints of difficulty falling asleep
Awakening earlier or later than desired
Interrupted sleep
Verbal complaints of not feeling well rested
Remaining awake 30 minutes after going to bed
[Awakening very early in the morning and being unable to go back to sleep]
[Excessive yawning and desire to nap during the day]
[Hypersomnia; using sleep as an escape]

Goals/Objectives

Short-Term Goal

Client will be able to sleep 4 to 6 hours with the aid of a sleeping medication within 5 days.

Long-Term Goal

Client will be able to fall asleep within 30 minutes of retiring and obtain 6 to 8 hours of uninterrupted sleep each night without medication by discharge from treatment.

Interventions with *Selected Rationales*

1. Keep strict records of sleeping patterns. ***Accurate baseline data are important in planning care to assist client with this problem.***
2. Discourage sleep during the day ***to promote more restful sleep at night.***
3. Administer antidepressant medication at bedtime ***so client does not become drowsy during the day.***
4. Assist with measures that may promote sleep, such as warm, nonstimulating drinks, light snacks, warm baths, back rubs.
5. Performing relaxation exercises to soft music may be helpful prior to sleep.
6. Limit intake of caffeinated drinks, such as tea, coffee, and colas. ***Caffeine is a CNS stimulant that may interfere with the client's achievement of rest and sleep.***
7. Administer sedative medications, as ordered, ***to assist client to achieve sleep until normal sleep pattern is restored.***
8. For client experiencing hypersomnia, set limits on time spent in room. Plan stimulating diversionary activities on a structured, daily schedule. Explore fears and feelings that sleep is helping to suppress.

Outcome Criteria

1. Client is sleeping 6 to 8 hours per night without medication.
2. Client is able to fall asleep within 30 minutes of retiring.
3. Client is dealing with fears and feelings rather than escaping from them through excessive sleep.

■ BIPOLAR DISORDER, MANIA

Predisposing Factors

1. **Physiological**
   a. ***Genetics:*** Studies indicate that there is an increased incidence of bipolar disorder in first-degree relatives of individuals with the disorder than in the general population. If one identical twin has bipolar disorder, the possibility is as high as 80 percent that the other will also develop the disorder (Kelsoe, 1991). Bipolar disorder appears to be equally common in men and women (APA, 1994). Increasing evidence continues to support the role of genetics in the predisposition to bipolar disorder.

b. ***Biochemical:*** Just as there is an indication of lowered levels of norepinephrine and dopamine during an episode of depression, the opposite appears to be true of an individual experiencing a manic episode (Kaplan and Sadock, 1989). Thus, the behavioral responses of elation and euphoria may be caused by an excess of these biogenic amines in the brain. It has also been suggested that manic individuals have increased intracellular sodium and calcium. These electrolyte imbalances may be related to abnormalities in cellular membrane function in bipolar disorder.

2. **Psychosocial**

NOTE: The credibility of psychosocial theories has declined in recent years. Conditions such as schizophrenia and bipolar disorder are now viewed by many clinicians as disorders of the brain with biological etiologies. The etiology of these illnesses remains unclear, however, and it may be possible that both biological and psychosocial factors are influential. For this reason, a discussion of the psychosocial theory of bipolar disorder is included.

a. ***Theory of Family Dynamics:*** A study by Cohen and coworkers (1954) found that the individual with bipolar disorder most likely began life in a loving, nurturing environment. All physical and emotional needs were fulfilled by the primary caregiver, who assumed the image of "goodness" in the mind of the infant. As the child developed and became increasingly independent, some of the nurturing was withdrawn. The child, who had not yet achieved object constancy, was unable to incorporate the concepts of both "good" and "bad" in the primary caregiver. A feeling of ambivalence developed toward the primary caregiver as the child learned the necessity of fulfilling expectations in order to gain affection, even at the expense of negating his or her own needs and desires.

As the child matured, he or she had a tendency to be particularly sensitive, and to crave approval, support, and affection from others. Gibson and colleagues (1959) found that the childhood family of the manic-depressive had been characterized by a striving for social prestige and that as a child the client had borne the brunt of this expectation, with heavy pressure from one or both parents to succeed in social life. The family showed little interest in the child in his or her own right, but only in the role as carrier of prestige. Parental approval depended not on "who you are" but on "what you do." Expectations were often unrealistic, and the child's social and psychological life became greatly restricted, resulting in the development of rigid behavior patterns. A love-hate relationship was established as resentment toward the parents continued to grow, even though the child strongly desired and continued to try to please them.

The child's ego development is disrupted in this dysfunctional family system, and the adult bipolar client's gratification and security are strongly tied to unfulfilled needs for approval. The depressive and manic episodes are precipitated by a loss in which the client feels rejected, rebuked, or not appreciated (Aleksandrowicz, 1980). The loss need not be a conspicuous and obviously stressful life event. Cohen and associates (1954) pointed out that even a change in the client's appraisal of existing relationships may be subjectively experienced as loss of love.

Because there is weak ego development, the response to loss is directed by influences from the id or superego component of the personality. If the superego becomes punitive, the individual turns anger inward on the self and experiences depression. When the depression subsides, the ego may still be too weak to control the impulsive, excessive behavior dominated by the id, and the symptoms of mania are manifested (Aleksandrowicz, 1980).

Symptomatology (Subjective and Objective Data)

1. The affect of a manic individual is one of elation and euphoria—a continuous "high." However, the affect is very labile and may change quickly to hostility, particularly in response to attempts at limit setting, or to sadness, ruminating about past failures.
2. Alterations in thought processes and communication patterns are manifested by the following:
   a. ***Flight of Ideas:*** There is a continuous, rapid shift from one topic to another.
   b. ***Loquaciousness:*** The pressure of the speech is

so forceful and strong that it is difficult to interrupt maladaptive thought processes.

c. ***Delusions of Grandeur:*** The individual believes he or she is all important, all powerful, with feelings of greatness and magnificence.

d. ***Delusions of Persecution:*** The individual believes someone or something desires to harm or violate him or her in some way.

3. Motor activity is constant. The individual is literally moving at all times.
4. Dress is often inappropriate: bright colors that do not match; clothing inappropriate for age or stature; excessive makeup and jewelry.
5. The individual has a meager appetite, despite excessive activity level. He or she is unable or unwilling to stop moving to eat.
6. Sleep patterns are disturbed. Client becomes oblivious to feelings of fatigue, and rest and sleep are abandoned for days or weeks.
7. Spending sprees are common. Individual spends large amounts of money, which is not available, on numerous items, which are not needed.
8. Usual inhibitions are discarded in favor of sexual and behavioral indiscretions.
9. Manipulative behavior and limit testing are common in the attempt to fulfill personal desires. Verbal or physical hostility may follow his of her failure in these attempts.
10. Projection is a major defense mechanism. The individual refuses to accept responsibility for the negative consequences of personal behavior.
11. There is an inability to concentrate because of a limited attention span. The individual is easily distracted by even the slightest stimulus in the environment.
12. Alterations in sensory perception may occur, and the individual may experience hallucinations.
13. As agitation increases, symptoms intensify. Unless the client is placed in a protective environment, death can occur from exhaustion or injury.

Common Nursing Diagnoses and Interventions for Mania

(Interventions are applicable to various health-care settings, such as inpatient and partial hospitalization, community outpatient clinic, home health, and private practice.)

RISK FOR INJURY

Definition: A state in which the individual is at risk of injury as a result of environmental conditions interacting with the individual's adaptive and defensive resources.

Related/Risk Factors ("related to")

[Extreme hyperactivity]
[Destructive behaviors]
[Anger directed at the environment]
[Hitting head (hand, arm, foot, etc.) against wall when angry]
[Temper tantrums—becomes destructive of inanimate objects]
[Increased agitation and lack of control over purposeless, and potentially injurious, movements]

Goals/Objectives

Short-Term Goal

Client will no longer exhibit potentially injurious movements after 24 hours with administration of tranquilizing medication.

Long-Term Goal

Client will experience no physical injury.

Interventions with *Selected Rationales*

1. Reduce environmental stimuli. Assign private room, if possible, with soft lighting, low noise level, and simple room decor. *In hyperactive state, client is extremely distractible, and responses to even the slightest stimuli are exaggerated.*
2. Assign to quiet unit, if possible. *Milieu unit may be too distracting.*
3. Limit group activities. Help client try to establish one or two close relationships. *Client's ability to interact with others is impaired. He or she feels more secure in a one-to-one relationship that is consistent over time.*
4. Remove hazardous objects and substances from client's environment (including smoking materials). *Client's rationality is impaired, and he or she may harm self inadvertently. Client safety is a nursing priority.*
5. Stay with the client *to offer support and provide a feeling of security* as agitation grows and hyperactivity increases.
6. Provide structured schedule of activities that includes established rest periods throughout the day. *A structured schedule provides a feeling of security for the client.*

7. Provide physical activities as a substitution for purposeless hyperactivity. (Examples: brisk walks, housekeeping chores, dance therapy, aerobics). ***Physical exercise provides a safe and effective means of relieving pent-up tension.***
8. Administer tranquilizing medication, as ordered by physician. Antipsychotic drugs, such as chlorpromazine (Thorazine) or haloperidol (Haldol), are commonly prescribed for rapid relief of agitation and hyperactivity. Observe for effectiveness and evidence of adverse side effects.

Outcome Criteria

1. Client is no longer exhibiting signs of physical agitation.
2. Client exhibits no evidence of physical injury obtained while experiencing hyperactive behavior.

■ RISK FOR VIOLENCE: SELF-DIRECTED OR DIRECTED AT OTHERS

Definition: Behaviors in which an individual demonstrates that he/she can be physically, emotionally, and/or sexually harmful either to self or to others.

Related/Risk Factors ("related to")

Manic excitement
[Dysfunctional grieving—denial of depression]
[Hereditary factors]
[Biochemical alterations]
[Threat to self-concept]
[Suspicion of others]
[Paranoid ideation]
[Delusions]
[Hallucinations]
[Rage reactions]
Body language—rigid posture, clenching of fists and jaw, hyperactivity, pacing, breathlessness, and threatening stances.
[History of threats of violence toward self or others or of destruction to the property of others]
Impulsivity
Suicidal ideation, plan, available means
Repetition of verbalizations (continuous complaints, requests, and demands)

Goals/Objectives

Short-Term Goal

Client's agitation will be maintained at manageable level with the administration of tranquilizing medication during first week of treatment (decreasing risk of violence to self or others).

Long-Term Goal

Client will not harm self or others.

Interventions with *Selected Rationales*

1. Maintain low level of stimuli in client's environment (low lighting, few people, simple decor, low noise level). ***Anxiety and agitation rise in a stimulating environment. Individuals may be perceived as threatening by a suspicious, agitated client.***
2. Observe client's behavior frequently (every 15 minutes). ***Close observation is required so that intervention can occur if required to ensure client's (and others') safety.***
3. Remove all dangerous objects from client's environment (sharp objects, glass or mirrored items, belts, ties, smoking materials) ***so that in his or her agitated, hyperactive state, client may not use them to harm self or others.***
4. Try to redirect the violent behavior with physical outlets for the client's hostility (e.g., punching bags). ***Physical exercise is a safe and effective way of relieving pent-up tension.***
5. Staff should maintain and convey a calm attitude to the client. Respond matter of factly to verbal hostility. ***Anxiety is contagious and can be transmitted from staff to client.***
6. Have sufficient staff available to indicate a show of strength to client if necessary. ***This conveys to the client evidence of control over the situation and provides some physical security for staff.***
7. Administer tranquilizing medications as ordered by physician. Monitor medication for effectiveness and for adverse side effects.
8. If the client is not calmed by "talking down" or by medication, use mechanical restraints as necessary. Be sure to have sufficient staff available to assist. Follow protocol established by the institution. Most states require that the physician reevaluate and issue a new order for restraints every 3 hours, except between midnight and 8:00 AM. If the client has refused medication, administer after restraints have been applied. Most states consider this intervention appropriate in emergency situations or in the event that a client would likely harm self or others.
9. Observe the client in restraints every 15 minutes (or ac-

cording to institutional policy). Ensure that circulation to extremities is not compromised (check temperature, color, pulses). Assist client with needs related to nutrition, hydration, and elimination. Position client so that comfort is facilitated and aspiration can be prevented. ***Client safety is a nursing priority.***

10. As agitation decreases, assess client's readiness for restraint removal or reduction. Remove one restraint at a time, while assessing client's response. ***This procedure minimizes the risk of injury to client and staff.***

Outcome Criteria

1. Client is able to verbalize anger in an appropriate manner.
2. There is no evidence of violent behavior to self or others.
3. Client is no longer exhibiting hyperactive behaviors.

ALTERED NUTRITION, LESS THAN BODY REQUIREMENTS

Definition: The state in which an individual experiences an intake of nutrients insufficient to meet metabolic needs.

Possible Etiologies ("related to")

[Refusal or inability to sit still long enough to eat meals]
[Lack of appetite]
[Excessive physical agitation]
[Physical exertion in excess of energy produced through caloric intake]
Lack of interest in food

Defining Characteristics ("evidenced by")

Loss of weight
Pale conjunctiva and mucous membranes
Poor muscle tone
[Amenorrhea]
[Poor skin turgor]
[Anemias]
[Electrolyte imbalances]

Goals/Objectives

Short-Term Goal

Client will consume sufficient finger foods and between-meal snacks to meet recommended daily allowances of nutrients.

Long-Term Goal

Client will exhibit no signs or symptoms of malnutrition.

Interventions with *Selected Rationales*

1. In collaboration with dietitian, determine number of calories required to provide adequate nutrition for maintenance or realistic (according to body structure and height) weight gain.
2. Provide client with high-protein, high-calorie, nutritious finger foods and drinks that can be consumed "on the run." ***Because of hyperactive state, client has difficulty sitting still long enough to eat a meal. The likelihood is greater that he or she will consume food and drinks that can be carried around and eaten with little effort.***
3. Have juice and snacks available on the unit at all times. ***Nutritious intake is required on a regular basis to compensate for increased caloric requirements due to hyperactivity.***
4. Maintain accurate record of intake, output, and calorie count. ***This information is necessary to make an accurate nutritional assessment and maintain client's safety.***
5. Weigh client daily. ***Weight loss or gain is important nutritional assessment information.***
6. Determine client's likes and dislikes, and collaborate with dietitian to provide favorite foods. ***Client is more likely to eat foods that he or she particularly enjoys.***
7. Administer vitamin and mineral supplements, as ordered by physician, ***to improve nutritional state.***
8. Pace or walk with client as finger foods are taken. As agitation subsides, sit with client during meals. Offer support and encouragement. Assess and record amount consumed. ***Presence of a trusted individual may provide feeling of security and decrease agitation. Encouragement and positive reinforcement increase self-esteem and foster repetition of desired behaviors.***
9. Monitor laboratory values, and report significant changes to physician. ***Laboratory values provide objective nutritional assessment data.***
10. Explain the importance of adequate nutrition and fluid intake. ***Client may have inadequate or inaccurate knowledge regarding the contribution of good nutrition to overall wellness.***

Outcome Criteria

1. Client has gained (maintained) weight during hospitalization.

2. Vital signs, blood pressure, and laboratory serum studies are within normal limits.
3. Client is able to verbalize importance of adequate nutrition and fluid intake.

ALTERED THOUGHT PROCESSES

Definition: A state in which an individual experiences a disruption in cognitive operations and activities.

Possible Etiologies ("related to")

[Hereditary factors]
[Biochemical alterations]
[Unmet dependency needs]
[Unresolved grief—denial of depression]

Defining Characteristics ("evidenced by")

Inaccurate interpretation of environment
Hypervigilance
[Altered attention span]—distractibility
Egocentricity
[Decreased ability to grasp ideas]
[Inability to follow]
[Impaired ability to make decisions, problem-solve, reason]
[Delusions of grandeur]
[Delusions of persecution]
[Suspiciousness]

Goals/Objectives

Short-Term Goal

Within 1 week, client will be able to recognize and verbalize when thinking is non–reality-based.

Long-Term Goal

Client will experience no delusional thinking by discharge from treatment.

Interventions with *Selected Rationales*

1. Convey your acceptance of client's need for the false belief, while letting him or her know that you do not share the delusion. ***A positive response would convey to the client that you accept the delusion as reality.***
2. Do not argue or deny the belief. Use *reasonable doubt* as a therapeutic technique: "I find that hard to believe." ***Arguing with the client or denying the belief serves no***

useful purpose, because delusional ideas are not eliminated by this approach, and the development of a trusting relationship may be impeded.

3. Use the techniques of *consensual validation* and *seeking clarification* when communication reflects alteration in thinking. (Examples: "Is it that you mean . . . ?" or "I don't understand what you mean by that. Would you please explain?") ***These techniques reveal to the client how he or she is being perceived by others, and the responsibility for not understanding is accepted by the nurse.***
4. Reinforce and focus on reality. Talk about real events and real people. Use real situations and events to divert client away from long, tedious, repetitive verbalizations of false ideas.
5. Give positive reinforcement as client is able to differentiate between reality-based and non–reality-based thinking. ***Positive reinforcement enhances self-esteem and encourages repetition of desirable behaviors.***
6. Teach client to intervene, using thought-stopping techniques, when irrational thoughts prevail. Thought stopping involves using the command "Stop!" or a loud noise (such as hand clapping) to interrupt unwanted thoughts. ***This noise or command distracts the individual from the undesirable thinking, which often precedes undesirable emotions or behaviors.***
7. Use touch cautiously, particularly if thoughts reveal ideas of persecution. ***Clients who are suspicious may perceive touch as threatening and may respond with aggression.***

Outcome Criteria

1. Thought processes reflect an accurate interpretation of the environment.
2. Client is able to recognize thoughts that are not based in reality and intervene to stop their progression.

SENSORY-PERCEPTUAL ALTERATION

Definition: A state in which an individual experiences a change in the amount or patterning of incoming stimuli [either internally or externally initiated] accompanied by a diminished, exaggerated, distorted, or impaired response to such stimuli.

Possible Etiologies ("related to")

[Hereditary factors]
Biochemical imbalance
Electrolyte imbalance
[Unmet dependency needs]
[Unresolved grief—denial of depression]
[Sleep deprivation]

Defining Characteristics ("evidenced by")

Change in usual response to stimuli
Hallucinations
Disorientation
Inappropriate responses
[Rapid mood swings]
[Exaggerated emotional responses]
[Visual and auditory distortions]
[Talking and laughing to self]
[Listening pose (tilting head to one side as if listening)]
[Stops talking in middle of sentence to listen]

Goals/Objectives

Short-Term Goal

Client will be able to recognize and verbalize when he or she is interpreting the environment inaccurately.

Long-Term Goal

Client will be able to define and test reality, eliminating the occurrence of sensory misperceptions.

Interventions with *Selected Rationales*

1. Observe client for signs of hallucinations (listening pose, laughing or talking to self, stopping in midsentence). *Early intervention may prevent aggressive responses to command hallucinations.*
2. Avoid touching the client before warning him or her that you are about to do so. *Client may perceive touch as threatening and respond in an aggressive manner.*
3. An attitude of acceptance will encourage the client to share the content of the hallucination with you. *This is important to prevent possible injury to the client or others from command hallucinations.*
4. Do not reinforce the hallucination. Use "the voices" instead of words like "they" that imply validation. Let the client know that you do not share the perception. Say, "Even though I realize that the voices are real to you, I do

not hear any voices speaking." ***The nurse must be honest with the client so that he or she may realize that the hallucinations are not real.***

5. Try to connect the times of the misperceptions to times of increased anxiety. Help client to understand this connection. ***If client can learn to interrupt the escalating anxiety, reality orientation may be maintained.***
6. Try to distract the client away from the misperception. ***Involvement in interpersonal activities and explanation of the actual situation may bring the client back to reality.***

Outcome Criteria

1. Client is able to differentiate between reality and unrealistic events or situations.
2. Client is able to refrain from responding to false sensory perceptions.

IMPAIRED SOCIAL INTERACTION

Definition: The state in which an individual participates in an insufficient or excessive quantity or ineffective quality of social exchange.

Possible Etiologies ("related to")

Altered thought processes
[Strong dependency needs]
[Delusions of grandeur]
[Delusions of persecution]
[Underdeveloped ego]
[Low self-esteem]

Defining Characteristics ("evidenced by")

Verbalized or observed discomfort in social situations
Verbalized or observed inability to receive or communicate a satisfying sense of belonging, caring, interest, or shared history
Observed use of unsuccessful social interaction behaviors
Dysfunctional interaction with peers, family, and others
[Excessive use of projection—does not accept responsibility for own behavior]
[Verbal manipulation]
[Inability to delay gratification]

Goals/Objectives

Short-Term Goal

Client will verbalize which of his or her interaction behaviors are appropriate and which are inappropriate within 1 week.

Long-Term Goal

Client will demonstrate use of appropriate interaction skills as evidenced by lack of, or marked decrease in, manipulation of others to fulfill own desires.

Interventions with *Selected Rationales*

1. Recognize the purpose these behaviors serve for the client: to reduce feelings of insecurity by increasing feelings of power and control. ***Understanding the motivation behind the manipulation may facilitate acceptance of the individual and his or her behavior.***
2. Set limits on manipulative behaviors. Explain to client what you expect and what the consequences are if the limits are violated. Limits must be agreed upon by all staff who will be working with the client. ***Client is unable to establish own limits, so this must be done for him or her. Unless administration of consequences for violation of limits is consistent, manipulative behavior will not be eliminated.***
3. Do not argue, bargain, or try to reason with the client. Merely state the limits and expectations. Be sure to follow through with consequences if limits are violated. ***Consistency is essential for success of this intervention.*** Do not let this "charmer" talk you out of it. ***Ignoring these attempts may work to decrease manipulative behaviors.***
4. Provide positive reinforcement for nonmanipulative behaviors. Explore feelings, and help the client seek more appropriate ways of dealing with them. ***Positive reinforcement enhances self-esteem and promotes repetition of desirable behaviors.***
5. Help client recognize consequences of own behaviors and refrain from attributing them to others. ***Client must accept responsibility for own behaviors before adaptive change can occur.***
6. Help client identify positive aspects about self, recognize accomplishments, and feel good about them. ***As self-esteem is increased, client will feel less need to manipulate others for own gratification.***

Outcome Criteria

1. Client is able to verbalize positive aspects about self.
2. Client accepts responsibility for own behaviors.
3. Client does not manipulate others for gratification of own needs.

SLEEP PATTERN DISTURBANCE

Definition: Time-limited disruption of sleep (natural, periodic suspension of consciousness) amount and quality.

Possible Etiologies ("related to")

[Excessive hyperactivity]
[Agitation]
[Biochemical alterations]

Defining Characteristics ("evidenced by")

[Pacing in hall during sleeping hours]
Sleep onset greater than 30 minutes
[Sleeping only short periods at a time]
[Numerous periods of wakefulness during the night]
[Awakening and rising extremely early in the morning; exhibiting signs of restlessness]

Goals/Objectives

Short-Term Goal

With the aid of a sleeping medication, within 3 days, client will sleep 4 to 6 hours without awakening.

Long-Term Goal

By discharge from treatment, client will be able to acquire 6 to 8 hours of uninterrupted sleep without medication.

Interventions with *Selected Rationales*

1. Provide a quiet environment, with a low level of stimulation. ***Hyperactivity increases and ability to achieve sleep and rest are hindered in a stimulating environment.***
2. Monitor sleep patterns. Provide structured schedule of activities that includes established times for naps or rest. ***Accurate baseline data are important in planning care to assist client with this problem. A structured schedule, including time for naps, will help the hyperactive client achieve much-needed rest.***
3. Assess client's activity level. Client may ignore or be unaware of feelings of fatigue. Observe for signs such as increasing restlessness; fine tremors; slurred speech; and puffy, dark circles under eyes. ***Client can collapse from exhaustion if hyperactivity is uninterrupted and rest is not achieved.***
4. Before bedtime, provide nursing measures that promote

sleep, such as back rub; warm bath; warm, nonstimulating drinks; soft music; and relaxation exercises.

5. Prohibit intake of caffeinated drinks, such as tea, coffee, and colas. ***Caffeine is a CNS stimulant and may interfere with the client's achievement of rest and sleep.***
6. Administer sedative medications, as ordered, to assist client achieve sleep until normal sleep pattern is restored.

Outcome Criteria

1. Client is sleeping 6 to 8 hours per night without medication.
2. Within 30 minutes of retiring, client is able to fall asleep.
3. Client is dealing openly with fears and feelings rather than manifesting denial of them through hyperactivity.

■ INTERNET REFERENCES

Additional information about Mood Disorders, including psychosocial and pharmacological treatment of these disorders, may be located at the following Websites:

- http://pw2.netcom.com/~shakey/bipolar.html
- http://www.pslgroup.com/depression.htm
- http://depression.miningco.com/
- http://www.snap.com
- http://www.ndmda.org
- http://www.fadavis.com
- http://www.laurus.com

CHAPTER 8

*Anxiety Disorders**

BACKGROUND ASSESSMENT DATA

The characteristic features of this group of disorders are symptoms of anxiety and avoidance behavior. Anxiety disorders are categorized in the following manner:

Panic Disorder

300.01 Without Agoraphobia
300.21 With Agoraphobia

Panic disorder is characterized by recurrent panic attacks, the onset of which are unpredictable, and manifested by intense apprehension, fear, or terror, often associated with feelings of impending doom and accompanied by intense physical discomfort. The attacks usually last minutes or, more rarely, hours. If accompanied by agoraphobia, there is a fear of being in places or situations from which escape might be difficult or in which help might not be available in the event of a panic attack (APA, 1994). Common agoraphobic situations include being outside the home alone; being in a crowd or standing in a line; being on a bridge; and traveling in a bus, train, or car.

300.22 Agoraphobia Without History of Panic Disorder

This *DSM-IV* identifies the essential feature of this disorder as fear of being in places or situations from which escape might be difficult or in which help might not be

*Reprinted with permission from the *Diagnostic and Statistical Manual of Mental Disorders, Fourth Edition.* Copyright 1994 American Psychiatric Association, 1994.

available in the event of suddenly developing a symptom(s) that could be incapacitating or extremely embarrassing. Travel is restricted, or the individual needs a companion when away from home or else endures agoraphobic situations despite intense anxiety.

300.23 Social Phobia

Social phobia is characterized by a persistent fear of behaving or performing in the presence of others in a way that will be humiliating or embarrassing to the individual. The individual has extreme concerns about being exposed to possible scrutiny by others and fears social or performance situations in which embarrassment may occur (APA, 1994). Exposure to the phobic situation is avoided, or it is endured with intense anxiety. Common social phobias include speaking or writing in front of a group of people, eating in the presence of others, and using public restrooms.

300.29 Specific Phobia

Formerly called simple phobia, this disorder is characterized by persistent fears of specific objects or situations. These phobias are fairly widespread among the general population, the most common being fear of animals (zoophobia), fear of closed places (claustrophobia), and fear of heights (acrophobia). Exposure to the phobic stimulus is avoided or endured with intense anxiety.

300.3 Obsessive-Compulsive Disorder

This disorder is characterized by involuntary recurring thoughts or images that the individual is unable to ignore and by recurring impulse to perform a seemingly purposeless activity. These obsessions and compulsions serve to prevent extreme anxiety on the part of the individual.

309.81 Posttraumatic Stress Disorder

Posttraumatic stress disorder (PTSD) is characterized by the development of physiological and behavorial symptoms following a psychologically traumatic event that is generally outside the range of usual human experience. The stressor, which would be considered markedly distressing to almost anyone, has usually been experienced with intense fear, terror, and helplessness. If duration of the symptoms is 3 months or more, the diagnosis is specified as "chronic." If there is a delay of 6 months or more in the onset of symptoms, the diagnosis is specified as "delayed onset."

308.3 Acute Stress Disorder

Acute stress disorder is characterized by the development of physiological and behavioral symptoms similar to those of PTSD. The major difference in the diagnosis lies in the length of time the symptoms exist. With acute stress disorder, the symptoms must subside within 4 weeks of occurrence of the stressor. If they last longer than 4 weeks, the individual is given the diagnosis of PTSD.

300.02 Generalized Anxiety Disorder

This disorder is characterized by chronic, unrealistic, and excessive anxiety and worry. The symptoms must have occurred more days than not for at least 6 months and must cause clinically significant distress or impairment in social, occupational, or other important areas of functioning. Symptoms include restlessness, feeling "on edge," becoming easily fatigued, difficulty concentrating, and irritability.

293.89 Anxiety Disorder Due to a General Medical Condition

The symptoms of this disorder are judged to be the direct physiological consequence of a general medical condition. Symptoms may include prominent generalized anxiety symptoms, panic attacks, or obsessions or compulsions (APA, 1994). Medical conditions that have been known to cause anxiety disorders include endocrine, cardiovascular, respiratory, metabolic, and neurological disorders.

Substance-Induced Anxiety Disorder (Refer to Substance-Related Disorders for substance-specific codes)

The *DSM-IV* (APA, 1994) describes the essential features of this disorder as prominent anxiety symptoms that are judged to be caused by the direct physiological effects of a substance (i.e., a drug of abuse, a medication, or toxin exposure). The symptoms may occur during substance intoxication or withdrawal and may involve prominent anxiety, panic attacks, phobias, or obsessions or compulsions.

Predisposing Factors

1. **Physiological**
   a. ***Biochemical:*** Although biochemical and neurophysiological influences in the etiology of these disorders have been investigated, no definitive relationship has yet been established. Increased levels of norepinephrine have been noted in panic and generalized anxiety disorders. Decreased levels of serotonin have been implicated in the etiology of obsessive-compulsive disorder.
   b. ***Genetic:*** Studies suggest that anxiety disorders are prevalent within the general population. It has been shown that they are more common among first-degree biological relatives of people with the disorders than among the general population (APA, 1994).
   c. ***Medical or Substance-Induced:*** Anxiety disorders may be caused by a variety of medical conditions or the ingestion of various substances. (Refer to previous section on categories of anxiety disorders.)
2. **Psychosocial**
   a. ***Psychodynamic:*** This theory (Erikson, 1963) suggests a predisposition to anxiety disorders when tasks assigned to earlier developmental stages go unresolved. In response to stress, behaviors associated with these earlier stages appear, as the individual regresses to, or is fixated in, the earlier level of development.
   b. ***Interpersonal:*** Sullivan (1953) attributes the anxiety response to difficulty in interpersonal relationships that stem from the early mother (primary caregiver)-child relationship. The child does not receive the unconditional love and nurturing he or she requires. Futile attempts to "earn" this love result in a fragile ego and the persistent fear of disapproval from others throughout life.
   c. ***Sociocultural:*** Horney (1939) suggests that anxiety disorders are predisposed by a multitude of

contradictions occurring within our society that contribute to feelings of insecurity and helplessness. [Example: Teaching that "all men are created equal," as the child grows up observing numerous inequalities.)

Symptomatology (Subjective and Objective Data)

An individual may experience a panic attack under any of the following conditions:

- As the predominant disturbance, with no apparent precipitant
- When exposed to a phobic stimulus
- When attempts are made to curtail ritualistic behavior
- Following a psychologically traumatic event

Symptoms include the following (APA, 1994):

- Palpitations, pounding heart, or accelerated heart rate
- Sweating
- Trembling or shaking
- Sensations of shortness of breath or smothering
- Feeling of choking
- Chest pain or discomfort
- Nausea or abdominal distress
- Feeling dizzy, unsteady, lightheaded, or faint
- Derealization (feelings of unreality) or depersonalization (being detached from oneself)
- Fear of losing control or going crazy
- Fear of dying
- Paresthesias (numbness or tingling sensations)
- Chills or hot flashes

Other symptoms of anxiety disorders include the following:

1. Restlessness, feeling "on edge," excessive worry, being easily fatigued, difficulty concentrating, irritability, muscle tension, and sleep disturbances (generalized anxiety disorder).
2. Recurrent and intrusive recollections or dreams about the traumatic event, feeling of reliving the trauma (flashback episodes), difficulty feeling emotion (a "numbing" affect), insomnia, and irritability or outbursts of anger (PTSD).
3. Repetitive, obsessive thoughts, common ones being related to violence, contamination, and doubt; repeti-

tive, compulsive performance of purposeless activity, such as handwashing, counting, checking, touching (obsessive-compulsive disorder).
4. Marked and persistent fears of specific objects or situations (specific phobia), social or performance situations (social phobia), or being in a situation from which one has difficulty escaping (agoraphobia).

Common Nursing Diagnoses and Interventions

(Interventions are applicable to various health-care settings, such as inpatient and partial hospitalization, community outpatient clinic, home health, and private practice.)

■ ANXIETY (PANIC)

Definition: A vague uneasy feeling, of discomfort or dread accompanied by an autonomic response; the source is often nonspecific or unknown to the individual; a feeling of apprehension caused by anticipation of danger. It is an altering signal that warns of impending danger and enables the individual to take measures to deal with threat.

Possible Etiologies ("related to")

Unconscious conflict about essential values and goals of life
Situational and maturational crises
[Real or perceived] threat to self-concept
[Real or perceived] threat of death
Unmet needs
[Fixation in earlier level of development]
[Being exposed to a phobic stimulus]
[Attempts at interference with ritualistic behaviors]
[Traumatic experience]

Defining Characteristics ("evidenced by")

Increased respiration
Increased pulse
Decreased or increased blood pressure
Nausea
Confusion
Increased perspiration
Faintness
Trembling or shaking

Restlessness
Insomnia
[Nightmares or visual perceptions of traumatic event]
[Fear of dying, going crazy, or doing something uncontrolled during an attack]

Goals/Objectives

Short-Term Goal

Client will verbalize ways to intervene in escalating anxiety within 1 week.

Long-Term Goal

Client will be able to recognize symptoms of onset of anxiety and intervene before reaching panic stage by discharge from treatment.

Interventions with *Selected Rationales*

1. Maintain a calm, nonthreatening manner while working with client. ***Anxiety is contagious and may be transferred from staff to client or vice versa. Client develops feeling of security in presence of calm staff person.***
2. Reassure client of his or her safety and security. This can be conveyed by physical presence of nurse. Do not leave client alone at this time. ***Client may fear for his or her life. Presence of a trusted individual provides client with feeling of security and assurance of personal safety.***
3. Use simple words and brief messages, spoken calmly and clearly, to explain hospital experiences to client. ***In an intensely anxious situation, client is unable to comprehend anything but the most elemental communication.***
4. Keep immediate surroundings low in stimuli (dim lighting, few people, simple decor). ***A stimulating environment may increase level of anxiety.***
5. Administer tranquilizing medication, as ordered by physician. Assess medication for effectiveness and for adverse side effects.
6. When level of anxiety has been reduced, explore with client possible reasons for occurrence. ***Recognition of precipitating factor(s) is the first step in teaching the client to interrupt escalation of the anxiety.***
7. Encourage client to talk about traumatic experience under nonthreatening conditions. Help client work through feelings of guilt related to the traumatic event. Help client understand that this was an event to which most people would have responded in like manner. Support client during flashbacks of the experience. ***Verbalization of feel-***

ings in a nonthreatening environment may help client come to terms with unresolved issues.

8. Teach signs and symptoms of escalating anxiety, and ways to interrupt its progression (e.g., relaxation techniques, deep-breathing exercises, physical exercises, brisk walks, jogging, meditation).

Outcome Criteria

1. Client is able to maintain anxiety at level in which problem solving can be accomplished.
2. Client is able to verbalize signs and symptoms of escalating anxiety.
3. Client is able to demonstrate techniques for interrupting the progression of anxiety to the panic level.

FEAR

Definition: Fear is anxiety caused by consciously recognized and realistic danger. It is a perceived threat, real or imagined. Operationally, fear is the presence of immediate feeling of apprehension and fright; source known and specific; subjective responses that act as energizers but cannot be observed; and objective signs that are the result of the transformation of energy into relief behaviors and responses.

Possible Etiologies ("related to")

Phobic stimulus or phobia
[Being in place or situation from which escape might be difficult]
[Causing embarrassment to self in front of others]

Defining Characteristics ("evidenced by")

[Refuses to leave own home alone]
[Refuses to eat in public]
[Refuses to speak or perform in public]
[Refuses to expose self to (specify phobic object or situation)]
Subjective ability to identify fearful object or situation
[Symptoms of apprehension or sympathetic stimulation in presence of phobic object or situation]

Goals/Objectives

Short-Term Goal

Client will discuss phobic object or situation with nurse or therapist within 5 days.

Long-Term Goal

Client will be able to function in presence of phobic object or situation without experiencing panic anxiety by discharge from treatment.

Interventions with *Selected Rationales*

1. Reassure client of his or her safety and security. ***At panic level of anxiety, client may fear for own life.***
2. Explore client's perception of threat to physical integrity or threat to self-concept. ***It is important to understand the client's perception of the phobic object or situation to assist with the desensitization process.***
3. Discuss reality of the situation with client to recognize aspects that can be changed and those that cannot. ***Client must accept the reality of the situation (aspects that cannot change) before the work of reducing the fear can progress.***
4. Include client in making decisions related to selection of alternative coping strategies. (Example: Client may choose to either avoid the phobic stimulus or attempt to eliminate the fear associated with it.) ***Allowing the client choices provides a measure of control and serves to increase feelings of self-worth.***
5. If the client elects to work on elimination of the fear, techniques of desensitization may be employed. This is a systematic plan of behavior modification, designed to expose the individual gradually to the situation or object (either in reality or through fantasizing) until the fear in no longer experienced. This is also sometimes accomplished through implosion therapy, in which the individual is "flooded" with stimuli related to the phobic situation or object (rather than in gradual steps) until anxiety is no longer experienced in relation to the object or situation. ***Fear is decreased as the physical and psychological sensations diminish in response to repeated exposure to the phobic stimulus under nonthreatening conditions.***
6. Encourage client to explore underlying feelings that may be contributing to irrational fears. Help client to understand how facing these feelings, rather than suppressing them, can result in more adaptive coping abilities. ***Verbalization of feelings in a nonthreatening environment may help client come to terms with unresolved issues.***

Outcome Criteria

1. Client does not experience disabling fear when exposed to phobic object or situation, *or*

2. Client verbalizes ways in which he or she will be able to avoid the phobic object or situation with minimal change in lifestyle.
3. Client is able to demonstrate adaptive coping techniques that may be used to maintain anxiety at a tolerable level.

INEFFECTIVE INDIVIDUAL COPING

Definition: Inability to form a valid appraisal of the stressors, inadequate choices of practiced responses, and/or inability to use available resources.

Possible Etiologies ("related to")

[Fixation in earlier level of development]
[Underdeveloped ego; punitive superego]
[Fear of failure]
[Unmet dependency needs]
Situational crises
[Personal vulnerability]
[Inadequate support systems]
Maturational crises

Defining Characteristics ("evidenced by")

[Ritualistic behavior]
[Obsessive thoughts]
Inability to meet basic needs
Inability to meet role expectations
Inability to problem-solve
[Alteration in societal participation]

Goals/Objectives

Short-Term Goal

Within 1 week, client will decrease participation in ritualistic behavior to half of time being spent in ritualistic behavior on admission.

Long-Term Goal

By discharge from treatment, client will demonstrate ability to cope effectively without resorting to obsessive-compulsive behaviors or increased dependency.

Interventions with *Selected Rationales*

1. Assess client's level of anxiety. Try to determine the types of situations that increase anxiety and result in ritualistic

behaviors. ***Recognition of precipitating factors is the first step in teaching the client to interrupt the escalating anxiety.***

2. Initially meet client's dependency needs as required. Encourage independence and give positive reinforcement for independent behaviors. ***Sudden and complete elimination of all avenues for dependency would create intense anxiety on the part of the client. Positive reinforcement enhances self-esteem and encourages repetition of desired behaviors.***
3. In the beginning of treatment allow plenty of time for rituals. Do not be judgmental or verbalize disapproval of the behavior. ***To deny client this activity may precipitate panic level of anxiety.***
4. Support client's efforts to explore the meaning and purpose of the behavior. ***Client may be unaware of the relationship between emotional problems and compulsive behaviors. Recognition is important before change can occur.***
5. Provide structured schedule of activities for the client, including adequate time for completion of rituals. ***Structure provides a feeling of security for the anxious client.***
6. Gradually begin to limit amount of time allotted for ritualistic behavior as client becomes more involved in unit activities. ***Anxiety is minimized when client is able to replace ritualistic behaviors with more adaptive ones.***
7. Give positive reinforcement for nonritualistic behaviors. ***Positive reinforcement enhances self-esteem and encourages repetition of desired behaviors.***
8. Encourage recognition of situations that provoke obsessive thoughts or ritualistic behaviors. Explain ways of interrupting these thoughts and patterns of behavior (e.g., thought-stopping techniques, relaxation techniques, physical exercise, or other constructive activity with which client feels comfortable).

Outcome Criteria

1. Client is able to verbalize signs and symptoms of increasing anxiety and intervene to maintain anxiety at manageable level.
2. Client demonstrates ability to interrupt obsessive thoughts and refrain from ritualistic behaviors in response to stressful situations.

POWERLESSNESS

Definition: The perception that one's own action will not significantly affect an outcome; a perceived lack of control over a current situation or immediate happening.

Possible Etiologies ("related to")

Lifestyle of helplessness
[Fear of disapproval from others]
[Fixation in earlier level of development]
[Unmet dependency needs]
[Lack of positive feedback]
[Consistent negative feedback]

Defining Characteristics ("evidenced by")

Verbal expressions of having no control or influence over situation, outcome, or self-care
Nonparticipation in care or decision making when opportunities are provided
Expression of doubt regarding role performance
Reluctance to express true feelings, fearing alienation from caregivers
Apathy
Dependence on others that may result in irritability, resentment, anger, and guilt
Passivity

Goals/Objectives

Short-Term Goal

Client will participate in decision making regarding own care within 5 days.

Long-Term Goal

Client will be able to effectively problem-solve ways to take control of his or her life situation by discharge, thereby decreasing feelings of powerlessness.

Interventions with *Selected Rationales*

1. Allow client to take as much responsibility as possible for own self-care practices. ***Providing client with choices will increase his or her feelings of control.*** Examples are as follows:
   a. Include client in setting the goals of care he or she wishes to achieve.

   b. Allow client to establish own schedule for self-care activities.
   c. Provide client with privacy as need is determined.
   d. Provide positive feedback for decisions made. Respect client's right to make those decisions independently, and refrain from attempting to influence him or her toward those that may seem more logical.
2. Assist client to set realistic goals. ***Unrealistic goals set the client up for failure and reinforce feelings of powerlessness.***
3. Help identify areas of life situation that client can control. ***Client's emotional condition interferes with his or her ability to solve problems. Assistance is required to perceive the benefits and consequences of available alternatives accurately.***
4. Help client identify areas of life situation that are not within his or her ability to control. Encourage verbalization of feelings related to this inability ***in an effort to deal with unresolved issues and accept what cannot be changed.***
5. Identify ways in which client can achieve. Encourage participation in these activities, and provide positive reinforcement for participation, as well as for achievement. ***Positive reinforcement enhances self-esteem and encourages repetition of desirable behaviors.***

Outcome Criteria

1. Client verbalizes choices made in a plan to maintain control over his or her life situation.
2. Client verbalizes honest feelings about life situations over which he or she has no control.
3. Client is able to verbalize system for problem solving as required for adequate role performance.

SOCIAL ISOLATION

Definition: Condition of aloneness experienced by the individual and perceived as imposed by others and as a negative or threatened state.

Possible Etiologies ("related to")

[Panic level of anxiety]
[Regression to earlier level of development]
[Past experiences of difficulty in interactions with others]

[Need to engage in ritualistic behavior in order to keep anxiety under control]
[Repressed fears]

Defining Characteristics ("evidenced by")

[Stays alone in room]
Inability to communicate, withdrawal, lack of eye contact
Inappropriate or immature interests and activities for developmental age or stage
Preoccupation with own thoughts; repetitive, meaningless actions
Expression of feelings of rejection or of aloneness imposed by others
Experiencing feelings of difference from others
Insecurity in public

Goals/Objectives

Short-Term Goal

Client will willingly attend therapy activities accompanied by trusted support person within 1 week.

Long-Term Goal

Client will voluntarily spend time with other clients and staff members in group activities by discharge from treatment.

Interventions with *Selected Rationales*

1. Convey an accepting attitude by making brief, frequent contacts. *An accepting attitude increases feelings of self-worth and facilitates trust.*
2. Show unconditional positive regard. *Conveys your belief in the client as a worthwhile human being.*
3. Be with the client to offer support during group activities that may be frightening or difficult for him or her. *The presence of a trusted individual provides emotional security for the client.*
4. Be honest and keep all promises. *Honesty and dependability promote a trusting relationship.*
5. Be cautious with touch. Allow client extra space and an avenue for exit if he or she becomes too anxious. *A person in panic anxiety may perceive touch as a threatening gesture.*
6. Administer tranquilizing medications as ordered by physician. Monitor for effectiveness, as well as for adverse side effects. *Antianxiety medications, such as diazepam, chlordiazepoxide, or alprazolam, help to reduce level*

of anxiety in most individuals, thereby facilitating interactions with others.

7. Discuss with client the signs of increasing anxiety and techniques to interrupt the response (e.g., relaxation exercises, thought stopping). ***Maladaptive behaviors, such as withdrawal and suspiciousness, are manifested during times of increased anxiety.***
8. Give recognition and positive reinforcement for client's voluntary interactions with others. ***Positive reinforcement enhances self-esteem and encourages repetition of acceptable behaviors.***

Outcome Criteria

1. Client demonstrates willingness or desire to socialize with others.
2. Client voluntarily attends group activities.
3. Client approaches others in appropriate manner for one-to-one interaction.

■ SELF-CARE DEFICIT (Identify Specific Area)

Definition: A state in which the individual experiences an impaired ability to perform or complete [activities of daily living (ADLs) independently].

Possible Etiologies ("related to")

[Regression to an earlier level of development]
[Withdrawal; isolation from others]
[Unmet dependency needs]
[Excessive ritualistic behavior]
[Disabling anxiety]
[Irrational fears]

Defining Characteristics ("evidenced by")

[Unwillingness to bathe regularly]
[Uncombed hair; dirty clothes; offensive body and breath odor; disheveled appearance]
[Eating only a few bites of food from meal tray]
[Lack of interest in selecting appropriate clothing to wear, dressing, grooming, or maintaining appearance at a satisfactory level]
[Incontinence]

Goals/Objectives

Short-Term Goal

Client will verbalize desire to take control of self-care activities within 5 days.

Long-Term Goal

Client will be able to take care of own ADLs and demonstrate a willingness to do so by discharge from treatment.

Interventions with *Selected Rationales*

1. Urge client to perform normal ADLs to his or her level of ability. ***Successful performance of independent activities enhances self-esteem.***
2. Encourage independence, but intervene when client is unable to perform. ***Client comfort and safety are nursing priorities.***
3. Offer recognition and positive reinforcement for independent accomplishments. (Example: "Mrs. J., I see you have put on a clean dress and combed your hair.") ***Positive reinforcement enhances self-esteem and encourages repetition of desired behaviors.***
4. Show client how to perform activities with which he or she is having difficulty. ***When anxiety level is high, client may require simple, concrete demonstrations of activities that would be performed without difficulty under normal conditions.***
5. Keep strict records of food and fluid intake. ***This information is necessary to formulate an accurate nutritional assessment.***
6. Offer nutritious snacks and fluids between meals. ***Client may be unable to tolerate large amounts of food at mealtimes and may therefore require additional nourishment at other times during the day to achieve adequate nutrition.***
7. If client is incontinent, establish routine schedule for toileting needs. Assist client to bathroom on hourly or bi-hourly schedule, as need is determined, until he or she is able to fulfill this need without assistance.

Outcome Criteria

1. Client feeds self, leaving no more than a few bites of food on food tray.
2. Client selects appropriate clothing and dresses and grooms self daily.

3. Client maintains optimal level of personal hygiene by bathing daily and carrying out essential toileting procedures without assistance.

INTERNET REFERENCES

Additional information about Anxiety Disorders and medications to treat these disorders may be located at the following Websites:

- http://www.adaa.org
- http://www.mentalhealth.com
- http://www.psychweb.com/obsessiv.htm
- http://www.cmhc.com/articles/grohol/ocd.htm
- http://www.wvhealth.wvu.edu/mentalhealth/ansocial.htm
- http://www.nimh.nih.gov/events/socifact.htm
- http://www.anxietynetwork.com/pdhome.html
- http://www.uams.edu/department_of_psychiatry/syllabus/anxiolytics/anxiolytics.htm

CHAPTER 9

*Somatoform and Sleep Disorders**

■ BACKGROUND ASSESSMENT DATA

Somatoform disorders are identified by the presence of physical symptoms for which there are no demonstrable organic findings or known physiological mechanisms and for which there is evidence, or a strong presumption, that the symptoms are linked to psychological factors or conflicts. Disordered sleep is a problem that identifies abnormalities in the amount, quality, or timing of sleep and abnormal behavioral and physiological events occurring in association with sleep, specific sleep stages, or sleep-wake transitions. The *DSM-IV* (APA, 1994) identifies the following categories of somatoform and sleep disorders:

■ SOMATOFORM DISORDERS

300.81 Somatization Disorder

Somatization disorder is a chronic syndrome of multiple somatic symptoms that cannot be explained medically and are associated with psychosocial distress and long-term seeking of assistance from health-care professionals. Symptoms can represent virtually any organ system but commonly are expressed as neurological, gastrointestinal, psychosexual, or cardiopulmonary disorders. Onset of the disorder is usually in adolescence or early adulthood and is more common in women than in men.

---

*Reprinted with permission from the *Diagnostic and Statistical Manual of Mental Disorders, Fourth Edition*. Copyright 1994 American Psychiatric Association, 1994.

The disorder usually runs a fluctuating course, with periods of remission and exacerbation.

307.xx Pain Disorder

The essential feature of pain disorder is severe and prolonged pain that causes clinically significant distress or impairment in social, occupational, or other important areas of functioning (APA, 1994). This diagnosis is made when psychological factors have been judged to have a major role in the onset, severity, exacerbation, or maintenance of the pain, even when the physical examination reveals pathology that is associated with the pain.

300.7 Hypochondriasis

Hypochondriasis is an unrealistic preoccupation with the fear of having a serious illness. The *DSM-IV* suggests that this fear arises out of an unrealistic interpretation of physical signs and sensations. Occasionally medical disease may be present, but in the hypochondriacal individual, the symptoms are grossly disproportionate to the degree of pathology (Barsky, 1989). Individuals with hypochondriasis often have a long history of "doctor shopping" and are convinced that they are not receiving the proper care.

300.11 Conversion Disorder

Conversion disorder is a loss of or change in body function resulting from a psychological conflict, the physical symptoms of which cannot be explained by any known medical disorder or pathophysiological mechanism (Barsky, 1989). The most common conversion symptoms are those that suggest neurological disease such as paralysis, aphonia, seizures, coordination disturbance, akinesia, dyskinesia, blindness, tunnel vision, anosmia, anesthesia, and paresthesia.

300.7 Body Dysmorphic Disorder

This disorder, formerly called dysmorphophobia, is characterized by the exaggerated belief that the body is deformed or defected in some specific way. The most common complaints involve imagined or slight flaws of the face or head, such as thinning hair, acne, wrinkles, scars, vascular markings, facial swelling or asymmetry, or excessive facial hair (APA, 1994).

■ SLEEP DISORDERS

307.42 Insomnia

Insomnia is defined as difficulty with initiating or maintaining sleep. It is identified as *primary* when it is not associated with any other physical or mental illness and *secondary* when it is associated with another physical or mental illness.

307.44 Hypersomnia

Hypersomnia (sometimes called *somnolence*) is defined as excessive sleepiness or seeking excessive amounts of sleep. Primary hypersomnia refers to the condition when no other cause for the symptom can be found. With this disorder, individuals have difficulty staying awake during what would be considered the waking hours of the sleep-wake cycle.

347 Narcolepsy

Narcolepsy is a disorder similar to hypersomnia in that both produce excessive sleepiness. The characteristic manifestation of narcolepsy, however, is sleep attacks. When the attack occurs, the individual cannot prevent falling asleep, sometimes in the middle of a task or even in the middle of a sentence. Also associated with the sleep attack in 50 to 70 percent of the cases is *cataplexy,* a sudden loss of muscle tone, such as jaw drop, head drop, weakness of the knees, or paralysis of all skeletal muscles with collapse (Kaplan, Sadock, and Grebb, 1994).

307.47 Nightmare Disorder

Nightmares are frightening dreams that lead to awakenings from sleep (APA, 1994). Nightmare disorder is diagnosed when there is a repeated occurrence of the frightening dreams, which interferes with social or occupational functioning.

307.46 Sleep Terror Disorder

The manifestations of sleep terrors include abrupt arousal from sleep with a piercing scream or cry. The individual is difficult to awaken or comfort, and if wakefulness does occur, the individual is usually disoriented and expresses a sense of intense fear but cannot recall the dream episode. On awakening in the morning, the individual has amnesia of the whole experience.

307.46 Sleepwalking

The disorder of sleepwalking is characterized by the performance of motor activity initiated during sleep in which the individual may leave the bed and walk about, dress, go to the bathroom, talk, scream, or even drive (Kaplan, Sadock, and Grebb, 1994). Episodes may last from a few minutes to a half hour. Most often the person returns to bed and has no memory of the event on awakening. Should the individual awaken during the episode, he or she may experience several minutes of confusion and disorientation.

307.45 Circadian Rhythm Sleep Disorder

Sleep-wake schedule disturbances can be described as a misalignment between sleep and wake behaviors (Kaplan, Sadock, and Grebb, 1994). *Circadian rhythm sleep disorder* occurs when the normal sleep-wake schedule is disrupted from its usual circadian rhythm. The individual is unable to sleep (or be awake) when he or she wants to sleep (or be awake) but can do so at other times. Sleep-wake schedule disturbances are common among shift workers and airplane travelers (commonly called *jet lag*).

Predisposing Factors

1. **Physiological**
   a. ***Genetic:*** Studies have shown an increased incidence of somatization disorder and hypochondriasis in first-degree relatives, implying a possible inheritable predisposition (Kaplan and Sadock, 1998). Genetic or familial patterns are thought to play a contributing role in primary insomnia, primary hypersomnia, narcolepsy, sleep terror disorder, and sleepwalking.
   b. ***Biochemical:*** Decreased levels of serotonin and endorphins may play a role in the etiology of pain disorder.
   c. ***Medical Conditions:*** A number of medical conditions, including sleep apnea, endocrine or metabolic disorders, infectious or neoplastic disease, and CNS lesions, have been associated with insomnia and/or hypersomnia. Neurological abnormalities, particularly in the temporal lobe, may be related to precipitation of night terrors.
2. **Psychosocial**
   a. ***Psychodynamic:*** This theory emphasizes a distur-

bance in the early mother-child relationship. McCracken (1985) describes the mother as one who, because of her own conflicts regarding sexuality and dependency, alternately clings to and rejects the child. Out of this conditional nurturing by the mother, the child fails to develop feelings of self-security. He or she defends against this insecurity by learning to gain affection and care through illness.

Some psychodynamicists view hypochondriasis as an ego defense mechanism. Physical complaints are the expression of low self-esteem and feelings of worthlessness, because it is easier to feel something is wrong with the body than to feel something is wrong with the self (Barsky, 1989).

The psychodynamic theory of conversion disorder proposes that emotions associated with a traumatic event that the individual cannot express because of moral or ethical unacceptability are "converted" into physical symptoms. The unacceptable emotions are repressed and converted to a somatic hysterical symptom that is symbolic in some way of the original emotional trauma.

b. ***Family Dynamics:*** Some families have difficulty expressing emotions openly and resolving conflicts verbally. When this occurs, the child may become ill, and a shift in focus is made from the open conflict to the child's illness, leaving unresolved the underlying issues that the family cannot confront openly. Thus, somatization by the child brings some stability to the family, as harmony replaces discord and the child's welfare becomes the common concern. The child in turn receives positive reinforcement for the illness (Minuchin et al., 1975).
c. ***Sociocultural/Familial Factors:*** Somatic complaints are often reinforced when the sick role relieves the individual from the need to deal with a stressful situation, whether it be within society or within the family. When the sick person is allowed to avoid stressful obligations and postpone unwelcome challenges, is excused from toublesome duties, or becomes the prominent focus of attention because of the illness, positive reinforcement virtually guarantees repetition of the response.
d. ***Past Experience with Physical Illness:*** Personal experience, or the experience of close family members, with serious or life-threatening illness can predispose an individual to hypochondriasis. Once

an individual has experienced a threat to biological integrity, he or she may develop a fear of recurrence. The fear of recurring illness generates an exaggerated response to minor physical changes, leading to hypochondriacal behaviors.

Symptomatology (Subjective and Objective Data)

1. Virtually any physical symptom for which there is no organic basis but for which evidence exists for the implication of psychological factors.
2. Depressed mood is common.
3. Loss or alteration in physical functioning, with no organic basis. Examples include the following:
   a. Blindness or tunnel vision
   b. Paralysis
   c. Anosmia (inability to smell)
   d. Aphonia (inability to speak)
   e. Seizures
   f. Coordination disturbances
   g. Pseudocyesis (false pregnancy)
   h. Akinesia or dyskinesia
   i. Anesthesia or paresthesia
4. "La belle indifference"—a relative lack of concern regarding the severity of the symptoms just described (e.g., a person is suddenly blind but shows little anxiety over the situation).
5. "Doctor shopping."
6. Excessive use of analgesics.
7. Requests for surgery.
8. Assumption of an invalid role.
9. Impairment in social or occupational functioning because of preoccupation with physical complaints.
10. Psychosexual dysfunction (impotence, dyspareunia [painful coitus experienced by women], sexual indifference).
11. Excessive dysmenorrhea.
12. Excessive preoccupation with physical defect that is out of proportion to the actual condition.
13. Difficulty initiating or maintaining sleep.
14. Excessive sleepiness or seeking excessive amounts of sleep.
15. Sleep attacks.
16. Persistent, frightening nightmares.
17. Sleep terrors (abrupt arousal from sleep with a piercing scream or cry).

18. Physical motor activity initiated during sleep.
19. Inability to sleep (or be awake) when desiring to sleep (or be awake).

Common Nursing Diagnoses and Interventions

(Interventions are applicable to various health-care settings, such as inpatient and partial hospitalization, community outpatient clinic, home health, and private practice.)

CHRONIC PAIN

Definition: Sudden or slow onset of any intensity from mild to severe, constant or recurring without anticipated or predictable end, and a duration of greater than 6 months.

Possible Etiologies ("related to")

[Severe level of anxiety, repressed]
[Low self-esteem]
[Unmet dependency needs]
[Secondary gains from the sick role]

Defining Characteristics ("evidenced by")

[Verbal complaints of pain, in the absence of pathophysiological evidence]
[Social withdrawal]
Facial mask [of pain]
Guarding behaviors
[Demanding behaviors]
[Refuses to attend therapeutic activities because of pain]
[History of seeking assistance from numerous health-care professionals]
[Excessive use of analgesics, without relief of pain]
Self-focusing

Goals/Objectives

Short-Term Goal

Within 2 weeks, client will verbalize understanding of correlation between pain and psychological problems.

Long-Term Goal

By discharge from treatment, client will verbalize a noticeable, if not complete, relief from pain.

Interventions with *Selected Rationales*

1. Monitor physician's ongoing assessments and laboratory reports *to ascertain that organic pathology is clearly ruled out.*
2. Recognize and accept that the pain is indeed real to the individual, even though no organic etiology can be identified. *Denying the client's feelings is nontherapeutic and hinders the development of a trusting relationship.*
3. Observe and record the duration and intensity of the pain. Note factors that precipitate the onset of pain. *Identification of the precipitating stressor is important for assessment purposes. This information will be used to develop a plan for assisting the client to cope more adaptively.*
4. Provide pain medication as prescribed by physician. *Client comfort and safety are nursing priorities.*
5. Assist with comfort measures, such as back rub, warm bath, and heating pad. Be careful, however, not to respond in a way that reinforces the behavior. *Secondary gains from physical symptoms may prolong maladaptive behaviors.*
6. Offer your attention at times when client is not focusing on pain. *Positive reinforcement encourages repetition of adaptive behaviors.*
7. Identify activities that serve to distract client from focus on self and pain. *These distractors serve in a therapeutic manner as a transition from focus on self or physical manifestations to focus on unresolved psychological issues.*
8. Encourage verbalization of feelings. Explore meaning that pain holds for client. Help client to connect symptoms of pain to times of increased anxiety and to identify specific situations that cause anxiety to rise. *Verbalization of feelings in a nonthreatening environment facilitates expression and resolution of disturbing emotional issues.*
9. Encourage client to identify alternative methods of coping with stress. *These may avert the physical pain as a maladaptive response to stress.*
10. Explore with client ways to intervene as symptoms begin to intensify, so that pain does not become disabling. (Examples: visual or auditory distractions, guided imagery, breathing exercises, massage, application of heat or cold, relaxation techniques [Carpenito, 1993].)
11. Provide positive reinforcement for adaptive behaviors. *Positive reinforcement enhances self-esteem and encourages repetition of desired behaviors.*

Outcome Criteria

1. Client verbalizes that pain does not interfere with completion of daily activities.
2. Client verbalizes an understanding of the relationship between pain and emotional problems.
3. Client demonstrates ability to intervene as anxiety rises, to prevent the onset or increase in severity of pain.

INEFFECTIVE INDIVIDUAL COPING

Definition: Impairment of adaptive behaviors and abilities of a person in meeting life's demands and roles.

Possible Etiologies ("related to")

[Severe level of anxiety, repressed]
[Low self-esteem]
[Unmet dependency needs]
[History of self or loved one having experienced a serious illness or disease]
[Regression to, or fixation in , an earlier level of development]
[Retarded ego development]
[Inadequate coping skills]

Defining Characteristics ("evidenced by")

[Numerous physical complaints verbalized, in the absence of any pathophysiological evidence]
[Total focus on the self and physical symptoms]
[History of doctor shopping]
[Demanding behaviors]
[Refuses to attend therapeutic activities]
[Does not correlate physical symptoms with psychological problems]
Inability to meet the needs
Inability to meet role expectations
Inability to problem-solve

Goals/Objectives

Short-Term Goal

Within 2 weeks, client will verbalize understanding of correlation between physical symptoms and psychological problems.

Long-Term Goal

Client will demonstrate ability to cope with stress by means other than preoccupation with physical symptoms by discharge from treatment.

Interventions with *Selected Rationales*

1. Monitor physician's ongoing assessments, laboratory reports, and other data to maintain assurance that possibility of organic pathology is clearly ruled out. ***Knowledge of these data is vital for the provision of adequate and appropriate client care.***
2. Recognize and accept that the physical complaint is indeed real to the individual, even though no organic cause can be identified. ***Denial of the client's feelings is nontherapeutic and interferes with establishment of a trusting relationship.***
3. Identify gains that the physical symptom is providing for the client: increased dependency, attention, distraction from other problems. ***These are important assessment data to be used in assisting the client with problem resolution.***
4. Initially, fulfill client's most urgent dependency needs. ***Failure to do this may cause client to become extremely anxious, with an increase in maladaptive behaviors.***
5. Gradually withdraw attention to physical symptoms. Minimize time given in response to physical complaints. ***Lack of positive response will discourage repetition of undesirable behaviors.***
6. Explain to client that any new physical complaints will be referred to the physician and give no further attention to them. Be sure to note physician's assessment of the complaint. ***The possibility of organic pathology must always be taken into consideration. Failure to do so could jeopardize client's safety.***
7. Encourage client to verbalize fears and anxieties. Explain that attention will be withdrawn if rumination about physical complaints begins. Follow through. ***Without consistency of limit setting, change will not occur.***
8. Help client observe that physical symptoms occur because of, or are exacerbated by, specific stressors. Discuss alternative coping responses to these stressors.
9. Give positive reinforcement for adaptive coping strategies. ***Positive reinforcement encourages repetition of desired behaviors.***
10. Help client identify ways to achieve recognition from others without resorting to physical symptoms. ***Positive recognition from others enhances self-esteem and minimizes the need for attention through maladaptive behaviors.***

11. Discuss how interpersonal relationships are affected by client's narcissistic behavior. Explain how this behavior alienates others. ***Client may not realize how he or she is perceived by others.***
12. Provide instruction in relaxation techniques and assertiveness skills. ***These approaches decrease anxiety and increase self-esteem, which facilitate adaptive responses to stressful situations.***

Outcome Criteria

1. Client is able to demonstrate techniques that may be used in response to stress to prevent the occurrence or exacerbation of physical symptoms.
2. Client verbalizes an understanding of the relationship between emotional problems and physical symptoms.

BODY IMAGE DISTURBANCE

Definition: Disruption in the way one perceives one's body image.

Possible Etiologies ("related to")

[Severe level of anxiety, repressed]
[Low self-esteem]
[Unmet dependency needs]

Defining Characteristics ("evidenced by")

[Preoccupation with real or imagined change in bodily structure or function]
[Verbalizations about physical appearance that are out of proportion to any actual physical abnormality that may exist]
Fear of rejection or of reaction of others
Negative feelings about body
Change in social involvement

Goals/Objectives

Short-Term Goal

Client will verbalize understanding that changes in bodily structure or function are exaggerated out of proportion to the change that actually exists. (Time frame for this goal must be determined according to individual client's situation.)

Long-Term Goal

Client will verbalize perception of own body that is realistic to actual structure or function by discharge from treatment.

Interventions with *Selected Rationales*

1. Establish trusting relationship with client. ***Trust enhances therapeutic interactions between nurse and client.***
2. If there is actual change in structure or function, encourage client to progress through stages of grieving. Assess level of knowledge and provide information regarding normal grieving process and associated feelings. ***Knowledge of acceptable feelings facilitates progression through the grieving process.***
3. Identify misperceptions or distortions client has regarding body image. Correct inaccurate perceptions in a matter-of-fact, nonthreatening manner. Withdraw attention when preoccupation with distorted image persists. ***Lack of attention may encourage elimination of undesirable behaviors.***
4. Assist client to recognize personal body boundaries. ***Use of touch may help him or her recognize acceptance of the individual by others and reduce fear of rejection because of changes in bodily structure or function.***
5. Encourage independent self-care activities, providing assistance as required. ***Self-care activities accomplished independently enhance self-esteem and also create the necessity for client to confront reality of his or her bodily condition.***
6. Provide positive reinforcement for client's expressions of realistic bodily perceptions. ***Positive reinforcement enhances self-esteem and encourages repetition of desired behaviors.***

Outcome Criteria

1. Client verbalizes realistic perception of bodily condition.
2. Client demonstrates acceptance of changes in bodily structure or function, as evidenced by expression of positive feelings about body, ability or willingness to perform self-care activities independently, and a focus on personal achievements rather than preoccupation with distorted body image.

SENSORY-PERCEPTUAL ALTERATION

Definition: A state in which an individual experiences a change in the amount or patterning of incoming stimuli [either internally or externally initiated] accompanied by a diminished, exaggerated, distorted, or impaired response to such stimuli.

Possible Etiologies ("related to")

[Severe level of anxiety, repressed]
[Low self-esteem]
[Unmet dependency needs]
[Regression to, or fixation in, an earlier level of development]
[Retarded ego development]
[Inadequate coping skills]
Psychological stress [narrowed perceptual fields caused by anxiety]

Defining Characteristics ("evidenced by")

[Loss or alteration in physical functioning suggesting a physical disorder (often neurological in nature), but for which organic pathology is not evident. Common alterations include paralysis, anosmia, aphonia, deafness, blindness.]
[La belle indifference]

Goals/Objectives

Short-Term Goal

Client will verbalize understanding of emotional problems as a contributing factor to alteration in physical functioning within 10 days.

Long-Term Goal

Client will demonstrate recovery of lost function.

Interventions with *Selected Rationales*

1. Monitor physician's ongoing assessments, laboratory reports, and other data to maintain assurance that possibility of organic pathology is clearly ruled out. ***Failure to do so may jeopardize client's safety.***
2. Identify gains that the physical symptom is providing for the client: increased dependency, attention, distraction from other problems. ***These are important assessment data to be used in assisting the client with problem resolution.***
3. Fulfill client's needs related to ADLs with which the physical symptom is interfering. ***Client comfort and safety are nursing priorities.***
4. Do not focus on the disability, and allow client to be as independent as possible. Intervene only when client requires assistance. ***Positive reinforcement would encourage continual use of the maladaptive response for secondary gains, such as dependency.***
5. Encourage client to participate in therapeutic activities to

the best of his or her ability. Do not allow client to use the disability as a manipulative tool. Withdraw attention if client continues to focus on physical limitation. Reinforce reality as required, but ensure maintenance of a non-threatening environment.

6. Encourage client to verbalize fears and anxieties. Help client to recognize that the physical symptom appears at a time of extreme stress and is a mechanism used for coping. ***Client may be unaware of the relationship between physical symptom and emotional stress.***
7. Help client identify coping mechanisms that he or she could use when faced with stressful situations rather than retreating from reality with a physical disability.
8. Explain assertiveness techniques and practice use of same through role playing. ***Use of assertiveness techniques enhances self-esteem and minimizes anxiety in interpersonal relationships.***
9. Help client identify a satisfactory support system within the community from which he or she may seek assistance as needed to cope with overwhelming stress.

Outcome Criteria

1. Client is no longer experiencing symptoms of altered physical functioning.
2. Client verbalizes an understanding of the relationship between extreme psychological stress and loss of physical functioning.
3. Client is able to verbalize adaptive ways of coping with stress and identify community support systems to which he or she may go for help.

■ **SELF-CARE DEFICIT** (Identify Specific Area)

Definition: A state in which the individual experiences an impaired ability to perform or complete [activities of daily living independently].

Possible Etiologies ("related to")

[Paralysis of body part]
[Inability to see]
[Inability to hear]
[Inability to speak]
Pain, discomfort

Defining Characteristics ("evidenced by")

Inability to bring food from a receptacle to the mouth
Inability to wash body or body parts; obtain or get to water sources; regulate temperature or flow
Impaired ability to put on or take off necessary items of clothing; obtain or replace articles of clothing; fasten clothing; maintain appearance at a satisfactory level
Inability to get to toilet or commode [impaired mobility]
Inability to manipulate clothing for toileting
Inability to flush toilet or commode
Inability to sit on or rise from toilet or commode
Inability to carry out proper toilet hygiene

Goals/Objectives

Short-Term Goal

Client will perform self-care needs independently, to the extent that physical ability will allow, within 5 days.

Long-Term Goal

By discharge from treatment, client will be able to perform ADLs independently and demonstrate a willingness to do so.

Interventions with *Selected Rationales*

1. Assess client's level of disability; note areas of strength and impairment. ***This knowledge is required to develop adequate plan of care for client.***
2. Encourage client to perform normal ADLs to his or her level of ability. ***Successful performance of independent activities enhances self-esteem.***
3. Encourage independence, but intervene when client is unable to perform. ***Client comfort and safety are nursing priorities.***
4. Ensure that nonjudgmental attitude is conveyed as nursing assistance with self-care activities is provided. Remember that the physical symptom is real to the client. It is not within the client's conscious control. ***A judgmental attitude interferes with the nurse's ability to provide therapeutic care for this client.***
5. Feed client, if necessary, and provide assistance with containers, positioning, and other matters, as required. ***Client comfort and safety are nursing priorities.***
6. Bathe client, or assist with bath, depending on his or her level of ability. ***Client comfort and safety are nursing priorities.***
7. Assist client with dressing, oral hygiene, combing hair,

and applying makeup, as required. ***Client comfort and safety are nursing priorities.***

8. Provide bedpan, commode, or assistance to bathroom as determined by client's level of ability. ***Client comfort and safety are nursing priorities.***
9. Provide positive reinforcement for ADLs performed independently. ***Positive reinforcement enhances self-esteem and encourages repetition of desired behaviors.***
10. Take precautions against fostering dependency by intervening when client is capable of performing independently. Allow ample time to complete these activities to the best of his or her ability without assistance.
11. Encourage client to discuss feelings regarding the disability and the need for dependency it creates. Help client to see the purpose this disability is serving for him or her. ***Self-disclosure and exploration of feelings with a trusted individual may help client fulfill unmet needs and confront unresolved issues.***

Outcome Criteria

1. Client feeds self without assistance.
2. Client selects appropriate clothing and dresses and grooms self daily.
3. Client maintains level of personal hygiene by bathing daily and carrying out essential toileting procedures without assistance.

■ KNOWLEDGE DEFICIT (Psychological Causes for Physical Symptoms)

Definition: Absence or deficiency of cognitive information related to specific topic.

Possible Etiologies ("related to")

Lack of interest in learning
[Severe level of anxiety]

Defining Characteristics ("evidenced by")

[Denial of emotional problems]
[Statements such as, "I don't know why the doctor put me on the psychiatric unit. I have a physical problem."]
[History of "shopping" for a doctor who will substantiate symptoms as pathophysiological]
[Noncompliance with psychiatric treatment plan]

Goals/Objectives

Short-Term Goal

Client will verbalize an understanding that no pathophysiological condition exists to substantiate physical symptoms.

Long-Term Goal

By discharge from treatment, client will be able to verbalize psychological cause(s) for physical symptoms.

Interventions with *Selected Rationales*

1. Assess client's level of knowledge regarding effects of psychological problems on the body. ***An adequate database is necessary for the development of an effective teaching plan.***
2. Assess client's level of anxiety and readiness to learn. ***Learning does not occur beyond the moderate level of anxiety.***
3. Discuss physical examinations and laboratory tests that have been conducted. Explain purpose and results of each.
4. Explore feelings and fears held by client. Go slowly. These feelings may have been suppressed or repressed for a very long time and their disclosure will undoubtedly be a painful experience. Be supportive.
5. Have client keep a diary of appearance, duration, and intensity of physical symptoms. A separate record of situations that the client finds especially stressful should also be kept. ***Comparison of these records may provide objective data from which to observe the relationship between physical symptoms and stress.***
6. Help client identify needs that are being met through the sick role. Together, formulate a more adaptive means for fulfilling these needs. Practice by role playing.
7. Explain assertiveness techniques to the client. Discuss the importance of recognizing the differences among passive, assertive, and aggressive behaviors, and of respecting the human rights of others while protecting one's own basic human rights. ***Use of these techniques enhances self-esteem and facilitates client's interpersonal relationships.***
8. Discuss adaptive methods of stress management: relaxation techniques, physical exercise, meditation, breathing exercises, autogenics. ***These techniques may be employed in an attempt to relieve anxiety and discourage the use of physical symptoms as a maladaptive response.***

Outcome Criteria

1. Client verbalizes an understanding of the relationship between psychological stress and physical symptoms.
2. Client demonstrates the ability to use therapeutic techniques in the management of stress.

SLEEP PATTERN DISTURBANCE

Definition: Time-limited disruption of sleep (natural, periodic suspension of consciousness) amount and quality.

Possible Etiologies ("related to")

[A specific medical condition]
[Use of, or withdrawal from, substances]
Anxiety
Depression
Circadian rhythm disruption
[Familial patterns]

Defining Characteristics ("evidenced by")

[Insomnia]
[Hypersomnia]
[Nightmares]
[Sleep terrors]
[Sleepwalking]

Goals/Objectives

Short-Term Goal

Client will verbalize causal relationship of sleep disorder.

Long-Term Goal

Client will be able to achieve adequate, uninterrupted sleep.
Client will report feeling rested and demonstrate a sense of well-being.

Interventions with *Selected Rationales*

1. To promote sleep:
   a. Encourage activities that prepare one for sleep: soft music, relaxation exercises, warm bath. *These activities promote relaxation.*
   b. Discourage strenuous exercise within 1 hour of bedtime. *Strenuous exercise can be stimulating and keep one awake.*

c. Control intake of caffeine-containing substances within 4 hours of bedtime (e.g., coffee, tea, colas, chocolate, and certain analgesic medications). *Caffeine is a CNS stimulant and can interfere with the promotion of sleep.*
d. Provide a high-carbohydrate snack before bedtime. *Carbohydrates increase the levels of the amino acid tryptophan, a precursor to the neurotransmitter serotonin. Serotonin is thought to play a role in the promotion of sleep.*
e. Keep the temperature of the room between 68° and 72°F. *This range provides the temperature most conducive to sleep.*
f. Instruct the client not to use alcoholic beverages to relax. *Although alcohol may initially induce drowsiness and promote falling asleep, a rebound stimulation occurs in the CNS within several hours after drinking alcohol. The individual may fall asleep, only to be wide awake a few hours later.*
g. Discourage smoking and the use of other tobacco products near sleep time. *These products produce a stimulant effect on the CNS.*
h. Discourage daytime napping. Increase program of activities to keep the person busy. *Sleeping during the day can interfere with the ability to achieve sleep at night.*
i. Individuals with chronic insomnia should use sleeping medications judiciously. *Sedatives and hypnotics have serious side effects and are highly addicting. Life-threatening symptoms can occur with abrupt withdrawal, and discontinuation should be tapered under a physician's supervision. Long-term use can result in rebound insomnia.*

2. To prevent "jet lag" (circadian rhythm disruption):
   a. If time permits, use a preventive strategy of altering mealtimes and sleep times in the appropriate direction *to prepare the body for the oncoming change.*
   b. If preventive measures are impossible, increasing the amount of sleep on arrival sometimes helps *to reduce fatigue and restore the rested feeling.*
   c. Short-term use of sleep medication may be helpful.

Outcome Criteria

1. Client verbalizes a decrease in problems with sleep.
2. Client reports feeling rested and demonstrates a sense of well-being.

RISK FOR INJURY

Definition: A state in which the individual is at risk of injury as a result of environmental conditions interacting with the individual's adaptive and defensive resources.

Related/Risk Factors ("related to")

[Excessive sleepiness]
[Sleep terrors]
[Sleepwalking]
[Sleep deprivation]

Goals/Objectives

Short-Term and Long-Term Goal

Client will not experience injury.

Interventions with *Selected Rationales*

1. Ensure that side rails are up on the bed. *An individual who experiences serious nightmares or night terrors can fall from the bed during an episode.*
2. Keep the bed in a low position *to diminish the risk of injury by the person who gets out of bed during a sleepwalking episode.*
3. Equip the bed with a bell (or other noisemaker) that is activated when the bed is exited. *This may alert the caretaker so that supervision to prevent accidental injury can be instituted.*
4. Keep a night-light on and arrange the furniture in the bedroom in a manner that promotes safety *to provide a safe environment for the individual who awakens (fully or partially) during the night.*
5. Administer drug therapy as ordered. *Insomnia and parasomnias have been treated effectively with benzodiazepines. The usual treatment for hypersomnia and narcolepsy has been with CNS stimulants such as amphetamines. In some instances, the selective serotonin reuptake inhibitors (SSRIs) have also been helpful for these problems.*
6. For the child who experiences nightmares, encourage him or her to talk about the dream. Tell the child that all people have dreams. Validate his or her feeling of fearfulness while ensuring safety. Keep a light on in the room or give the child a flashlight. *Talking about the dream helps to promote the unreality of the dream and to differentiate between what is real and what is not real. Light*

gives the child a feeling of control over the darkness within the room.

Outcome Criteria

1. Client has not experienced injury from behaviors associated with sleep disorders.
2. Client is following medication regimen and is experiencing no adverse effects.

■ INTERNET REFERENCES

Additional information about Somatoform Disorders may be located at the following Websites:

- http://www.psyweb.com/Mdisord/somatd.html
- http://www.delmarnursing.com/frisch/web2.html#psychosomatic
- http://www.mc.vanderbilt.edu/peds/pidl/adolesc/convreac.htm
- http://www.emedicinc.com/EMERG/topic112.Htm
- http://www.lifewell.com/educenter/294.cfm
- http://www.yahoo.com/Health/Mental_Health/Diseases_and_Conditions/Hypochondria

Additional information about Sleep Disorders may be located at the following Websites:

- http://www.sleepnet.com/disorder.htm
- http://www.asda.org/
- http://www.sleepmedservices.com/

Information about medications for Sleep Disorders may be located at the following Websites:

- http://www.rxmed.com/prescribe.html
- http://www.mentalhealth.com/drug/

CHAPTER 10

*Dissociative Disorders**

■ BACKGROUND ASSESSMENT DATA

The essential feature of the dissociative disorders is a disruption in the usually integrated functions of consciousness, memory, identity, or perception of the environment (APA, 1994). During periods of intolerable stress, the individual blocks off part of his or her life from consciousness. The stressful emotion becomes a separate entity, as the individual "splits" from it and mentally drifts into a fantasy state. The following categories are defined in the *DSM-IV* (APA, 1994):

1. **300.12 Dissociative Amnesia:** An inability to recall important personal information, usually of a traumatic or stressful nature. The extent of the disturbance is too great to be explained by ordinary forgetfulness. Types of impairment in recall include the following:
   a. ***Localized Amnesia:*** Inability to recall all incidents associated with a traumatic event for a specific time period following the event (usually a few hours to a few days).
   b. ***Selective Amnesia:*** Inability to recall only certain incidents associated with a traumatic event for a specific time period following the event.
   c. ***Generalized Amnesia:*** Failure of recall encompassing one's entire life.
   d. ***Continuous Amnesia:*** Inability to recall events subsequent to a specific time up to and including the

*Reprinted with permission from the *Diagnostic and Statistical Manual of Mental Disorders, Fourth Edition*. Copyright 1994 American Psychiatric Association, 1994.

present. (The memory does not return after a short period of time, as in localized amnesia. The individual actually is unable to form new memories.)

e. ***Systematized Amnesia:*** With this type of amnesia, the individual cannot remember events that relate to a specific category of information, such as one's family, or to one particular person or event.

2. **300.13 Dissociative Fugue:** A sudden, unexpected travel away from home or customary work locale with assumption of a new identity and an inability to recall one's previous identity. Following recovery, there is no recollection of events that took place during the fugue. Course is typically brief—hours to days and, rarely, months. Recurrences are rare.
3. **300.14 Dissociative Identity Disorder (DID):** The existence within the individual of two or more distinct personalities, each of which is dominant at a particular time. The original personality usually is not aware (at least initially) of the existence of subpersonalities. When there are more than two subpersonalities, however, they are usually aware of each other. Transition from one personality to another is usually sudden and often associated with psychosocial stress. The course tends to be more chronic than in the other dissociative disorders.
4. **300.6 Depersonalization Disorder:** Depersonalization disorder is characterized by a temporary change in the quality of self-awareness, which often takes the form of feelings unreality, changes in body image, feelings of detachment from the environment, or a sense of observing oneself from outside the body (Marciniak, 1985).

Predisposing Factors

1. **Physiological**
   a. ***Genetics:*** The *DSM-IV* suggests that DID is more common in first-degree relatives of people with the disorder than in the general population. The disorder is often seen in more than one generation of a family.
   b. ***Neurobiological:*** Some clinicians have suggested a possible correlation between neurological alterations and dissociative disorders. Although available information is inadequate, it is possible that dissociative amnesia and dissociative fugue may be related to alterations in the ascending reticular activating system and thalamocortical projections (Nemiah, 1989).

Some studies have suggested a possible link between DID and certain neurological conditions, such as temporal lobe epilepsy, severe migraine headaches, cerebral cortical damage, and visual alterations. Electroencephalographic abnormalities have been observed in some clients with DID.

2. **Psychosocial**
   a. ***Psychodynamic Theory:*** Freud (1962) believed that dissociative behaviors occurred when individuals repressed distressing mental contents from conscious awareness. He believed that the unconscious was a dynamic entity in which repressed mental contents were stored and unavailable to conscious recall. Current psychodynamic explanations of dissociation are based on Freud's concepts.
   b. ***Psychological Trauma:*** A growing body of evidence points to the etiology of DID as a set of traumatic experiences that overwhelms the individual's capacity to cope by any means other than dissociation. These experiences usually take the form of severe physical, sexual, or psychological abuse by a parent or significant other in the child's life. DID is thought to serve as a survival strategy for the child in this traumatic environment, in which he or she creates a new being who is able to experience the overwhelming pain of the cruel reality, while the primary self can then escape awareness of the pain. Kluft (1984) suggests that the number of an individual's alternate personalities is related to the number of different types of abuse he or she suffered as a child.

Symptomatology (Subjective and Objective Data)

1. Impairment in recall.
   a. Inability to remember specific incidents.
   b. Inability to recall any of one's past life, including one's identity.
2. Sudden travel away from familiar surroundings; assumption of new identity, with inability to recall past.
3. Assumption of additional identities within the personality; behavior involves transition from one identity to another as a method of dealing with stressful situations.
4. Feeling of unreality; detachment from a stressful situ-

ation—may be accompanied by dizziness, depression, obsessive rumination, somatic concerns, anxiety, fear of going insane, and a disturbance in the subjective sense of time.

Common Nursing Diagnoses and Interventions

(Interventions are applicable to various health-care settings, such as inpatient and partial hospitalization, community outpatient clinic, home health, and private practice.)

INEFFECTIVE INDIVIDUAL COPING

Definition: Inability to form a valid appraisal of the stressors, inadequate choices of practiced responses, and/or inability to use available resources.

Possible Etiologies ("related to")

[Severe level of anxiety, repressed]
[Childhood trauma]
[Childhood abuse]
[Low self-esteem]
[Unmet dependency needs]
[Regression to, or fixation in, an earlier level of development]
[Retarded ego development]
[Inadequate coping skills]

Defining Characteristics ("evidenced by")

[Dissociating self from painful situation by experiencing:
Memory loss (partial or complete)
Sudden travel away from home with inability to recall previous identity
The presence of more than one personality within the individual
Detachment from reality]
Inability to problem-solve
Inability to meet role expectations
[Inappropriate use of defense mechanisms]

Goals/Objectives

Short-Term Goals

1. Client will verbalize understanding that he or she is employing dissociative behaviors in times of psychosocial stress.

2. Client will verbalize more adaptive ways of coping in stressful situations than resorting to dissociation.

Long-Term Goal

Client will demonstrate ability to cope with stress (employing means other than dissociation).

Interventions with *Selected Rationales*

1. Reassure client of safety and security through your presence. Dissociative behaviors may be frightening to the client. ***Presence of a trusted individual provides feeling of security and assurance of freedom from harm.***
2. Identify stressor that precipitated severe anxiety. ***This information is necessary to the development of an effective plan of client care and problem resolution.***
3. Explore feelings that client experienced in response to the stressor. Help client to understand that the disequilibrium felt is acceptable—indeed, even expected—in times of severe stress. ***Client's self-esteem is preserved by the knowledge that others may experience these behaviors under similar circumstances.***
4. As anxiety level decreases (and memory returns), use exploration and an accepting, nonthreatening environment to encourage client to identify repressed traumatic experiences that contribute to chronic anxiety.
5. Have client identify methods of coping with stress in the past and determine whether the response was adaptive or maladaptive. ***In times of extreme anxiety, client is unable to evaluate appropriateness of response. This information is necessary for client to develop a plan of action for the future.***
6. Help client define more adaptive coping strategies. Make suggestions of alternatives that might be tried. Examine benefits and consequences of each alternative. Assist client in the selection of those that are most appropriate for him or her. ***Depending on current level of anxiety, client may require assistance with problem solving and decision making.***
7. Provide positive reinforcement for client's attempts to change. ***Positive reinforcement enhances self-esteem and encourages repetition of desired behaviors.***
8. Identify community resources to which the individual may go for support if past maladaptive coping patterns return.

Outcome Criteria

1. Client is able to demonstrate techniques that may be used in response to stress to prevent dissociation.

2. Client verbalizes an understanding of the relationship between severe anxiety and the dissociative response.

ALTERED THOUGHT PROCESSES

Definition: A state in which an individual experiences a disruption in cognitive operations and activities.

Possible Etiologies ("related to")

[Severe level of anxiety, repressed]
[Childhood trauma]
[Childhood abuse]
[Threat to physical integrity]
[Threat to self-concept]

Defining Characteristics ("evidenced by")

[Memory loss—inability to recall selected events related to a stressful situation]
[Memory loss—inability to recall events associated with entire life]
[Memory loss—inability to recall own identity]

Goals/Objectives

Short-Term Goal

Client will verbalize understanding that loss of memory is related to stressful situation and begin discussing stressful situation with nurse or therapist.

Long-Term Goal

Client will recover deficits in memory and develop more adaptive coping mechanisms to deal with stressful situations.

Interventions with *Selected Rationales*

1. Obtain as much information as possible about client from family and significant others (likes, dislikes, important people, activities, music, pets). *A baseline assessment is important for the development of an effective plan of care.*
2. Do not flood client with data regarding his or her past life. *Individuals who are exposed to painful information from which the amnesia is providing protection may decompensate even further into a psychotic state.*
3. Instead, expose client to stimuli that represent pleasant experiences from the past, such as smells associated with enjoyable activities, beloved pets, and music known to have been pleasurable to client.

4. As memory begins to return, engage client in activities that may provide additional stimulation. ***Recall may occur during activities that simulate life experiences.***
5. Encourage client to discuss situations that have been especially stressful and to explore the feelings associated with those times. ***Verbalization of feelings in a nonthreatening environment may help client come to terms with unresolved issues that may be contributing to the dissociative process.***
6. Identify specific conflicts that remain unresolved, and assist client in identifying possible solutions. ***Unless these underlying conflicts are resolved, any improvement in coping behaviors must be viewed as only temporary.***
7. Provide instruction regarding more adaptive ways to respond to anxiety so that dissociative behaviors are no longer needed.

Outcome Criteria

1. Client is able to recall all events of past life.
2. Client is able to demonstrate adaptive coping strategies that may be used in response to severe anxiety to avert amnestic behaviors.

PERSONAL IDENTITY DISTURBANCE

Definition: Inability to distinguish between self and nonself.

Possible Etiologies ("related to")

[Severe level of anxiety, repressed]
[Childhood trauma]
[Childhood abuse]
[Threat to physical integrity]
[Threat to self-concept]
[Underdeveloped ego]

Defining Characteristics ("evidenced by")

[Presence of more than one personality within the individual]

Goals/Objectives

Short-Term Goal

Client will verbalize understanding of the existence of multiple personalities within the self and be able to recognize stressful situations that precipitate transition from one to another.

Long-Term Goal

Client will verbalize understanding of the need for, enter into, and cooperate with long-term therapy for this disorder, with the ultimate goal being integration into one personality.

Interventions with *Selected Rationales*

1. The nurse must develop a trusting relationship with the original personality and with each of the subpersonalities. ***Trust is the basis of a therapeutic relationship. Each of the personalities views itself as a separate entity and must initially be treated as such.***
2. Help the client understand the existence of the subpersonalities. ***Client may be unaware of this dissociative response to stressful situations.***
3. Help client identify the need each subpersonality serves in the personal identity of the individual. ***Knowledge of these unfulfilled needs is the first step toward integration of the personalities and the client's ability to face unresolved issues without dissociation.***
4. Help the client identify stressful situations that precipitate the transition from one personality to another. Carefully observe and record these transitions. ***This knowledge is required to assist the client in responding more adaptively and to eliminate the need for transition to another personality.***
5. Use nursing interventions necessary to deal with maladaptive behaviors associated with individual subpersonalities. For example, if one personality is suicidal, precautions must be taken to guard against client's self-harm. If another personality has a tendency toward physical hostility, precautions must be taken for the protection of others. ***Safety of the client and others is a nursing priority.***
6. Help subpersonalities to understand that their "being" will not be destroyed, but integrated into a unified identity within the individual. ***Because subpersonalities function as separate entities, the idea of total elimination generates fear and defensiveness.***
7. Provide support during disclosure of painful experiences and reassurance when the client becomes discouraged with lengthy treatment.

Outcome Criteria

1. Client recognizes the existence of more than one personality.

2. Client is able to verbalize the purpose these personalities serve.
3. Client verbalizes the intention of seeking long-term outpatient psychotherapy.

SENSORY-PERCEPTUAL ALTERATION (Kinesthetic)

Definition: A state in which an individual experiences a change in the amount or patterning of incoming stimuli [either internally or externally initiated] accompanied by a diminished exaggerated, distorted, or impaired response to such stimuli.

Possible Etiologies ("related to")

[Severe level of anxiety, repressed]
[Childhood trauma]
[Childhood abuse]
[Threat to physical integrity]
[Threat to self-concept]
[Underdeveloped ego]

Defining Characteristics ("evidenced by")

[Alteration in the perception or experience of the self]
[Loss of one's own sense of reality]
[Loss of the sense of reality of the external world]

Goals/Objectives

Short-Term Goal

Client will verbalize adapative ways of coping with stress.

Long-Term Goal

Client will demonstrate the ability to perceive stimuli correctly and maintain a sense of reality during stressful situations by discharge from treatment.

Interventions with *Selected Rationales*

1. Provide support and encouragement during times of depersonalization. The client manifesting these symptoms may express fear and anxiety at experiencing such behaviors. They do not understand the response and may express a fear of "going insane." ***Support and encouragement from a trusted individual provide a feeling of security when fears and anxieties are manifested.***

2. Explain the depersonalization behaviors and the purpose they usually serve for the client. ***This knowledge may help to minimize fears and anxieties associated with their occurrence.***
3. Explain the relationship between severe anxiety and depersonalization behaviors. ***The client may be unaware that the occurrence of depersonalization behaviors is related to severe anxiety.***
4. Help client relate these behaviors to times of severe psychological stress that he or she has experienced personally.
5. Explore past experiences and possibly repressed painful situations such as trauma or abuse. ***It is thought that traumatic experiences predispose individuals to dissociative disorders.***
6. Discuss these painful experiences with the client and encourage him or her to deal with the feelings associated with these situations. Work to resolve the conflicts these repressed feelings have nurtured. ***These interventions serve to decrease the need for the dissociative response to anxiety.***
7. Discuss ways the client may more adaptively respond to stress and role-play with him or her to practice using these new methods.

Outcome Criteria

1. Client perceives stressful situations correctly and is able to maintain a sense of reality.
2. Client demonstrates use of adaptive strategies for coping with stress.

■ INTERNET REFERENCES

Additional information about Dissociative Disorders may be located at the following Websites:

- http://www.human-nature.com/odmh/dissociative.html
- http://www.nami.org/helpline/whatdiss.htm
- http://www.voiceofwomen.com/VOW2_11950/center.html
- http://www.shakey.net/dissoc.html
- http://www.webcrawler.com/health/mental_health/dissociative_disorders
- http://www.issd.org/isdabout.htm
- http://www.lifewell.com/InfoSprings/spring14.cfm

CHAPTER 11

*Sexual and Gender Identity Disorders**

■ BACKGROUND ASSESSMENT DATA

The *DSM-IV* (APA, 1994) identifies two categories of sexual disorders: paraphilias and sexual dysfunctions. Paraphilias are characterized by recurrent, intense sexual urges, fantasies, or behaviors that involve unusual objects, activities, or situations (APA, 1994). Sexual dysfunction disorders can be described as an impairment or disturbance in any of the phases of the sexual response cycle. These include disorders of desire, arousal, orgasm, and disorders that relate to the experience of genital pain during intercourse. Gender identity disorders are characterized by strong and persistent cross-gender identification accompanied by persistent discomfort with one's assigned sex (APA, 1994).

Paraphilias

Abel (1989) identifies the term *paraphilia* as repetitive or preferred sexual fantasies or behaviors that involve any of the following:

1. The preference for use of a nonhuman object.
2. Repetitive sexual activity with humans involving real or simulated suffering or humiliation.
3. Repetitive sexual activity with nonconsenting partners.

Types of paraphilias include the following:

1. **302.4 Exhibitionism:** The major symptoms include

---

*Reprinted with permission from the *Diagnostic and Statistical Manual of Mental Disorders, Fourth Edition.* Copyright 1994 American Psychiatric Association, 1994.

recurrent, intense sexual urges, behaviors, or sexually arousing fantasies, of at least 6 months' duration, involving the exposure of one's genitals to an unsuspecting stranger (APA, 1994). Masturbation may occur during the exhibitionism. The condition apparently occurs only in men, and the victims are women in 99 percent of the cases (Kaplan, Sadock, and Grebb, 1994).

2. **302.81 Fetishism:** This is identified by recurrent, intense sexual urges or behaviors, or sexually arousing fantasies of at least 6 months' duration, involving the use of nonliving objects (APA, 1994). Common fetish objects include bras, women's underpants, stockings, shoes, boots, or other wearing apparel. The fetish object is generally used during masturbation or incorporated into sexual activity with another person to produce sexual excitation. When the fetish involves cross-dressing, the disorder is called **transvestic fetishism (302.3)**.
3. **302.89 Frotteurism:** This disorder is defined as the recurrent preoccupation with intense sexual urges or fantasies, of at least 6 months' duration, involving touching or rubbing against a nonconsenting person (APA, 1994). Sexual excitement is derived from the actual touching or rubbing, not from the coercive nature of the act.
4. **302.2 Pedophilia:** The *DSM-IV* describes the essential feature of this disorder as recurrent sexual urges, behaviors, or sexually arousing fantasies, of at least 6 months' duration, involving sexual activity with a prepubescent child. The age of the molester is 16 or older and is at least 5 years older than the child. This category of paraphilia is the most common of sexual assaults (Abel, 1989).
5. **302.83 Sexual Masochism:** The identifying feature of this disorder is recurrent, intense sexual urges, behaviors, or sexually arousing fantasies, of at least 6 months' duration, involving the act (real, not simulated) of being humiliated, beaten, bound, or otherwise made to suffer (APA, 1994). These masochistic activities may be fantasized, solitary, or with a partner. Examples include becoming sexually aroused by self-inflicted pain or being restrained, raped, or beaten by a sexual partner.
6. **302.84 Sexual Sadism:** The essential feature of this disorder is identified as recurrent, intense, sexual urges, behaviors, or sexually arousing fantasies, of at least 6 months' duration, involving acts (real, not sim-

ulated) in which the psychological or physical suffering (including humiliation) of the victim is sexually exciting (APA, 1994). The sadistic activities may be fantasized or acted on with a consenting or nonconsenting partner. In all instances, sexual excitation occurs in response to the suffering of the victim. Examples include rape, beating, torture, or even killing.

7. **302.82 Voyeurism:** This disorder is identified by recurrent, intense sexual urges, behaviors, or sexually arousing fantasies, of at least 6 months' duration, involving the act of observing an unsuspecting person who is naked, in the process of disrobing, or engaging in sexual activity (APA, 1994). Sexual excitement is achieved through the act of looking, and no contact with the person is attempted. Masturbation usually accompanies the "window peeping" but may occur later as the individual fantasizes about the voyeuristic act.

Predisposing Factors *(to Paraphilias)*

1. **Physiological**
   a. ***Physical Factors:*** Several physical factors have been implicated in the etiology of paraphilias. They include abnormalities in the limbic system of the brain, temporal lobe epilepsy, temporal lobe tumors, and abnormal levels of androgens (Bradford and McLean, 1984). The results of these studies are inconclusive at this time.
2. **Psychosocial**
   a. ***Psychoanalytical Theory:*** The psychoanalytical approach defines a paraphiliac as one who has failed the normal developmental process toward heterosexual adjustment (Abel, 1989). This occurs when the individual fails to resolve the oedipal crisis, thereby maintaining sexual feelings for the parent of the opposite gender. This creates intense anxiety, which leads the individual to seek sexual gratification in ways that provide a "safe substitution" for the parent (Becker and Kavoussi, 1988).

Symptomatology *(Subjective and Objective Data)*

1. Exposure of one's genitals to a stranger.
2. Sexual arousal in the presence of nonliving objects.

3. Touching and rubbing one's genitals against an unconsenting person.
4. Sexual attraction to, or activity with, a prepubescent child.
5. Sexual arousal from being humiliated, beaten, bound, or otherwise made to suffer (through fantasy, self-infliction, or by a sexual partner).
6. Sexual arousal by inflicting psychological or physical suffering on another individual (either consenting or nonconsenting).
7. Sexual arousal from dressing in the clothes of the opposite gender.
8. Sexual arousal from observing unsuspecting people either naked or engaged in sexual activity.
9. Masturbation often accompanies the activities described when they are performed solitarily.
10. The individual is markedly distressed by these activities.

Sexual Dysfunctions

Sexual dysfunctions may occur in any phase of the sexual response cycle. Types of sexual dysfunctions include the following:

1. **Sexual Desire Disorders**
   a. ***302.71 Hypoactive Sexual Desire Disorder:*** This disorder is defined by the *DSM-IV* (APA, 1994) as a persistent or recurrent deficiency or absence of sexual fantasies and desire for sexual activity. The complaint appears to be more common among women than men.
   b. ***302.79 Sexual Aversion Disorder:*** This disorder is characterized by a persistent or recurrent extreme aversion to, and avoidance of, all or almost all genital sexual contact with a sexual partner (APA, 1994).
2. **Sexual Arousal Disorders**
   a. ***302.72 Female Sexual Arousal Disorder:*** This disorder is identified in the *DSM-IV* (APA, 1994) as a persistent or recurrent inability to attain, or to maintain until completion of the sexual activity, an adequate lubrication or swelling response of sexual excitement.
   b. ***302.72 Male Erectile Disorder:*** This disorder is characterized by a persistent or recurrent inability

to attain, or to maintain until completion of the sexual activity, an adequate erection (APA, 1994).

3. **Orgasmic Disorders**
   a. ***302.73 Female Orgasmic Disorder (Anorgasmia):*** This disorder is defined by the *DSM-IV* as a persistent or recurrent delay in, or absence of, orgasm following a normal sexual excitement phase.
   b. ***302.74 Male Orgasmic Disorder (Retarded Ejaculation):*** With this disorder, the man is unable to ejaculate, even though he has a firm erection and has had more than adequate stimulation (Hyde, 1986). The severity of the problem may range from only occasional problems ejaculating to a history of never having experienced on orgasm.
   c. ***302.75 Premature Ejaculation:*** The *DSM-IV* describes this disorder as persistent or recurrent ejaculation with minimal sexual stimulation, or before, on, or shortly after penetration and before the person wishes it.
4. **Sexual Pain Disorders**
   a. ***302.76 Dyspareunia:*** This disorder is defined as recurrent or persistent genital pain associated with sexual intercourse, in either a man or a woman, that is not caused by vaginismus, lack of lubrication, other general medical condition, or the physiological effects of substance use (APA, 1994).
   b. ***306.51 Vaginismus:*** This disorder is characterized by an involuntary constriction of the outer one-third of the vagina, which prevents penile insertion and intercourse (Sadock, 1989).

***Predisposing Factors** (to Sexual Dysfunctions)*

1. **Physiological Factors**
   a. ***Hypoactive Sexual Desire Disorders:*** These have been linked to low levels of serum testosterone in men (Sadock, 1989) and to elevated levels of serum prolactin in both men and women (Segraves, 1988). Various medications, such as antihypertensives, antipsychotics, antidepressants, anxiolytics, and anticonvulsants, as well as chronic use of drugs such as alcohol and cocaine, have also been implicated in sexual desire disorders (Abel, 1985).
   b. ***Sexual Arousal Disorders:*** These may occur in response to decreased estrogen levels in postmenopausal women. Medications such as antihis-

tamines and cholinergic blockers may produce similar results. Erectile dysfunctions in men may be attributed to arteriosclerosis, diabetes, temporal lobe epilepsy, multiple scleorsis, some medications (antihypertensives, tranquilizers), spinal cord injury, pelvic surgery, and chronic use of alcohol.

c. ***Orgasmic Disorders:*** In women these may be attributed to some medical conditions (hypothyroidism, diabetes, and hyperprolactinemia), and certain medications (antihypertensives, antidepressants). Medical conditions that may interfere with male orgasm include genitourinary surgery (e.g., prostatectomy), Parkinson's disease, and diabetes. Various medications have also been implicated, including antihypertensives, anticholinergics, and antipsychotics.

d. ***Sexual Pain Disorders:*** In women these can be caused by disorders of the vaginal entrance, irritation or damage to the clitoris, vaginal or pelvic infections, endometriosis, tumors, or cysts. Painful intercourse in men may be attributed to penile infections, phimosis, urinary tract infections, or prostate problems.

2. **Psychosocial Factors**

a. ***Sexual Desire Disorders:*** These may be attributed to a number of early developmental conflicts that have left the individual with unconscious connections between the sexual impulse and overwhelming feelings of shame and guilt (Sadock, 1989). Childhood sexual assault or abuse, as well as repeated painful coital experiences, mental depression, aging-related concerns, and relationship difficulties may also be implicated.

b. ***Sexual Arousal Disorders:*** In the female these may be attributed to doubts, fears, guilt, anxiety, shame, conflict, embarrassment, tension, disgust, resentment, grief, anger toward the partner, and puritanical or moralistic upbringing. A history of sexual abuse may also be an important etiologic factor (Becker, 1989). In men, erectile disorder may be related to an inability to express the sexual impulse because of fear, anxiety, anger, or moral prohibition (Sadock, 1989). Early developmental factors that promote feelings of inadequacy and a sense of being unloving or unlovable may also result in impotence. Difficulties in the relationship may also be a contributing factor.

c. ***Orgasmic Disorders:*** A number of factors have been implicated in the etiology of female orgasm disorders. They include fear of becoming pregnant, hostility toward men, negative cultural conditioning, childhood exposure to rigid religious orthodoxy, and traumatic sexual experiences during childhood or adolescence. Orgasm disorders in men may be related to a rigid, puritanical background in which sex was perceived as sinful and the genitals as dirty; or interpersonal difficulties such as ambivalence about commitment, fear of pregnancy, or unexpressed hostility may be implicated.

d. ***Sexual Pain Disorders:*** Vaginismus may occur after having experienced painful intercourse for any organic reason, after which involuntary constriction of the vagina occurs in anticipation and fear of recurring pain. Other psychosocial factors that have been implicated in the etiology of vaginismus include negative childhood conditioning of sex as dirty, sinful, and shameful; early childhood sexual trauma; homosexual orientation; traumatic experience with an early pelvic examination; pregnancy phobia; venereal disease phobia; or cancer phobia (Kolodny et al., 1979, Kaplan and Sadock, 1998).

Symptomatology *(Subjective and Objective Data)*

1. Absence of sexual fantasies and desire for sexual activity.
2. Discrepancy between partners' levels of desire for sexual activity.
3. Feelings of disgust, anxiety, or panic responses to genital contact.
4. Inability to produce adequate lubrication for sexual activity.
5. Absence of a subjective sense of sexual excitement during sexual activity.
6. Failure to attain or maintain penile erection until completion of sexual activity.
7. Inability to achieve orgasm (in men, to ejaculate) following a period of sexual excitement judged adequate in intensity and duration to produce such a response.
8. Ejaculation occurs with minimal sexual stimulation or before, on, or shortly after penetration and before the individual wishes it.

9. Genital pain occurring before, during, or after sexual intercourse.
10. Constriction of the outer one-third of the vagina prevents penile penetration.

Common Nursing Diagnoses and Interventions

(Interventions are applicable to various health-care settings, such as inpatient and partial hospitalization, community outpatient clinic, home health, and private practice.)

SEXUAL DYSFUNCTION

Definition: The state in which an individual experiences a change in sexual function that is viewed as unsatisfying, unrewarding, or inadequate.

Possible Etiologies ("related to")

Ineffectual or absent role models
Physical [or sexual] abuse
Psychosocial abuse
Values conflict
Lack of privacy
Lack of significant other
Altered body structure or function (pregnancy, recent childbirth, drugs, surgery, anomalies, disease process, trauma, radiation)
Misinformation or lack of knowledge
[Depression]
[Pregnancy phobia]
[Venereal disease phobia]
[Cancer phobia]
[Previous painful experience]
[Severe anxiety]
[Relationship difficulties]

Defining Characteristics ("evidenced by")

Verbalization of problem:

- [Absence of desire for sexual activity
- Feelings of disgust, anxiety, or panic responses to genital contact
- Absence of lubrication or subjective sense of sexual excitement during sexual activity

- Failure to attain or maintain penile erection during sexual activity
- Inability to achieve orgasm or ejaculation
- Premature ejaculation
- Genital pain during intercourse
- Constriction of the vagina that prevents penile penetration]

Verbalization of inability to achieve desired sexual satisfaction

Goals/Objectives

Short-Term Goals

1. Client will identify stressors that may contribute to loss of sexual function within 1 week *or*
2. Client will discuss pathophysiology of disease process that contributes to sexual dysfunction within 1 week.

For client with permanent dysfunction due to disease process:

3. Client will verbalize willingness to seek professional assistance from a sex therapist to learn alternative ways of achieving sexual satisfaction with partner by (time dimension is individually determined).

Long-Term Goal

Client will resume sexual activity at level satisfactory to self and partner by (time dimension determined by individual situation).

Interventions with *Selected Rationales*

1. Assess client's sexual history and previous level of satisfaction in sexual relationship. ***This establishes a data base from which to work and provides a foundation for goal setting.***
2. Assess client's perception of the problem. ***Client's idea of what constitutes a problem may differ from the nurse's. It is the client's perception on which the goals of care must be established.***
3. Help client determine time dimension associated with the onset of the problem and discuss what was happening in life situation at that time. ***Stress in any areas of life can affect sexual functioning. Client may be unaware of correlation between stress and sexual dysfunction.***
4. Assess client's mood and level of energy. ***Depression and fatigue decrease desire and enthusiasm for participation in sexual activity.***
5. Review medication regimen; observe for side effects. ***Many medications can affect sexual functioning. Evaluation of drug and individual response is important to ascertain whether drugs may be contributing to the problem.***

6. Encourage client to discuss disease process that may be contributing to sexual dysfunction. Ensure that client is aware that alternative methods of achieving sexual satisfaction exist and can be learned through sex counseling if he or she and partner desire to do so. *Client may be unaware that satisfactory changes can be made in his or her sex life. He or she may also be unaware of the availability of sex counseling.*
7. Encourage client to ask questions regarding sexuality and sexual functioning that may be troubling him or her. *Increasing knowledge and correcting misconceptions can decrease feelings of powerlessness and anxiety and facilitate problem resolution.*
8. Make referral to sex therapist, if necessary. Client may even request that an initial appointment be made for him or her. *Complex problems are likely to require assistance from an individual who is specially trained to treat problems related to sexuality. Client and partner may be somewhat embarrassed to seek this kind of assistance. Support from a trusted nurse can provide the impetus for them to pursue the help that they need.*

Outcome Criteria

1. Client is able to correlate physical or psychosocial factors that interfere with sexual functioning.
2. Client is able to communicate with partner about their sexual relationship without discomfort.
3. Client and partner verbalize willingness and desire to seek assistance from professional sex therapist *or*
4. Client verbalizes resumption of sexual activity at level satisfactory to self and partner.

ALTERED SEXUALITY PATTERNS

Definition: The state in which an individual expresses concern regarding his or her sexuality.

Possible Etiologies ("related to")

Lack of significant other
Ineffective or absent role models
[Illness-related alterations in usual sexuality patterns]
Conflicts with sexual orientation or variant preferences
[Unresolved oedipal conflict]
[Delayed sexual adjustment]

Defining Characteristics ("evidenced by")

Reported difficulties, limitations, or changes in sexual behaviors or activities

[Expressed dissatisfaction with sexual behaviors]

[Reports that sexual arousal can be achieved only through variant practices, such as pedophilia, fetishism, masochism, sadism, frotteurism, exhibitonism, voyeurism]

[Desires to experience satisfying sexual relationship with another individual without need for arousal through variant practices]

Goals/Objectives

(Time elements to be determined by individual situation.)

Short-Term Goals

1. Client will verbalize aspects about sexuality that he or she would like to change.
2. Client and partner will communicate with each other ways in which each believes their sexual relationship could be improved.

Long-Term Goals

1. Client will express satisfaction with own sexuality pattern.
2. Client and partner will express satisfaction with sexual relationship.

Interventions with *Selected Rationales*

1. Take sexual history, noting client's expression of areas of dissatisfaction with sexual pattern. *Knowledge of what client perceives as the problem is essential for providing the type of assistance he or she may need.*
2. Assess areas of stress in client's life and examine relationship with sexual partner. *Variant sexual behaviors are often associated with added stress in the client's life. Relationship with partner may deteriorate as individual eventually gains sexual satisfaction only from variant practices.*
3. Note cultural, social, ethnic, racial, and religious factors that may contribute to conflicts regarding variant sexual practices. *Client may be unaware of the influence these factors exert in creating feelings of discomfort, shame, and guilt regarding sexual attitudes and behavior.*
4. Be accepting and nonjudgmental. *Sexuality is a very personal and sensitive subject. The client is more likely to*

share this information if he or she does not fear being judged by the nurse.

5. Assist therapist in plan of behavior modification to help client who desires to decrease variant sexual behaviors. ***Individuals with paraphilias are treated by specialists who have experience in modifying variant sexual behaviors. Nurses can intervene by providing assistance with implementation of the plan for behavior modification.***
6. If altered sexuality patterns are related to illness or medical treatment, provide information to client and partner regarding the correlation between the illness and the sexual alteration. Explain possible modifications in usual sexual patterns that client and partner may try in an effort to achieve a satisfying sexual experience in spite of the limitation. ***Client and partner may be unaware of alternate possibilities for achieving sexual satisfaction, or anxiety associated with the limitation may interfere with rational problem solving.***
7. Explain to client that sexuality is a normal human response and is not synonymous with any one sexual act; it involves complex interrelationships among one's self-concept, body image, personal history, family and cultural influences, and all interactions with others (VandeVusse and Simandl, 1992). ***If client feels "abnormal" or very unlike everyone else, the self-concept is likely to be very low—he or she may even feel worthless. To increase the client's feelings of self-worth and desire to change behavior, help him or her see that even though the behavior is variant, feelings and motivations are common.***

Outcome Criteria

1. Client is able to verbalize fears about abnormality and inappropriateness of sexual behaviors.
2. Client expresses desire to change variant sexual behavior and cooperates with plan of behavior modification.
3. Client and partner verbalize modifications in sexual activities in response to limitations imposed by illness or medical treatment.
4. Client expresses satisfaction with own sexuality pattern or satisfying sexual relationship with another.

Gender Identity Disorders

Gender identity is the sense of knowing to which gender one belongs—that is, the awareness of one's masculinity or femininity. Gender identity disorders occur when there is incongruity between anatomic sex and gender identity. An individual with gender identity disorder has an intense desire to be, or insists that he or she is, of the other gender. The *DSM-IV* (APA, 1994) identifies two categories of the disorder:

1. **302.6 Gender Identity Disorder in Children**
2. **302.85 Gender Identity Disorder in Adolescents and Adults**

Kaplan, Sadock, and Gregg (1994) report that intervention with adolescents and adults with gender identity disorder is difficult. Adolescents commonly act out and rarely have the motivation required to alter their cross-gender roles. Adults generally seek therapy to learn how to cope with their altered sexual identity, not to correct it.

Treatment of children with the disorder is aimed at helping them to become more comfortable with their assigned gender and to avoid the possible development of gender dissatisfaction in adulthood.

Predisposing Factors *(to Gender Identity Disorder)*

1. **Physiological**
   a. Studies of genetics and physiological alterations have been conducted in an attempt to determine whether a biological predisposition to gender identity disorder exists. To date, no clear evidence has been demonstrated.
2. **Psychosocial**
   a. ***Family Dynamics:*** Dynamics within a family may have a role in the etiology of gender identity disorder. In Green's (1976, 1985) studies with feminine boys, he found the following:
      (1) Parental indifference to feminine behavior
      (2) Parental encouragement of feminine behavior
      (3) Maternal overprotection of a son and prohibition of "rough, boyish" play
      (4) Excessive maternal attention and physical contact, resulting in lack of separation and individuation of the boy from his mother
      (5) Absence of, or rejection by, the father
      (6) Physical beauty of a boy, influencing adults to treat him in a feminine manner

(7) Lack of male playmates during early years of socialization

Pauly (1974) found that a disturbed parental relationship was also commonly reported by a substantial majority of adult women with gender identity disorder. The dynamics often included a weak or depressive mother or an aggressive, excessively masculine and often alcoholic father. Encouragement by both parents of masculinity in the daughter was common.

b. ***Psychoanalytical Theory:*** This theory suggests that gender identity problems begin during the struggle of the oedipal conflict. Problems may reflect both real family events and those created in the imagination of the child. These conflicts, whether real or imagined, interfere with the child's loving of the opposite-gender parent and identifying with the same-gender parent, and ultimately with normal gender identity.

Symptomatology *(Subjective and Objective Data)*

In children or adolescents:

1. Repeatedly stating intense desire to be of the opposite gender.
2. Insistence that one is of the opposite gender.
3. Preference in males for cross-dressing or simulating female attire.
4. Insistence by females on wearing only stereotypical masculine clothing.
5. Fantasies of being of the opposite gender.
6. Intense desire to participate in the stereotypical games and pastimes of the opposite gender.
7. Strong preference for playmates (peers) of the opposite gender.

In adults:

1. A stated desire to be of the opposite gender.
2. Frequently passing as the opposite gender.
3. Desire to live or to be treated as the opposite gender.
4. Stated conviction that one has the typical feelings and reactions of the opposite gender.
5. Persistent discomfort with or sense of inappropriateness in the assigned gender role.
6. Request for opposite-gender hormones or surgery to alter sexual characteristics.

Common Nursing Diagnoses and Interventions

(Interventions are applicable to various health-care settings, such as inpatient and partial hospitalization, community outpatient clinic, home health, and private practice.)

NOTE: Because adults and adolescents rarely have the desire or motivation to modify their gender identity, nursing interventions in this section are focused on working with gender-disordered children.

PERSONAL IDENTITY DISTURBANCE

Definition: Inability to distinguish between self and nonself.

Possible Etiologies ("related to")

[Parenting patterns that encourage culturally unacceptable behaviors for assigned gender]
[Unresolved oedipal conflict]

Defining Characteristics ("evidenced by")

[Statements of desire to be opposite gender]
[Statements that one is the opposite gender]
[Cross-dressing, or passing as the opposite gender]
[Strong preference for playmates (peers) of the opposite gender]
[Stated desire to be treated as the opposite gender]
[Statements of having feelings and reactions of the opposite gender]

Goals/Objectives

Short-Term Goals

Client will verbalize knowledge of behaviors that are appropriate and culturally acceptable for assigned gender.
Client will verbalize desire for congruence between personal feelings and behavior and assigned gender.

Long-Term Goals

Client will demonstrate behaviors that are appropriate and culturally acceptable for assigned gender.
Client will express personal satisfaction and feelings of being comfortable in assigned gender.

Interventions with *Selected Rationales*

1. Spend time with client and show positive regard. ***Trust and unconditional acceptance are essential to the establishment of a therapeutic nurse-client relationship.***
2. Be aware of own feelings and attitudes toward this client and his or her behavior. ***Attitudes influence behavior. The nurse must not allow negative attitudes to interfere with the effectiveness of interventions.***
3. Allow client to describe his or her perception of the problem. ***It is important to know how the client perceives the problem before attempting to correct misperceptions.***
4. Discuss with the client the types of behaviors that are more culturally acceptable. Practice these behaviors through role playing or with play therapy strategies (e.g., male and female dolls). Positive reinforcement or social attention may be given for use of appropriate behaviors. No response is given for opposite-sex-stereotype behaviors. ***The goal is to enhance culturally appropriate same-sex behaviors, but not necessarily to extinguish all coexisting opposite-sex behaviors (Rosen et al., 1978).***

Outcome Criteria

1. Client demonstrates behaviors that are culturally appropriate for assigned gender.
2. Client verbalizes and demonstrates self-satisfaction with assigned gender role.
3. Client demonstrates development of a close relationship with the parent of the same gender.

IMPAIRED SOCIAL INTERACTION

Definition: The state in which an individual participates in an insufficient or excessive quantity or ineffective quality of social exchange.

Possible Etiologies ("related to")

[Socially and culturally unacceptable behavior]
[Negative role modeling]
[Low self-esteem]

Defining Characteristics ("evidenced by")

Verbalized or observed discomfort in social situations
Verbalized or observed inability to receive or communicate a

satisfying sense of belonging, caring, interest, or shared history
Observed use of unsuccessful social interaction behaviors
Dysfunctional interaction with peers, family, or others

Goals/Objectives

Short-Term Goal

Client will verbalize possible reasons for ineffective interactions with others.

Long-Term Goals

Client will interact with others using culturally acceptable behaviors.

Interventions with *Selected Rationales*

1. Once client feels comfortable with the new behaviors in role playing or one-to-one nurse-client interactions, they may be tried in group situations. If possible, remain with the client during initial interactions with others. ***Presence of a trusted individual provides security for the client in a new situation. It also provides the potential for feedback to the client about his or her behavior.***
2. Observe client behaviors and the responses he or she elicits from others. Give social attention (e.g., smile, nod) to desired behaviors. Follow up these "practice" sessions with one-to-one processing of the interaction. Give positive reinforcement for efforts. ***Positive reinforcement encourages repetition of desirable behaviors. One-to-one processing provides time for discussing the appropriateness of specific behaviors and why they should or should not be repeated.***
3. Offer support if client is feeling hurt from peer ridicule. Matter of factly discuss the behaviors that elicited the ridicule. Offer no personal reaction to the behavior. ***Personal reaction from the nurse would be considered judgmental. Validation of client's feelings is important, yet it is important that client understand why his or her behavior was the subject of ridicule and how to avoid it in the future.***

Outcome Criteria

1. Client interacts appropriately with others demonstrating culturally acceptable behaviors.
2. Client verbalizes and demonstrates comfort in assigned gender role in interactions with others.

SELF-ESTEEM DISTURBANCE

Definition: Negative self-evaluation and feelings about self or self-capabilities, which may be directly or indirectly expressed.

Possible Etiologies ("related to")

[Rejection by peers]
[Lack of positive feedback]
[Repeated negative feedback, resulting in diminished self-worth]
[Dysfunctional family system]
[Lack of personal satisfaction with assigned gender]

Defining Characteristics ("evidenced by")

[Inability to form close, personal relationships]
[Negative view of self]
[Expressions of worthlessness]
[Social isolation]
Hypersensitivity to slight or criticism
Expressions of shame or guilt
Self-negating verbalizations
[Lack of eye contact]

Goals/Objectives

Short-Term Goal

Client will verbalize positive statements about self, including past accomplishments and future prospects.

Long-Term Goal

Client will verbalize and demonstrate behaviors that indicate self-satisfaction with assigned gender, ability to interact with others, and a sense of self as a worthwhile person.

Interventions with *Selected Rationales*

1. *To enhance the child's self-esteem:*
   a. Encourage the child to engage in activities in which he or she is likely to achieve success.
   b. Help the child to focus on aspects of his or her life for which positive feelings exist. Discourage rumination about situations that are perceived as failures or over which the client has no control. Give positive feedback for these behaviors.
2. Help the client identify behaviors or aspects of life he or she

would like to change. If realistic, assist the child in problem-solving ways to bring about the change. ***Having some control over his or her life may decrease feelings of powerlessness and increase feelings of self-worth.***

3. Offer to be available for support to the child when he or she is feeling rejected by peers. ***Having an available support person who does not judge the child's behavior and who provides unconditional acceptance assists the child to progress toward acceptance of self as a worthwhile person.***

Outcome Criteria

1. Client verbalizes positive perception of self.
2. Client verbalizes self-satisfaction about accomplishments and demonstrates behaviors that reflect self-worth.

■ INTERNET REFERENCES

Additional information about Sexual Disorders may be located at the following Websites:

- http://www.sexualhealth.com/
- http://www.sexualhealthinstitute.com/
- http://www-hsl.mcmaster.ca/tomflem/sexual.html

Additional information about Gender Identity Disorders may be located at the following Websites:

- http://www.avitale.com/
- http://english-www.hss.cmu.edu/gender/

Additional information about Sexually Transmitted Diseases may be located at the following Website:

- http://www.nau.edu/~fronske/stdintro.html

CHAPTER 12

Eating Disorders

BACKGROUND ASSESSMENT DATA

The *DSM-IV* (APA, 1994) identifies eating disorders as those characterized by severe disturbances in eating behavior. Two such disorders are described in the *DSM-IV:* anorexia nervosa and bulimia nervosa. Obesity is not classified as a psychiatric disorder per se; however, because of the strong emotional factors associated with it, the *DSM-IV* suggests that obesity may be considered within the category of *Psychological Factors Affecting Medical Condition.*

307.1 Anorexia Nervosa*

Defined

Anorexia nervosa is a clinical syndrome in which the person has a morbid fear of obesity. It is characterized by the individual's gross distortion of body image, preoccupation with food, and refusal to eat. The *DSM-IV* lists the following criteria that must be present to confirm the diagnosis of anorexia nervosa:

1. Refusal to maintain body weight at or above a minimally normal weight for age and height (e.g., weight loss leading to maintenance of body weight less than 85 percent of that expected; or failure to make expected weight gain during period of growth, leading to body weight less than 85 percent of that expected).
2. Intense fear of gaining weight or becoming fat, even though underweight.

---

*Reprinted with permission from the *Diagnostic and Statistical Manual of Mental Disorders, Fourth Edition.* Copyright 1994 American Psychiatric Association, 1994.

3. Disturbance in the way one's body weight or shape is experienced, undue influence of body weight or shape on self-evaluation, or denial of the seriousness of the current low body weight.
4. In postmenarcheal females, amenorrhea, that is, absence of a least three consecutive menstrual cycles.

The disorder occurs predominantly in females aged 12 to 30 years. Without intervention, death from starvation can occur.

Symptomatology *(Subjective and Objective Data)*

1. Morbid fear of obesity. Preoccupied with body size. Reports "feeling fat" even when in an emaciated condition.
2. Refusal to eat. Reports "not being hungry," although it is thought that the actual feelings of hunger do not cease until late in the disorder.
3. Preoccupation with food. Thinks and talks about food at great length. Prepares enormous amounts of food for friends and family members but refuses to eat any of it.
4. Amenorrhea is common, often appearing even before noticeable weight loss has occurred.
5. Delayed psychosexual development.
6. Compulsive behavior, such as excessive handwashing, may be present.
7. Extensive exercising is common.
8. Feelings of depression and anxiety often accompany this disorder.
9. May engage in the binge-and-purge syndrome from time to time (see section on Bulimia Nervosa).

307.51 Bulimia Nervosa*

Defined

Bulimia nervosa is an eating disorder (commonly called "the binge-and-purge syndrome") characterized by extreme overeating, followed by self-induced vomiting and abuse of laxatives and diuretics. Diagnostic criteria for bulimia, as identified by the *DSM-IV,* include the following:

---

*Reprinted with permission from the *Diagnostic and Statistical Manual of Mental Disorders, Fourth Edition.* Copyright 1994 American Psychiatric Association, 1994.

1. Recurrent episodes of binge eating that is characterized by the following:
   a. Eating, within a discrete period of time (e.g., within any 2-hour period), an amount of food that is definitely larger than most people would eat during a similar period and under similar circumstances.
   b. A sense of lack of control over eating during the episode (e.g., a feeling that one cannot stop eating or control what or how much one is eating).
2. Recurrent, inappropriate compensatory behavior intended to prevent weight gain, such as self-induced vomiting; misuse of laxatives, diuretics, enemas, or other medications; fasting; or excessive exercise.
3. The binge eating and inappropriate compensatory behaviors both occur, on average, at least twice a week for 3 months.
4. Self-evaluation is unduly influenced by body shape and weight.
5. The disturbance does not occur exclusively during episodes of anorexia nervosa.

The disorder occurs predominantly in females and begins in adolescence or early adult life.

Symptomatology *(Subjective and Objective Data)*

1. Binges are usually solitary and secret, and the individual may consume thousands of calories in one episode.
2. After the binge has begun, there is often a feeling of loss of control or inability to stop eating.
3. Eating binges may be viewed as pleasurable but are followed by intense self-criticism and depressed mood.
4. Bulimics are usually within normal weight range, some a few pounds underweight, some a few pounds overweight.
5. Obsession with body image and appearance is a predominant feature of this disorder. Individuals with bulimia display undue concern with sexual attractiveness and how they will appear to others.
6. Binges usually alternate with periods of normal eating and fasting.
7. Excessive vomiting may lead to problems with dehydration and electrolyte imbalance. Gastric acid in the vomitus also contributes to the erosion of tooth enamel.

Predisposing Factors to Anorexia Nervosa and Bulimia Nervosa

1. **Physiological Factors**
   a. ***Genetics:*** A hereditary predisposition to eating disorders has been hypothesized on the basis of family histories and an apparent association with other disorders for which the likelihood of genetic influences exists. Anorexia nervosa is more common among sisters and mothers of those with the disorder than among the general population.
   b. ***Neuroendocrine Abnormalities:*** Some speculation has occurred regarding a primary hypothalamic dysfunction in anorexia nervosa. Studies consistent with this theory have revealed elevated cerebrospinal fluid cortisol levels and a possible impairment of dopaminergic regulation in anorectic individuals (Eckert and Mitchell, 1994).
2. **Psychosocial Factors**
   a. ***Psychodynamic Theory:*** The psychodynamic theory suggests that behaviors associated with eating disorders reflect a developmental arrest in the very early years of childhood caused by disturbances in mother-infant interactions. The tasks of trust, autonomy, and separation-individuation go unfulfilled, and the individual remains in the dependent position. Ego development is retarded.
   b. ***Family Dynamics:*** This theory proposes that the issue of control becomes the overriding factor in the family of the individual with an eating disorder. These families often consist of a passive father, a domineering mother, and an overly dependent child. A high value is placed on perfectionism in this family, and the child feels he or she must satisfy these standards.

      Parental criticism promotes an increase in obsessive and perfectionistic behavior on the part of the child, who continues to seek love, approval, and recognition. Feelings of helplessness and ambivalence toward the parents eventually develop. In adolescence, these distorted eating patterns may be a rebellion against the parents, viewed by the child as a means of gaining, and remaining in, control. The symptoms are often triggered by a stressor that the adolescent perceives as a loss of control in some aspect of his or her life.

Obesity

Defined

The following formula is used to determine the degree of obesity in an individual:

$$\text{Body mass index} = \frac{\text{weight (kg)}}{\text{height (m)}^2}$$

The body mass index (BMI) range for normal weight is 20 to 24.9. Studies by the National Center for Health Statistics indicate that *overweight* is defined as a BMI of 25.0 to 29.9 (based on U.S. Dietary Guidelines for Americans) and *obesity* is defined as a BMI of 30.0 or greater (based on criteria of the World Health Organization) [American Heart Association, 1999]. These guidelines, which were released by the National Heart, Lung, and Blood Institute in June 1998, have been received by the medical community with a great deal of controversy. This change in guidelines increased the number of individuals in the United States considered to be obese from one-third to approximately one-half. The average American woman has a BMI of 26, and fashion models typically have BMIs of 18.

Obesity is known to contribute to a number of health problems, including hyperlipidemia, diabetes mellitus, osteoarthritis, and increased workload on the heart and lungs.

Predisposing Factors to Obesity

1. **Physiological Factors**
   a. ***Genetics:*** Genetics have been implicated in the development of obesity, in that 80 percent of children born of two overweight parents will also be overweight. This hypothesis has also been supported by studies of twins reared by normal weight, as well as by overweight, parents.
   b. ***Physical Factors:*** Overeating and/or obesity has also been associated with lesions in the appetite and satiety centers of the hypothalamus, hypothyroidism, decreased insulin production in diabetes mellitus, and increased cortisone production in Cushing's disease.
2. **Psychosocial Factors**
   a. ***Psychoanalytical Theory:*** This theory suggests

that obesity is the result of unresolved dependency needs, with the individual being fixed in the oral stage of psychosexual development. The symptoms of obesity are viewed as depressive equivalents, attempts to regain "lost" or frustrated nurturance and care.

Common Nursing Diagnoses and Interventions (for Anorexia and Bulimia)

(Interventions are applicable to various health-care settings such as inpatient and partial hospitalization, community outpatient clinic, home health, and private practice.)

■ ALTERED NUTRITION: LESS THAN BODY REQUIREMENTS

Definition: The state in which an individual experiences an intake of nutrients insufficient to meet metabolic needs.

Possible Etiologies ("related to")

[Refusal to eat]
[Ingestion of large amounts of food, followed by self-induced vomiting]
[Abuse of laxatives, diuretics, and/or diet pills]
[Physical exertion in excess of energy produced through caloric intake]

Defining Characteristics ("evidenced by")

[Loss of 15 percent of expected body weight (anorexia nervosa)]
Pale conjunctiva and mucous membranes
Poor muscle tone
Excessive loss of hair [or increased growth of hair on body (lanugo)]
[Amenorrhea]
[Poor skin turgor]
[Electrolyte imbalances]
[Hypothermia]
[Bradycardia]
[Hypotension]
[Cardiac irregularities]
[Edema]

Goals/Objectives

Short-Term Goal

Client will gain _____ pounds per week (amount to be established by client, nurse, and dietitian)

Long-Term Goal

By discharge from treatment, client will exhibit no signs or symptoms of malnutrition.

Interventions with *Selected Rationales*

1. If client is unable or unwilling to maintain adequate oral intake, physician may order a liquid diet to be administered via nasogastric tube. Nursing care of the individual receiving tube feedings should be administered according to established hospital procedures. ***The client's physical safety is a nursing priority, and without adequate nutrition, a life-threatening situation exists.***
   For oral diet:
2. In collaboration with dietitian, determine number of calories required to provide adequate nutrition and realistic (according to body structure and height) weight gain.
3. Explain to client details of behavior modification program as outlined by physician. Explain benefits of compliance with prandial routine and consequences for noncompliance. ***Behavior modification bases privileges granted or restricted directly on weight gain and loss. Focus is placed on emotional issues, rather than on food and eating specifically.***
4. Sit with client during mealtimes for support and to observe amount ingested. A limit (usually 30 minutes) should be imposed on time allotted for meals. ***Without a time limit, meals can become lengthy, drawn-out sessions, providing client with attention based on food and eating.***
5. Client should be observed for at least 1 hour following meals. ***Otherwise, this time may be used by client to discard food stashed from tray or to engage in self-induced vomiting.***
6. Client may need to be accompanied to bathroom if self-induced vomiting is suspected.
7. Strict documentation of intake and output. ***This information is required to promote client safety and plan nursing care.***
8. Weigh client daily immediately on arising and following first voiding. Always use same scale, if possible. ***Client***

care, privileges, and restrictions will be based on accurate daily weights.

9. Do not discuss food or eating with client, once protocol has been established. Do, however, offer support and positive reinforcement for obvious improvements in eating behaviors. ***Discussing food with client provides positive feedback for maladaptive behaviors.***
10. Client must understand that if, because of poor oral intake, nutritional status does not improve, tube feedings will be initiated ***to ensure client's safety.*** Staff must be consistent and firm with this action, using a matter-of-fact approach regarding the tube insertion and subsequent feedings.
11. As nutritional status improves and eating habits are established, begin to explore with client the feelings associated with his or her extreme fear of gaining weight. ***Emotional issues must be resolved if maladaptive responses are to be eliminated.***

Outcome Criteria

1. Client has achieved and maintained at least 85 percent of expected body weight
2. Vital signs, blood pressure, and laboratory serum studies are within normal limits.
3. Client verbalizes importance of adequate nutrition.

FLUID VOLUME DEFICIT

Definition: The state in which an individual experiences vascular, cellular, or intracellular dehydration.

Possible Etiologies ("related to")

[Decreased fluid intake]
[Abnormal fluid loss caused by self-induced vomiting]
[Excessive use of laxatives or enemas]
[Excessive use of diuretics]
[Electrolyte or acid-base imbalance brought about by malnourished condition of self-induced vomiting]

Defining Characteristics ("evidenced by")

Decreased urine output
Output greater than intake
Concentrated urine
Hemoconcentration
Hypotension

Increased pulse rate
Increased body temperature
Dry skin
Decreased skin turgor
Weakness
Change in mental state
Dry mucous membranes

Goals/Objectives

Short-Term Goal

Client will drink 125 mL of fluid each hour during waking hours.

Long-Term Goal

By discharge from treatment, client will exhibit no signs or symptoms of dehydration (as evidenced by quantity of urinary output sufficient to individual client; normal specific gravity; vital signs within normal limits; moist, pink mucous membranes; good skin turgor; and immediate capillary refill).

Interventions with *Selected Rationales*

1. Keep strict record of intake and output. Teach client importance of daily fluid intake of 2000 to 3000 mL. ***This information is required to promote client safety and plan nursing care.***
2. Weigh client daily immediately on arising and following first voiding. Always use same scale, if possible. ***An accurate daily weight is needed to plan nursing care for the client.***
3. Assess and document condition of skin turgor and any changes in skin integrity. ***Condition of skin provides valuable data regarding client hydration.***
4. Discourage client from bathing every day if skin is very dry. ***Hot water and soap are drying to the skin.***
5. Monitor laboratory serum values, and notify physician of significant alterations. ***Laboratory data provide an objective measure for evaluating adequate hydration.***
6. Client should be observed for at least 1 hour following meals and may need to be accompanied to the bathroom if self-induced vomiting is suspected. ***Vomiting causes active loss of body fluids and can precipitate fluid volume deficit.***
7. Assess and document moistness and color of oral mucous membranes. ***Dry, pale mucous membranes may be indicative of malnutrition or dehydration.***
8. Encourage frequent oral care ***to moisten mucous membranes, reducing discomfort from dry mouth, and to decrease bacterial count, minimizing risk of tissue infection.***

9. Help client identify true feelings and fears that contribute to maladaptive eating behaviors. *Emotional issues must be resolved if maladaptive behaviors are to be eliminated.*

Outcome Criteria

1. Client's vital signs, blood pressure, and laboratory serum studies are within normal limits.
2. No abnormalities of skin turgor and dryness of skin and oral mucous membranes are evident.
3. Client verbalizes knowledge regarding consequences of fluid loss due to self-induced vomiting and importance of adequate fluid intake.

INEFFECTIVE INDIVIDUAL COPING

Definition: Inability to form a valid appraisal of the stressors, inadequate choices of practiced responses, and/or inability to use available resources.

Possible Etiologies ("related to")

[Retarded ego development]
[Unfulfilled tasks of trust and autonomy]
[Dysfunctional family system]
[Unmet dependency needs]
[[Feelings of helplessness and lack of control in life situation]
[Possible chemical imbalance caused by malfunction of the hypothalamus]
[Unrealistic perceptions]

Defining Characteristics ("evidenced by")

[Preoccupation with extreme fear of obesity, and distortion of own body image]
[Refusal to eat]
[Obsessed with talking about food]
[Compulsive behavior (e.g., excessive handwashing)]
[Excessive overeating, followed by self-induced vomiting and/or abuse of laxatives and diuretics]
[Poor self-esteem]
[Chronic fatigue]
[Chronic anxiety]
[Chronic depression]
Inability to problem-solve
Inability to meet role expectations
Destructive behavior toward self

Goals/Objectives

Short-Term Goal

Within 7 days, client will eat regular meals and attend activities without discussing food or physical appearance.

Long-Term Goal

Client will be able to verbalize adaptive coping mechanisms that can be realistically incorporated into his or her lifestyle, thereby eliminating the need for maladaptive eating behaviors.

Interventions with *Selected Rationales*

1. Establish a trusting relationship with client by being honest, accepting, and available and keeping all promises. ***The therapeutic nurse-client relationship is built on trust.***
2. Acknowledge client's anger at feelings of loss of control brought about by established eating regimen (refer to Interventions for Alteration in Nutrition).
3. When nutritional status has improved, begin to explore with client the feelings associated with his or her extreme fear of gaining weight. ***Emotional issues must be resolved if maladaptive behaviors are to be eliminated.***
4. Explore family dynamics. Help client to identify his or her role contributions and their appropriateness within the family system. Assist client to identify specific concerns within the family structure and ways to help relieve those concerns. Also, discuss importance of client's separation of self as individual within the family system as well as identification of independent emotions and acceptance of them as his or her own. ***Client must recognize how maladaptive eating behaviors are related to emotional problems—often issues of control within the family structure.***
5. Initially, allow client to maintain dependent role. ***To deprive the individual of this role, at this time, could cause his or her anxiety to rise to an unmanageable level.*** As trust is developed and physical condition improves, encourage client to be as independent as possible in self-care activities. Offer positive reinforcement for independent behaviors and problem solving and decision making. ***Client must learn to function independently. Positive reinforcement increases self-esteem and encourages the client to use behaviors that are more acceptable.***
6. Explore with client ways in which he or she may feel in control within the environment, without resorting to maladaptive eating behaviors.

Outcome Criteria

1. Client is able to assess maladaptive coping behaviors accurately.
2. Client is able to verbalize adaptive coping strategies that can be used in the home environment.

ANXIETY (Moderate to Severe)

Definition: A vague uneasy feeling of discomfort or dread accompanied by an autonomic response; the source is often nonspecific or unknown to the individual; a feeling of apprehension caused by anticipation of danger. It is an altering signal that warns of impending danger and enables the individual to take measures to deal with threat.

Possible Etiologies ("related to")

Situational and maturational crises
[Unmet dependency needs]
[Low self-esteem]
[Dysfunctional family system]
[Feelings of helplessness and lack of control in life situation]
[Unfulfilled tasks of trust and autonomy]

Defining Characteristics ("evidenced by")

[Increased tension]
Increased helplessness
Overexcited
Apprehensive; fearful
Restlessness
Poor eye contact
[Increased difficulty taking oral nourishment]
[Inability to learn]

Goals/Objectives

Short-Term Goal

Client will demonstrate use of relaxation techniques to maintain anxiety at manageable level within 7 days.

Long-Term Goal

By discharge from treatment, client will be able to recognize events that precipitate anxiety and intervene to prevent disabling behaviors.

Interventions with *Selected Rationales*

1. Be available to stay with client. Remain calm and provide reassurance of safety. ***Client safety and security is a nursing priority.***
2. Help client identify the situation that precipitated onset of anxiety symptoms. ***Client may be unaware that emotional issues are related to symptoms of anxiety. Recognition may be the first step in elimination of this maladaptive response.***
3. Review client's methods of coping with similar situations in the past. ***In seeking to create change, it would be helpful for client to identify past responses and determine whether they were successful and whether they could be employed again. Client strengths should be identified and used to his or her advantage.***
4. Provide quiet environment. Reduce stimuli: low lighting, few people. ***Anxiety level may be decreased in calm atmosphere with few stimuli.***
5. Administer antianxiety medications, as ordered by physician. Monitor for effectiveness of medication as well as for adverse side effects. ***Antianxiety medications (e.g., diazepam, chlordiazepoxide, alprazolam) provide relief from the immobilizing effects of anxiety and may facilitate client's cooperation with therapy.***
6. Teach client to recognize signs of increasing anxiety and ways to intervene for maintaining the anxiety at a manageable level (e.g., exercise, walking, jogging, relaxation techniques). ***Anxiety and tension can be reduced safely and with benefit to the client through physical activities.***

Outcome Criteria

1. Client is able to verbalize events that precipitate anxiety and demonstrate techniques for its reduction.
2. Client is able to verbalize ways in which he or she may gain more control of the environment and thereby reduce feelings of helplessness.

BODY IMAGE/SELF-ESTEEM DISTURBANCE

Definition: Confusion in mental picture of one's physical self. Negative self-evaluation and feelings about self-capabilities, which may be directly or indirectly expressed.

Possible Etiologies ("related to")

[Lack of positive feedback]
[Perceived failures]
[Unrealistic expectations (on the part of self and others)]
[Retarded ego development]
[Unmet dependency needs]
[Threat to security caused by dysfunctional family dynamics]
[Morbid fear of obesity]
[Perceived loss of control in some aspect of life]

Defining Characteristics ("evidenced by")

[Distorted body image, views self as fat, even in the presence of normal body weight or severe emaciation]
[Denial that problem with low body weight exists]
[Difficulty accepting positive reinforcement]
[Not taking responsibility for self-care (self-neglect)]
[Nonparticipation in therapy]
[Self-destructive behavior (self-induced vomiting; abuse of laxatives or diuretics; refusal to eat)]
[Lack of eye contact]
[Depressed mood and self-deprecating thoughts following episode of binging and purging]
[Preoccupation with appearance and how others perceive them]

Goals/Objectives

Short-Term Goal

Client will verbally acknowledge misperception of body image as "fat" within specified time (depending on severity and chronicity of condition).

Long-Term Goal

Client will demonstrate an increase in self-esteem as manifested by verbalizing positive aspects of self and exhibiting less preoccupation with own appearance as a more realistic body image is developed by discharge.

Interventions with *Selected Rationales*

1. Assist client to re-examine negative perceptions of self and to recognize positive attributes. ***Client's own identification of strengths and positive attributes can increase sense of self-worth.***
2. Offer positive reinforcement for independently made decisions influencing client's life. ***Positive reinforcement en-***

hances self-esteem and may encourage client to continue functioning more independently.

3. Offer positive reinforcement when honest feelings related to autonomy and dependence issues remain separated from maladaptive eating behaviors.
4. Help client to develop a realistic perception of body image and relationship with food. *Client needs to recognize that his or her perception of body image is unhealthy and that maintaining control through maladaptive eating behaviors is dangerous—even life-threatening.*
5. Promote feelings of control within the environment through participation and independent decision making. Through positive feedback, help client learn to accept self as is, including weaknesses as well as strengths. *Client must come to understand that he or she is a capable, autonomous individual who can perform outside the family unit and who is not expected to be perfect. Control of his or her life must be achieved in other ways besides dieting and weight loss.*
6. Help client realize that perfection is unrealistic, and explore this need with him or her. *As client begins to feel better about self and identifies positive self-attributes, as well as develops the ability to accept certain personal inadequacies, the need for unrealistic achievements should diminish.*
7. Help client claim ownership of angry feelings and recognize that expressing them is acceptable if done so in an appropriate manner. Be an effective role model. *Unexpressed anger is often turned inward on the self, resulting in a depreciation of self-esteem.*

Outcome Criteria

1. Client is able to verbalize positive aspects about self.
2. Client expresses interest in welfare of others and less preoccupation with own appearance.
3. Client verbalizes that image of body as "fat" was misperception and demonstrates ability to take control of own life without resorting to maladaptive eating behaviors.

Common Nursing Diagnoses and Interventions (for Obesity)

(Interventions are applicable to various health-care settings, such as inpatient and partial hospitalization, community outpatient clinic, home health, and private practice.)

ALTERED NUTRITION: MORE THAN BODY REQUIREMENTS

Definition: The state in which an individual is experiencing an intake of nutrients that exceeds metabolic needs.

Possible Etiologies ("related to")

[Compulsive eating]
[Excessive intake in relation to metabolic needs]
[Sedentary lifestyle]
[Genetics]
[Unmet dependency needs—fixation in oral developmental stage]

Defining Characteristics ("evidenced by")

[Weight more than 20 percent over expected body weight for age and height]
[Body mass index of 30 or more]

Goals/Objectives

Short-Term Goal

Client will verbalize understanding of what must be done to lose weight.

Long-Term Goal

Client will demonstrate change in eating patterns resulting in a steady weight loss.

Interventions with *Selected Rationales*

1. Encourage the client to keep a diary of food intake. *This provides the opportunity for the client to gain a realistic picture of the amount of food ingested and provides a database on which to tailor the dietary program.*
2. Discuss feelings and emotions associated with eating. *This helps to identify when client is eating to satisfy an emotional need rather than a physiological one.*
3. With input from the client, formulate an eating plan that includes food from the basic food groups with emphasis on low-fat intake. It is helpful to keep the plan as similar to the client's usual eating pattern as possible. *Diet must eliminate calories while maintaining adequate nutrition. Client is more likely to stay on the eating plan if he or*

she is able to participate in its creation and it deviates as little as possible from usual types of foods.

4. Identify realistic increment goals for weekly weight loss. *Reasonable weight loss (1–2 lb/wk) results in more lasting effects. Excessive, rapid weight loss may result in fatigue and irritability and may ultimately lead to failure in meeting goals for weight loss. Motivation is more easily sustained by meeting "stair- step" goals.*
5. Plan progressive exercise program tailored to individual goals and choice. *Exercise may enhance weight loss by burning calories and reducing appetite, increasing energy, toning muscles, and enhancing sense of well-being and accomplishment. Walking is an excellent choice for overweight individuals.*
6. Discuss the probability of reaching plateaus when weight remains stable for extended periods. *Client should know that this is likely to happen as changes in metabolism occur. Plateaus cause frustration, and client may need additional support during these times to remain on the weight loss program.*
7. Administer medications to assist with weight loss if ordered by the physician. *Appetite-suppressant drugs (e.g., phentermine and sibutramine) may be helpful to someone who is morbidly obese. They should be used for this purpose for only a short period while the individual attempts to adjust to the new pattern of eating.*

Outcome Criteria

1. Client has established a healthy pattern of eating for weight control with weight loss progressing toward a desired goal.
2. Client verbalizes plans for future maintenance of weight control.

BODY IMAGE/SELF-ESTEEM DISTURBANCE

Definition: Confusion in mental picture of one's physical self. Negative self-evaluation and feelings about self-capabilities, which may be directly or indirectly expressed.

Possible Etiologies ("related to")

[Dissatisfaction with appearance]
[Unmet dependency needs]
[Lack of adequate nurturing by maternal figure]

Defining Characteristics ("evidenced by")

Negative feelings about body (e.g., feelings of helplessness, hopelessness, or powerlessness)
[Verbalization of desire to lose weight]
[Failure to take responsibility for self-care (self-neglect)]
[Lack of eye contact]
[Expressions of low self-worth]

Goals/Objectives

Short-Term Goal

Client will begin to accept self based on self-attributes rather than on appearance.

Long-Term Goal

Client will pursue loss of weight as desired.

Interventions with *Selected Rationales*

1. Assess client's feelings and attitudes about being obese. *Fat and compulsive eating behaviors may have deep-rooted psychological implications, such as compensation for lack of love and nurturing or a defense against intimacy.*
2. Ensure that the client has privacy during self-care activities. *The obese individual may be sensitive or self-conscious about his or her body.*
3. Have client recall coping patterns related to food in family of origin and explore how these may affect current situation. *Parents are role models for their children. Maladaptive eating behaviors are learned within the family system and are supported through positive reinforcement. Food may be substituted by the parent for affection and love, and eating is associated with a feeling of satisfaction, becoming the primary defense.*
4. Determine client's motivation for weight loss and set goals. *The individual may harbor repressed feelings of hostility, which may be expressed inward on the self. Because of a poor self-concept, the person often has difficulty with relationships. When the motivation is to lose weight for someone else, successful weight loss is less likely to occur.*
5. Help client identify positive self-attributes. Focus on strengths and past accomplishments unrelated to physical appearance. *It is important that self-esteem not be tied solely to size of the body. Client needs to recognize that obesity need not interfere with positive feelings regarding self-concept and self-worth.*

6. Refer client to support or therapy group. ***Support groups can provide companionship, increase motivation, decrease loneliness and social ostracism, and give practical solutions to common problems. Group therapy can be helpful in dealing with underlying psychological concerns.***

Outcome Criteria

1. Client has established a healthy pattern of eating for weight control with weight loss progressing toward a desired goal.
2. Client verbalizes plans for future maintenance of weight control.

■ INTERNET REFERENCES

Additional information about Anorexia Nervosa and Bulimia Nervosa may be located at the following Websites:

- http://members.aol.com/amanbu/
- http://www.psych.org/public_info/eating.html
- http://www.mentalhealth.com/dis/p20-et01.html
- http://www.anred.com/
- http://www.mentalhealth.com/dis/p20-et02.html
- http://www.nimh.nih.gov/publicat/eatdis.htm
- http://medlineplus.nlm.nih.gov/medlineplus/eatingdisorders.html

Additional information about Obesity may be located at the following Websites:

- http://www.shapeup.org/bmi/index.html
- http://www.obesity.org/
- http://medlineplus.nlm.nih.gov/medlineplus/obesity.html
- http://www.asbp.org/bariatrics/obesity.htm
- http://www.niddk.nih.gov/health/nutrit/pubs/binge.htm

CHAPTER 13

*Adjustment Disorders**

BACKGROUND ASSESSMENT DATA

The essential feature of adjustment disorder is a maladaptive reaction to an identifiable psychosocial stressor that occurs within 3 months after the onset of the stressor and has persisted for no longer than 6 months (APA, 1994). The response is considered maladaptive either because there is impairment in social or occupational functioning or because the behaviors are exaggerated beyond the usual, expected response to such a stressor. The impairment is corrected with the disappearance of, or adaptation to, the stressor. The following categories are defined:

1. **309.0 Adjustment Disorder with Depressed Mood:** This category is the most commonly diagnosed adjustment disorder. The major symptoms include depressed mood, tearfulness, and hopelessness. A differential diagnosis with the affective disorders must be considered.
2. **309.24 Adjustment Disorder with Anxiety:** The predominant manifestation of this adjustment disorder is anxiety. Major symptoms include nervousness, worry, and jitteriness. A differential diagnosis with the anxiety disorders must be considered.
3. **309.28 Adjustment Disorder with Mixed Anxiety and Depressed Mood:** The predominant manifestation of this adjustment disorder is a combination of de-

---

*Reprinted with permission from the *Diagnostic and Statistical Manual of Mental Disorders, Fourth Edition.* Copyright 1994 American Psychiatric Association, 1994.

pression and anxiety. A differential diagnosis must be made considering the affective and anxiety disorders.

4. **309.3 Adjustment Disorder with Disturbance of Conduct:** The major response involves conduct in which there is violation of the rights of others or of major age-appropriate societal norms and rules. A differential diagnosis with conduct disorder or antisocial personality disorder must be considered.
5. **309.4 Adjustment Disorder with Mixed Disturbance of Emotions and Conduct:** The predominant manifestations are both emotional symptoms (e.g., depression, anxiety) and disturbances in conduct.
6. **309.9 Adjustment Disorder Unspecified:** This diagnosis is used when the maladaptive reaction is not consistent with any of the other categories of adjustment disorder. Manifestations may include physical complaints, social withdrawal, or work or academic inhibition, without significant depressed or anxious mood.

Predisposing Factors

1. **Physiological**
   a. ***Developmental Impairment:*** The presence of chronic disorders, such as organic mental disorder or mental retardation, is thought to limit the general adaptive capacity of an individual (DeWitt, 1984).
2. **Psychosocial Theories**
   a. ***Psychodynamic Theory:*** Erikson (1963) has proposed a systematic development of the personality through the achievement of specific tasks at each stage of the life cycle. Difficulties with adjustment occur when the individual is unable to successfully complete age-appropriate tasks and becomes fixed in a lower developmental level. There is often retarded ego development and the inability to use ego defense mechanisms appropriately. Freud (1964) theorized that traumatic childhood experiences created points of fixation to which the individual, during times of stress, would be likely to regress. This might also apply to other unresolved conflicts or developmental issues.
   b. ***Cognitive Model:*** DeWitt (1984) describes the predisposition to adjustment disorder as an inability to complete the grieving process in response to a painful life change. She describes the presumed cause of this inability to adapt as *psychic overload,*

"a level of intrapsychic strain that exceeds the individual's ability to cope and may therefore disrupt normal functioning and cause psychological or somatic symptoms." Some individuals remain in denial, acting as though the event never occurred. In others, intrusive symptoms may predominate. In all instances, however, it is the persistence of unwanted emotions and images, and the feeling of being powerless to stop them, that precludes the dysfunctional response. Popkin (1989) believes that in adjustment disorder, a specific meaningful stress has found the point of vulnerability in a person of otherwise adequate ego strength.

c. ***Stress-Adaptation Model:*** This model considers the type of stressor the individual experiences, the situational context in which it occurs, and intrapersonal factors in the predisposition to adjustment disorder. Andreasen and Wasek (1980) found that continuous stressors (those to which an individual is exposed over an extended period of time) were more commonly cited than sudden-shock stressors (those that occur without warning) as precipitants to maladaptive functioning.

The situational context in which the stressor occurs may include factors such as personal and general economic conditions; occupational and recreational opportunities; the availability of social supports, such as family, friends, and neighbors; and the availability of cultural or religious support groups.

Intrapersonal factors that have been implicated in the predisposition to adjustment disorder include birth temperament, learned social skills and coping strategies, presence of psychiatric illness, degree of flexibility, and level of intelligence.

Symptomatology (Subjective and Objective Data)

1. Depressed mood.
2. Tearfulness.
3. Hopelessness.
4. Nervousness.
5. Worry.
6. Jitteriness.
7. Ambivalence.

8. Anger, expressed inappropriately.
9. Increased dependency.
10. Violation of the rights of others.
11. Violation of societal norms and rules, such as truancy, vandalism, reckless driving, fighting.
12. Inability to function occupationally or academically.
13. Manipulative behavior.
14. Social isolation.
15. Physical complaints, such as headache, backache, other aches and pains, fatigue.

Common Nursing Diagnoses and Interventions

(Interventions are applicable to various health-care settings, such as inpatient and partial hospitalization, community outpatient clinic, home health, and private practice.)

RISK FOR VIOLENCE: SELF-DIRECTED OR DIRECTED AT OTHERS

Definition: Behaviors in which an individual demonstrates that he/she can be physically, emotionally, and/or sexually harmful either to self or to others.

Related/Risk Factors ("related to")

[Fixation in earlier level of development]
[Negative role modeling]
[Dysfunctional family system]
[Low self-esteem]
[Unresolved grief]
[Psychic overload]
[Extended exposure to stressful situation]
[Lack of support systems]
[Biological factors, such as organic changes in the brain]
Body language—rigid posture, clenching of fists and jaw, hyperactivity, pacing, breathlessness, and threatening stances
[History of threats of violence toward self or others or of destruction to the property of others]
Impulsivity
Suicidal ideation, plan, available means
[Anger; rage]
[Increasing anxiety level]
[Depressed mood]

Goals/Objectives

Short-Term Goals

1. Client will seek out staff member when hostile or suicidal feelings occur.
2. Client will verbalize adaptive coping strategies for use when hostile or suicidal feelings occur.

Long-Term Goals

1. Client will demonstrate adaptive coping strategies for use when hostile or suicidal feelings occur.
2. Client will not harm self or others.

Interventions with *Selected Rationales*

1. Observe client's behavior frequently. Do this through routine activities and interactions; avoid appearing watchful and suspicious. ***Close observation is required so that intervention can occur if required to ensure client's (and others') safety.***
2. Observe for suicidal behaviors: verbal statements, such as "I'm going to kill myself" and "Very soon my mother won't have to worry herself about me any longer," and nonverbal behaviors, such as giving away cherished items and mood swings. ***Clients who are contemplating suicide often give clues regarding their potential behavior. The clues may be very subtle and require keen assessment skills on the part of the nurse.***
3. Determine suicidal intent and available means. Ask direct questions, such as "Do you plan to kill yourself?" and "How do you plan to do it?" ***The risk of suicide is greatly increased if the client has developed a plan and particularly if means exist for the client to execute the plan.***
4. Obtain verbal or written contract from client agreeing not to harm self and to seek out staff in the event that suicidal ideation occurs. ***Discussion of suicidal feelings with a trusted individual provides a degree of relief to the client. A contract gets the subject out in the open and places some of the responsibility for his or her safety with the client. An attitude of acceptance of the client as a worthwhile individual is conveyed.***
5. Assist client to recognize when anger occurs and to accept those feelings as his or her own. Have client keep an "anger notebook," in which feelings of anger experi-

enced during a 24-hour period are recorded. Information regarding source of anger, behavioral response, and client's perception of the situation should also be noted. Discuss entries with client and suggest alternative behavioral responses for those identified as maladaptive.

6. Act as a role model for appropriate expression of angry feelings and give positive reinforcement to client for attempting to conform. ***It is vital that the client express angry feelings, because suicide and other self-destructive behaviors are often viewed as a result of anger turned inward on the self.***
7. Remove all dangerous objects from client's environment (e.g., sharp items, belts, ties, straps, breakable items, smoking materials). ***Client safety is a nursing priority.***
8. Try to redirect violent behavior with physical outlets for the client's anxiety (e.g., punching bag, jogging). ***Physical exercise is a safe and effective way of relieving pent-up tension.***
9. Be available to stay with client as anxiety level and tensions begin to rise. ***Presence of a trusted individual provides a feeling of security and may help to prevent rapid escalation of anxiety.***
10. Staff should maintain and convey a calm attitude to client. ***Anxiety is contagious and can be transmitted from staff members to client.***
11. Have sufficient staff available to indicate a show of strength to client if necessary. ***This conveys to the client evidence of control over the situation and provides some physical security for staff.***
12. Administer tranquilizing medications as ordered by physician or obtain an order if necessary. Monitor client response for effectiveness of the medication and for adverse side effects. ***Tranquilizing medications such as anxiolytics or antipsychotics have the capability of inducing a calming effect on the client and may prevent aggressive behaviors.***
13. Use of mechanical restraints or isolation room may be required if less restrictive interventions are unsuccessful. Follow policy and procedure prescribed by the institution in executing this intervention. Most states require that the physician re-evaluate the client and issue a new order for restraints every 3 hours, except between the hours of midnight and 8:00 AM. If the client has previously refused medication, administer after restraints have been applied. Most states consider this intervention appropriate in

emergency situations or in the event that a client would likely harm self or others.

14. Observe the client in restraints every 15 minutes (or according to institutional policy). Ensure that circulation to extremities is not compromised (check temperature, color, pulses). Assist client with needs related to nutrition, hydration, and elimination. Position client so that comfort is facilitated and aspiration can be prevented. ***Client safety is a nursing priority.***
15. As agitation decreases, assess client's readiness for restraint removal or reduction. Remove one restraint at a time, while assessing client's response. ***This minimizes risk of injury to the client and staff.***

Outcome Criteria

1. Anxiety is maintained at a level at which client feels no need for aggression.
2. Client denies any ideas of self-destruction.
3. Client demonstrates use of adaptive coping strategies when feelings of hostility or suicide occur.
4. Client verbalizes community support systems from whom assistance may be requested when personal coping strategies are not successful.

ANXIETY (Moderate to Severe)

Definition: A vague uneasy feeling of discomfort or dread accompanied by an autonomic response; the source is often nonspecific or unknown to the individual; a feeling of apprehension caused by anticipation of danger. It is an altering signal that warns of impending danger and enables the individual to take measures to deal with threat.

Possible Etiologies ("related to"):

Situational and maturational crises
[Low self-esteem]
[Dysfunctional family system]
[Feelings of powerlessness and lack of control in life situation]
[Retarded ego development]
[Fixation in earlier level of development]

Defining Characteristics ("evidenced by"]

Increased tension
Increased helplessness

Overexcited
Apprehensive; fearful
Restlessness
Poor eye contact
Feelings of inadequacy
Insomnia
Focus on the self
Increased cardiac and respiratory rates
[Difficulty learning]

Goals/Objectives

Short-Term Goal

Client will demonstrate use of relaxation techniques to maintain anxiety at manageable level within 7 days.

Long-Term Goal

By discharge from treatment, client will be able to recognize events that precipitate anxiety and intervene to prevent disabling behaviors.

Interventions with *Selected Rationales*

1. Be available to stay with client. Remain calm and provide reassurance of safety. ***Client safety and security is a nursing priority.***
2. Help client identify situation that precipitated onset of anxiety symptoms. ***Client may be unaware that emotional issues are related to symptoms of anxiety. Recognition may be the first step in elimination of this maladaptive response.***
3. Review client's methods of coping with similar situations in the past. Discuss ways in which client may assume control over these situations. ***In seeking to create change, it would be helpful for client to identify past responses and to determine whether they were successful and whether they could be employed again. A measure of control reduces feelings of powerlessness in a situation, ultimately decreasing anxiety. Client strengths should be identified and used to his or her advantage.***
4. Provide quiet environment. Reduce stimuli: low lighting, few people. ***Anxiety level may be decreased in calm atmosphere with few stimuli.***
5. Administer antianxiety medications as ordered by physician, or obtain order if necessary. Monitor client's response for effectiveness of the medication as well as for adverse side effects. ***Antianxiety medications (e.g., diazepam, chlordiazepoxide, alprazolam) provide relief from the***

immobilizing effects of anxiety and may facilitate client's cooperation with therapy.

6. Discuss with client signs of increasing anxiety and ways of intervening to maintain the anxiety at a manageable level (e.g., exercise, walking, jogging, relaxation techniques). *Anxiety and tension can be reduced safely and with benefit to the client through physical activities.*

Outcome Criteria

1. Client is able to verbalize events that precipitate anxiety and demonstrate techniques for its reduction.
2. Client is able to verbalize ways in which he or she may gain more control of the environment and thereby reduce feelings of powerlessness.

INEFFECTIVE INDIVIDUAL COPING

Definition: Inability to form a valid appraisal of the stressors, inadequate choices of practiced responses, and/or inability to use available resources.

Possible Etiologies ("related to")

Situational crises
Maturational crises
[Inadequate support systems]
[Negative role modeling]
[Retarded ego development]
[Fixation in earlier level of development]
[Dysfunctional family system]
[Low self-esteem]
[Unresolved grief]

Defining Characteristics ("evidenced by")

Inability to meet role expectations
[Alteration in societal participation]
[Increased dependency]
[Manipulation of others in the environment for purposes of fulfilling own desires]
[Refusal to follow rules]
Inadequate problem solving

Goals/Objectives

Short-Term Goal

By the end of 1 week, client will comply with rules of therapy and refrain from manipulating others to fulfill own desires.

Long-Term Goal

By discharge from treatment, client will identify, develop, and use socially acceptable coping skills.

Interventions with *Selected Rationales*

1. Discuss with client the rules of therapy and consequences of noncompliance. Carry out the consequences matter of factly if rules are broken. ***Negative consequences may work to decrease manipulative behaviors.***
2. Do not debate, argue, rationalize, or bargain with the client regarding limit setting on manipulative behaviors. ***Ignoring these attempts may work to decrease manipulative behaviors. Consistency among all staff members is vital if this intervention is to be successful.***
3. Encourage discussion of angry feelings. Help client identify the true object of the hostility. Provide physical outlets for healthy release of the hostile feelings (e.g., punching bags, pounding boards). ***Verbalization of feelings with a trusted individual may help client work through unresolved issues. Physical exercise provides a safe and effective means of releasing pent-up tension.***
4. Take care not to reinforce dependent behaviors. Encourage client to perform as independently as possible and provide positive feedback. ***Independent accomplishment and positive reinforcement enhance self-esteem and encourage repetition of desirable behaviors.***
5. Help client recognize some aspects of his or her life over which a measure of control is maintained. ***Recognition of personal control, however minimal, diminishes the feeling of powerlessness and decreases the need for manipulation of others.***
6. Identify the stressor that precipitated the maladaptive coping. If a major life change has occurred, encourage client to express fears and feelings associated with the change. Assist client through the problem-solving process:
   a. Identify possible alternatives that indicate positive adaptation.
   b. Discuss benefits and consequences of each alternative.
   c. Select the most appropriate alternative.
   d. Implement the alternative.
   e. Evaluate the effectiveness of the alternative.
   f. Recognize areas of limitation and make modifications. Request assistance with this process, if needed.
7. Provide positive reinforcement for application of adaptive coping skills and evidence of successful adjustment. ***Positive reinforcement enhances self-esteem and encourages repetition of desirable behaviors.***

Outcome Criteria

1. Client is able to verbalize alternative, socially acceptable, and lifestyle-appropriate coping skills he or she plans to use in response to stress.
2. Client is able to solve problems and fulfill ADLs independently.
3. Client does not manipulate others for own gratification.

IMPAIRED ADJUSTMENT*

Definition: Inability to modify lifestyle behavior in a manner consistent with a change in health status.

Possible etiologies ("related to")

Low state of optimism
Intense emotional state
Negative attitudes toward health behavior
Failure to intend to change behavior
Multiple stressors
Absence of social support for changed beliefs and practices
Disability or health status change requiring change in lifestyle
Lack of motivation to change behaviors

Defining Characteristics ("evidenced by")

Denial of health status change
Failure to achieve optimal sense of control
Failure to take actions that would prevent further health problems
Demonstration of nonacceptance of health status change

Goals/Objectives

Short-Term Goals

1. Client will discuss with primary nurse the kinds of lifestyle changes that will occur because of the change in health status.
2. With the help of primary nurse, client will formulate a plan of action for incorporating those changes into his or her lifestyle.
3. Client will demonstrate movement toward independence, considering change in health status.

*According to the North American Nursing Diagnosis Association definition, this diagnosis would only be appropriate for the person with adjustment disorder if the precipitating stressor was a change in health status.

Long-Term Goal

Client will demonstrate competence to function independently to his or her optimal ability, considering change in health status, by discharge from treatment.

Interventions with *Selected Rationales*

1. Encourage client to talk about lifestyle prior to the change in health status. Discuss coping mechanisms that were used at stressful times in the past. ***It is important to identify the client's strengths so that they may be used to facilitate adaptation to the change or loss that has occurred.***
2. Encourage client to discuss the change or loss and particularly to express anger associated with it. ***Some individuals may not realize that anger is a normal stage in the grieving process. If it is not released in an appropriate manner, it may be turned inward on the self, leading to pathological depression.***
3. Encourage client to express fears associated with the change or loss, or the alteration in lifestyle that the change or loss has created. ***Change often creates a feeling of disequilibrium and the individual may respond with fears that are irrational or unfounded. He or she may benefit from feedback that corrects misperceptions about how life will be with the change in health status.***
4. Provide assistance with ADLs as required, but encourage independence to the limit that client's ability will allow. Give positive feedback for activities accomplished independently. ***Independent accomplishments and positive feedback enhance self-esteem and encourage repetition of desired behaviors. Successes also provide hope that adaptive functioning is possible and decrease feelings of powerlessness.***
5. Help client with decision making regarding incorporation of change or loss into lifestyle. Identify problems that the change or loss is likely to create. Discuss alternative solutions, weighing potential benefits and consequences of each alternative. Support client's decision in the selection of an alternative. ***The high degree of anxiety that usually accompanies a major lifestyle change often interferes with an individual's ability to solve problems and to make appropriate decisions. Client may need assistance with this process in an effort to progress toward successful adaptation.***
6. Use role playing ***to decrease anxiety*** as client anticipates stressful situations that might occur in relation to the

health status change. ***Role playing decreases anxiety and provides a feeling of security by preparing the client with a plan of action to respond in an appropriate manner when a stressful situation occurs.***

7. Ensure that client and family are fully knowledgeable regarding the physiology of the change in health status and its necessity for optimal wellness. Encourage them to ask questions, and provide printed material explaining the change to which they may refer following discharge.
8. Help client identify resources within the community from which he or she may seek assistance in adapting to the change in health status. Examples include self-help or support groups and public health nurse, counselor, or social worker. Encourage client to keep follow-up appointments with physician or to call physician's office prior to follow-up date if problems or concerns arise.

Outcome Criteria

1. Client is able to perform ADLs independently.
2. Client is able to make independent decisions regarding lifestyle, considering change in health status.
3. Client is able to express hope for the future, with consideration of change in health status.

DYSFUNCTIONAL GRIEVING

Definition: Extended, unsuccessful use of intellectual and emotional responses by which individuals (families, communities) attempt to work through the process of modifying self-concept based upon the perception of [actual or] potential loss.

Possible Etiologies ("related to")

[Real or perceived loss of any concept of value to the individual]
[Bereavement overload (cumulative grief from multiple unresolved losses)]
[Thwarted grieving response to a loss]
[Absence of anticipatory grieving]
[Feelings of guilt generated by ambivalent relationship with lost concept]

Defining Characteristics ("evidenced by")

Verbal expression of distress at loss
Idealization of lost [concept]
Denial of loss

[Excessive anger, expressed inappropriately]
Developmental regression
Alterations in concentration or pursuit of tasks
Difficulty in expressing loss
Labile affect
Interference with life functioning
Repetitive use of ineffectual behaviors associated with attempts to reinvest in relationships
Reliving of past experiences with little or no reduction of intensity of the grief
Prolonged interference with life functioning, with onset or exacerbation of somatic or psychosomatic responses

Goals/Objectives

Short-Term Goal

By end of 1 week, client will express anger toward lost concept.

Long-Term Goal

Client will be able to verbalize behaviors associated with the normal stages of grief and identify own position in grief process, while progressing at own pace toward resolution.

Interventions with *Selected Rationales*

1. Determine stage of grief in which client is fixed. Identify behaviors associated with this stage. ***Accurate baseline assessment data are necessary to plan effective care for the grieving client.***
2. Develop trusting relationship with client. Show empathy and caring. Be honest and keep all promises. ***Trust is the basis for a therapeutic relationship.***
3. Convey an accepting attitude so that the client is not afraid to express feelings openly. ***An accepting attitude conveys to the client that you believe he or she is a worthwhile person. Trust is enhanced.***
4. Allow client to express anger. Do not become defensive if initial expression of anger is displaced on nurse or therapist. Assist client in exploring angry feelings so that they may be directed toward the intended object or person. ***Verbalization of feelings in a nonthreatening environment may help client come to terms with unresolved issues.***
5. Assist client in discharging pent-up anger through participation in large motor activities (e.g., brisk walks, jogging, physical exercises, volleyball, punching bag, exercise bike). ***Physical exercise provides a safe and effective method for discharging pent-up tension.***

6. Explain to client the normal stages of grief and the behaviors associated with each stage. Help client to understand that feelings such as guilt and anger toward the lost concept are appropriate and acceptable during the grief process. ***Knowledge of the acceptability of the feelings associated with normal grieving may help to relieve some of the guilt that these responses generate.***
7. Encourage client to review relationship with lost concept. With support and sensitivity, point out reality of the situation in areas in which misrepresentations are expressed. ***Client must give up idealized perception and be able to accept both positive and negative aspects about the lost concept before the grief process is complete.***
8. Communicate to client that crying is acceptable. Use of touch is therapeutic and appropriate with most clients. Knowledge of cultural influences specific to the client is important before employing this technique.
9. Assist client in solving problems as he or she attempts to determine methods for more adaptive coping with the experienced loss. Provide positive feedback for strategies identified and decisions made. ***Positive reinforcement enhances self-esteem and encourages repetition of desirable behaviors.***
10. Encourage client to reach out for spiritual support during this time in whatever form is desirable to him or her. Assess spiritual needs of client and assist as necessary in the fulfillment of those needs.

Outcome Criteria

1. Client is able to verbalize normal stages of grief process and behaviors associated with each stage.
2. Client is able to identify own position within the grief process and express honest feelings related to the lost concept.
3. Client is no longer manifesting exaggerated emotions and behaviors related to dysfunctional grieving and is able to carry out ADLs independently.

SELF-ESTEEM DISTURBANCE

Definition: Negative self-evaluation and feelings about self or self-capabilities, which may be directly or indirectly expressed.

Possible Etiologies ("related to")

[Lack of positive feedback]

[Unmet dependency needs]
[Retarded ego development]
[Repeated negative feedback, resulting in diminished self-worth]
[Personal or situational factors such as dysfunctional family system or absence of social support]

Defining Characteristics ("evidenced by")

[Difficulty accepting positive reinforcement]
[Nonparticipation in therapy]
Self-negating verbalizations
Evaluation of self as unable to deal with events
Hesitant to try new things or situations [because of fear of failure]
Projection of blame or responsibility for problems
Rationalization of personal failures
Hypersensitivity to slight or criticism
Grandiosity
[Lack of eye contact]
[Manipulation of one staff member against another in an attempt to gain special privileges]
[Inability to form close, personal relationships]
[Degradation of others in an attempt to increase own feelings of self-worth]

Goals/Objectives

Short-Term Goals

1. Client will discuss fear of failure with nurse within (realistic time period).
2. Client will verbalize things he or she likes about self within (realistic time period).

Long-Term Goals

1. Client will exhibit increased feelings of self-worth as evidenced by verbal expression of positive aspects about self, past accomplishments, and future prospects.
2. Client will exhibit increased feelings of self-worth by setting realistic goals and trying to reach them, thereby demonstrating a decrease in fear of failure.

Interventions with *Selected Rationales*

1. Ensure that goals are realistic. It is important for client to achieve something, so plan for activities in which success is likely. *Success enhances self-esteem.*
2. Convey unconditional positive regard for the client. Promote understanding of your acceptance of him or her as a worthwhile human being.

3. Spend time with the client, both on a one-to-one basis and in group activities. ***This conveys to client that you feel he or she is worth your time.***
4. Assist client in identifying positive aspects of self and in developing plans for changing the characteristics he or she views as negative. ***Individuals with low self-esteem often have difficulty recognizing their positive attributes. They may also lack problem-solving ability and require assistance in formulating a plan for implementing the desired changes.***
5. Encourage and support client in confronting the fear of failure by attending therapy activities and undertaking new tasks. Offer recognition of successful endeavors and positive reinforcement for attempts made. ***Recognition and positive reinforcement enhance self-esteem.***
6. Do not allow client to ruminate about past failures. Withdraw attention if he or she persists. ***Lack of attention to these behaviors may discourage their repetition. Client must focus on positive attributes if self-esteem is to be enhanced.***
7. Minimize negative feedback to client. Enforce limit setting in matter-of-fact manner, imposing previously established consequences for violations. ***Negative feedback can be extremely threatening to a person with low self-esteem, possibly aggravating the problem. Consequences should convey unacceptability of the BEHAVIOR, but not the PERSON.***
8. Encourage independence in the performance of personal responsibilities, as well as in decision making related to own self-care. Offer recognition and praise for accomplishments. ***The ability to perform self-care activities independently enhances self-esteem. Positive reinforcement encourages repetition of the desirable behavior.***
9. Help client increase level of self-awareness through critical examination of feelings, attitudes, and behaviors. Help him or her to understand that it is perfectly acceptable for one's attitudes and behaviors to differ from others' as long as they do not become intrusive. ***As the client achieves self-awareness and self-acceptance, the need for judging the behavior of others will diminish.***

Outcome Criteria

1. Client verbalizes positive perception of self.
2. Client demonstrates ability to manage own self-care, make independent decisions, and use problem-solving skills.
3. Client sets goals that are realistic and works to achieve those goals without evidence of fear of failure.

IMPAIRED SOCIAL INTERACTION

Definition: The state in which an individual participates in an insufficient or excessive quantity or ineffective quality of social exchange.

Possible Etiologies ("related to")

[Retarded ego development]
[Fixation in an earlier level of development]
[Negative role modeling]
[Low self-esteem]

Defining Characteristics ("evidenced by")

Verbalized or observed discomfort in social situations
Verbalized or observed inability to receive or communicate a satisfying sense of belonging, caring, interest, or shared history
Observed use of unsuccessful social interaction behaviors
Dysfunctional interaction with peers, family, or others
[Exhibiting behaviors unacceptable for age, as defined by dominant cultural group]

Goals/Objectives

Short-Term Goal

Client will develop trusting relationship with staff member within (realistic time period), seeking that staff member out for one-to-one interaction.

Long-Term Goals

1. Client will be able to interact with others on a one-to-one basis with no indication of discomfort.
2. Client will voluntarily spend time with others in group activities demonstrating acceptable, age-appropriate behavior.

Interventions with *Selected Rationales*

1. Develop trusting relationship with client. Be honest; keep all promises; convey acceptance of person, separate from unacceptable behaviors ("It is not *you,* but *your behavior,* that is unacceptable.") ***Unconditional acceptance of the client increases his or her feelings of self-worth.***
2. Offer to remain with client during initial interactions with others on the unit. ***Presence of a trusted individual provides a feeling of security.***
3. Provide constructive criticism and positive reinforcement for efforts. ***Positive reinforcement enhances self-esteem and encourages repetition of desirable behaviors.***

4. Confront client and withdraw attention when interactions with others are manipulative or exploitative. ***Attention to the unacceptable behavior may reinforce it.***
5. Act as role model for client through appropriate interactions with him or her, other clients, and staff members.
6. Provide group situations for client. ***It is through these group interactions, with positive and negative feedback from his or her peers, that client will learn socially acceptable behavior.***

Outcome Criteria

1. Client seeks out staff member for social as well as therapeutic interaction.
2. Client has formed and satisfactorily maintained one interpersonal relationship with another client.
3. Client willingly and appropriately participates in group activities.
4. Client verbalizes reasons for inability to form close interpersonal relationships with others in the past.

RELOCATION STRESS SYNDROME*

Definition: A state in which an individual experiences physiological or psychosocial disturbances as a result of transfer from one environment to another.

Possible Etiologies ("related to")

Change in environment or location
Past, concurrent, and recent losses
Losses involved with decision to move
Feeling of powerlessness
Lack of adequate support system
Little or no preparation for the impending move
Moderate to high degree of environmental change
History and types of previous transfers
Impaired psychosocial health status
Decreased physical health status

Defining Characteristics ("evidenced by")

Anxiety; restlessness
Apprehension

*This diagnosis would be appropriate for the individual with adjustment disorder if the precipitating stressor was relocation to a new environment.

Depression; sad effect
Loneliness
Verbalization of [opposition] to relocate
Sleep disturbance
Change in eating habits; weight change
Dependency; increased verbalization of needs
Gastrointestinal disturbances
Insecurity in new surroundings; lack of trust
Verbalization of being concerned/upset about [relocation]
Withdrawal; [social isolation]

Goals/Objectives

Short-Term Goal

Client will verbalize at least one positive aspect regarding relocation to new environment within (realistic time period).

Long-Term Goal

Client will demonstrate positive adaptation to new environment, as evidenced by involvement in activities, expression of satisfaction with new acquaintances, and elimination of previously evident physical and psychological symptoms associated with the relocation (time dimension to be determined individually).

Interventions with *Selected Rationales*

1. Encourage individual to discuss feelings (concerns, fears, anger) regarding relocation. ***Exploration of feelings with a trusted individual may help the individual perceive the situation more realistically and come to terms with the inevitable change.***
2. Encourage individual to discuss how the change will affect his or her life. Ensure that the individual is involved in decision making and problem solving regarding the move. ***Taking responsibility for making choices regarding the relocation will increase feelings of control and decrease feelings of powerlessness.***
3. Assist the individual in identifying positive aspects about the move. ***Anxiety associated with the opposed relocation may interfere with the individual's ability to recognize anything positive about it. Assistance may be required.***
4. Assist the individual in identifying resources within the new community from whom assistance with various types of services may be obtained. ***Because of anxiety and depression, the individual may not be able to identify these resources alone. Assistance with problem solving may be required.***

5. Identify groups within the community that specialize in helping individuals adapt to relocation. Examples include Newcomers's Club, Welcome Wagon Club, senior citizens' groups, as well as school and church organizations. *These groups offer support from individuals who have often encountered similar experiences. Adaptation may be enhanced by the reassurance, encouragement, and support of peers who exhibit positive adaptation to relocation stress.*
6. Refer individual or family for professional counseling if deemed necessary. *An individual who is experiencing dysfunctional grieving over loss of previous residence may require therapy to achieve resolution of the problem. It may be that other unresolved issues are interfering with successful adaptation to the relocation.*

Outcome Criteria

1. The individual no longer exhibits signs of anxiety, depression, or somatic symptoms.
2. The individual verbalizes satisfaction with new environment.
3. The individual willingly participates in social and vocational activities within his or her new environment.

■ INTERNET REFERENCES

Additional information about Adjustment Disorder may be located at the following Websites:

- http://www.mentalhealth.com/rx/p23-aj01.html
- http://www.cmhc.com/disorders/sx6.htm
- http://www.mentalhealth.com/mag1/p5h-adj1.html

CHAPTER 14

*Impulse Control Disorders**

■ BACKGROUND ASSESSMENT DATA

Impulse control disorders are characterized by a need or desire that must be satisfied immediately, regardless of the consequences (Booth, 1984). Many of the behaviors have adverse or even destructive consequences for the individuals affected, and seldom do these individuals know why they do what they do or why it is pleasurable.

The *DSM-IV* (APA, 1994) describes the essential features of impulse control disorders as follows:

1. Failure to resist an impulse, drive, or temptation to perform some act that is harmful to the person or others.
2. An increasing sense of tension or arousal before committing the act.
3. An experience of either pleasure, gratification, or relief at the time of committing the act. Following the act, there may or may not be regret, self-reproach, or guilt.

The *DSM-IV* (APA, 1994) describes the following categories of impulse control disorders:

312.34 Intermittent Explosive Disorder

This disorder is characterized by discrete episodes of failure to resist aggressive impulses, resulting in serious assaults or destruction of property (APA, 1994). Some clients report changes in sensorium, such as confusion

---

*Reprinted with permission from the *Diagnostic and Statistical Manual of Mental Disorders, Fourth Edition.* Copyright 1994 American Psychiatric Association, 1994.

during an episode or amnesia of events that occurred during an episode. Symptoms usually appear suddenly without apparent provocation and terminate abruptly, lasting only minutes to a few hours, followed by feelings of genuine remorse and self-reproach about the behavior.

312.32 Kleptomania

Kleptomania is described by the *DSM-IV* as "the recurrent failure to resist impulses to steal items not needed for personal use or for their monetary value" (APA, 1994). Often the stolen items (for which the individual usually has enough money to pay) are given away, discarded, returned, or kept and hidden. The individual with kleptomania steals purely for the sake of stealing and for the sense of relief and gratification that follows an episode.

312.31 Pathological Gambling

The *DSM-IV* defines pathological gambling as "persistent and recurrent maladaptive gambling behavior that disrupts personal, family, or vocational pursuits" (APA, 1994). The preoccupation with gambling, and impulse to gamble, intensifies when the individual is under stress. Many pathological gamblers exhibit characteristics associated with narcissism and grandiosity and often have difficulties with intimacy, empathy, and trust (Booth, 1984).

312.33 Pyromania

Pyromania is the inability to resist the impulse to set fires (Booth, 1984). The act itself is preceded by tension or affective arousal, and the individual experiences intense pleasure, gratification, or relief when setting the fires, witnessing their effects, or participating in their aftermath (APE, 1994). Motivation for the behavior is self-gratification, and even though some individuals with pyromania may take precautions to avoid apprehension, many are totally indifferent to the consequences of their behavior.

312.39 Trichotillomania

This disorder is defined by the *DSM-IV* as "the recurrent pulling out of one's own hair that results in noticeable hair loss" (APA, 1994). The impulse is preceded by an increasing sense of tension, and the individual experiences a sense of release or gratification from pulling out the hair.

Predisposing Factors

1. **Physiological**
   a. ***Genetics:*** A familial tendency appears to be a factor in some cases of intermittent explosive disorder, pathological gambling, and trichotillomania.
   b. ***Physical Factors:*** Brain trauma or dysfunction and mental retardation have also been implicated in the predisposition to impulse control disorders (Kaplan, Sadock, and Grebb, 1994).
2. **Psychosocial**
   a. ***Family Dynamics:*** Various dysfunctional family patterns have been suggested as contributors in the predisposition to impulse control disorders. These include the following:
      - Child abuse or neglect
      - Parental rejection or abandonment
      - Harsh or inconsistent discipline
      - Emotional deprivation
      - Parental substance abuse
      - Parental unpredictability

Symptomatology (Subjective and Objective Data)

1. Sudden inability to control violent, aggressive impulses.
2. Aggressive behavior accompanied by confusion or amnesia.
3. Feelings of remorse following aggressive behavior.
4. Inability to resist impulses to steal.
5. Increasing tension before committing the theft, followed by pleasure or relief during and following the act.
6. Sometimes discards, returns, or hides stolen items.
7. Inability to resist impulses to gamble.
8. Preoccupation with ways to obtain money with which to gamble.
9. Increasing tension that is relieved only by placing a bet.
10. The need to gamble or the loss of money interferes with social and occupational functioning.

11. Inability to resist the impulse to set fires.
12. Increasing tension that is relieved only by starting a fire.
13. Inability to resist impulses to pull out one's own hair.
14. Increasing tension followed by a sense of release or gratification from pulling out the hair.
15. Hair pulling may be accompanied by other types of self-mutilation (e.g., head banging, biting, scratching).

Common Nursing Diagnoses and Interventions

(Interventions are applicable to various health-care settings, such as inpatient and partial hospitalization, community outpatient clinic, home health, and private practice.)

RISK FOR VIOLENCE: DIRECTED TOWARD OTHERS

Definition: Behaviors in which an individual demonstrates that he/she can be physically, emotionally, and/or sexually harmful to others.

Related/Risk Factors ("related to")

[Possible familial tendency]
[Central nervous system trauma]
[Dysfunctional family system, resulting in behaviors such as the following:
- Child abuse or neglect
- Parental rejection or abandonment
- Harsh or inconsistent discipline
- Emotional deprivation
- Parental substance abuse
- Parental unpredictability]

Body language—rigid posture, clenching of fists and jaw, hyperactivity, pacing, breathlessness, and threatening stances
[History or threats of violence toward others or of destruction to the property of others]
Impulsivity

Goals/Objectives

Short-Term Goal

Client will recognize signs of increasing tension, anxiety, and agitation, and report to staff (or others) for assistance with intervention (time dimension to be individually determined).

Long-Term Goal

Client will not harm others or the property of others (time dimension to be individually determined).

Interventions with *Selected Rationales*

1. Convey an accepting attitude toward the client. Feelings of rejection are undoubtedly familiar to him or her. Work on the development of trust. Be honest, keep all promises, and convey the message that it is not *him* or *her* but the *behavior* that is unacceptable. ***An attitude of acceptance promotes feelings of self-worth. Trust is the basis of a therapeutic relationship.***
2. Maintain low level of stimuli in client's environment (low lighting, few people, simple decor, low noise level). ***A stimulating environment may increase agitation and promote aggressive behavior. Make the client's environment as safe as possible*** by removing all potentially dangerous objects.
3. Help client identify the true object of his or her hostility. ***Because of weak ego development, client may be unable to use ego defense mechanisms correctly. Helping him or her recognize this in a nonthreatening manner may help reveal unresolved issues so that they may be confronted.***
4. Staff should maintain and convey a calm attitude. ***Anxiety is contagious and can be transferred from staff to client. A calm attitude provides the client with a feeling of safety and security.***
5. Help the client recognize signs that tension is increasing and ways in which violence can be averted. ***Activities that require physical exertion are helpful in relieving pent-up tension.***
6. Explain to the client that should explosive behavior occur, staff will intervene in whatever way is required (e.g., tranquilizing medication, restraints, isolation) to protect client and others. ***This conveys to the client evidence of control over the situation and provides a feeling of safety and security.***

Outcome Criteria

1. Anxiety is maintained at a level at which client feels no need for aggression.

2. The client is able to verbalize the symptoms of increasing tension and adaptive ways of coping with it.
3. The client is able to inhibit the impulse for violence and aggression.

RISK FOR SELF-MUTILATION

Definition: A state in which an individual is at risk to perform an act on the self to injure, not kill, which produces tissue damage and tension relief.

Related/Risk Factors ("related to")

[Possible familial tendency]
[Central nervous system trauma]
[Mental retardation]
[Early emotional deprivation]
[Parental rejection or abandonment]
[Child abuse or neglect]
[History of self-mutilative behaviors in response to increasing anxiety: hair pulling, biting, head banging, scratching]

Goals/Objectives

Short-Term Goal

Client will cooperate with plan of behavior modification in an effort to respond more adaptively to stress (time dimension ongoing).

Long-Term Goal

Client will not harm self.

Interventions with *Selected Rationales*

1. Intervene to protect client when self-mutilative behaviors, such as head banging or hair pulling, become evident. ***The nurse is responsible for ensuring client safety.***
2. A helmet may be used to protect against head banging, hand mitts to prevent hair pulling, and appropriate padding to protect extremities from injury during hysterical movements.
3. Try to determine whether self-mutilative behaviors occur in response to increasing anxiety and, if so, to what the anxiety may be attributed. ***Self-mutilative behaviors may be averted if the cause can be determined.***
4. Work on one-to-one basis with client ***to establish trust.***

5. Assist with plan for behavior modification *in an effort to teach the client more adaptive ways of responding to stress.*
6. Encourage client to discuss feelings, particularly anger, *in an effort to confront unresolved issues and expose internalized rage that may be triggering self-mutilative behaviors.*
7. Offer self to client during times of increasing anxiety, *to provide feelings of security and decrease need for self-mutilative behaviors.*

Outcome Criteria

1. Anxiety is maintained at a level at which client feels no need for self-mutilation.
2. Client demonstrates ability to use adaptive coping strategies in the face of stressful situations.

INEFFECTIVE INDIVIDUAL COPING

Definition: Inability to form a valid appraisal of the stressors, inadequate choices of practiced responses, and/or inability to use available resources.

Possible Etiologies ("related to")

[Possible hereditary factors]
[Brain trauma or dysfunction]
[Mental retardation]
[Dysfunctional family system, resulting in behaviors such as the following:
Child abuse or neglect
Parental rejection or abandonment
Harsh or inconsistent discipline
Emotional deprivation
Parental substance abuse
Parental unpredictability]

Defining Characteristics ("evidenced by")

[Inability to control impulse of violence or aggression]
[Inability to control impulse to steal]
[Inability to control impulse to gamble]
[Inability to control impulse to set fires]
[Inability to control impulse to pull out own hair]
[Feeling of intense anxiety and tension that precedes, and is relieved by, engaging in these impulsive behaviors]

Goals/Objectives

Short-Term Goal

Client will verbalize adaptive ways to cope with stress by means other than impulsive behaviors (time dimension to be individually determined).

Long-Term Goal

Client will be able to delay gratification and use adaptive coping strategies in response to stress (time dimension to be individually determined).

Interventions with *Selected Rationales*

1. Help client gain insight into his or her own behaviors. Often these individuals rationalize to such an extent that they deny that what they have done is wrong. ***Client must come to understand that certain behaviors will not be tolerated within the society and that severe consequences will be imposed on those individuals who refuse to comply. Client must WANT to become a productive member of society before he or she can be helped.***
2. Talk about past behaviors with client. Discuss behaviors that are acceptable by societal norms and those that are not. Help client identify ways in which he or she has exploited others. Encourage client to explore how he or she would feel if the circumstances were reversed. ***An attempt may be made to enlighten the client to the sensitivity of others by promoting self-awareness in an effort to assist the client in gaining insight into his or her own behavior.***
3. Throughout relationship with client, maintain attitude of "It is not *you* but *your behavior,* that is unacceptable." ***An attitude of acceptance promotes feelings of dignity and self-worth.***
4. Work with client to increase the ability to delay gratification. Reward desirable behaviors and provide immediate positive feedback. ***Rewards and positive feedback enhance self-esteem and encourage repetition of desirable behaviors.***
5. Help client identify and practice more adaptive strategies for coping with stressful life situations. ***The impulse to perform the maladaptive behavior may be so great that the client is unable to see any other alternatives to relieve stress.***

Outcome Criteria

1. Client is able to demonstrate techniques that may be used

in response to stress to prevent resorting to maladaptive impulsive behaviors.

2. Client verbalizes understanding that behavior is unacceptable and accepts responsibility for own behavior.

■ INTERNET REFERENCES

Additional information about Impulse Control Disorders may be located at the following Websites:

- http://www.cmhc.com/disordcrs/sx23.htm
- http://www.ncpgambling.org/index.html
- http://www.gamblersanonymous.org/
- http://www.cmhc.com/disorders/sx51.htm

CHAPTER 15

*Psychological Factors Affecting Medical Condition**

■ BACKGROUND ASSESSMENT DATA

The *DSM-IV* (APA, 1994) identifies *Psychological Factors Affecting Medical Condition* as the presence of one or more specific psychological or behavioral factors that adversely affect a general medical condition. These factors can adversely affect the medical condition in several ways:

1. By influencing the course of the medical condition (i.e., contributing to the development or exacerbation of, or delayed recovery from, the medical condition).
2. By interfering with treatment of the medical condition.
3. By constituting an additional health risk for the individual (e.g., the individual who has peptic ulcers but continues to drink and smoke).

316 Psychological Factors Affecting Medical Condition

Defined

The *DSM-IV* (APA, 1994) designates this diagnosis when there is evidence of a physical symptom(s) or a physical disorder that is adversely affected by psychological factors. Common examples of medical conditions for which this category may be appropriate include, but are not

*Reprinted with permission from the *Diagnostic and Statistical Manual of Mental Disorders, Fourth Edition*. Copyright 1994 American Psychiatric Association, 1994.

limited to, tension headache, migraine headache, cardiospasm, pylorospasm, rheumatoid arthritis, asthma, ulcers, ulcerative colitis, regional enteritis, hypertension, nausea and vomiting, tachycardia, arrhythmia, acne, angina pectoris, painful menstruation, frequency of micturition, neurodermatitis, and sacroiliac pain. Kaplan (1989) states, "All disease is influenced by psychological factors." Virtually any organic disorder can be considered psychophysiological.

This category differs from somatoform disorders and conversion disorders in that there is evidence of either demonstrable organic pathology (such as the inflammation associated with rheumatoid arthritis) or a known pathophysiological process (such as the cerebral vasodilation of migraine headaches).

Several types of psychological factors are implicated by the *DSM-IV* as those that can affect a general medical condition. They include the following:

1. Mental disorders (e.g., major depression).
2. Psychological symptoms (e.g., depressed mood or anxiety).
3. Personality traits or coping style (e.g., denial of the need for medical care).
4. Maladaptive health behaviors (e.g., smoking or overeating).
5. Stress-related physiological responses (e.g., tension headaches).

Predisposing Factors

1. **Physiological**
   a. ***Physical Factors:*** Selye (1956) believes that psychophysiological disorders occur when the body is exposed to prolonged stress, producing a number of physiological effects under direct control of the pituitary-adrenal axis. He also suggests that genetic predisposition influences which organ system will be affected and determines the type of psychophysiological disorder the individual will develop.
2. **Psychosocial**
   a. ***Emotional Response Pattern:*** Alexander (1950) proposed that individuals exhibit specific physiological responses to certain emotions. For example, in response to the emotion of anger, one person may experience peripheral vasoconstriction, resulting in an increase in blood pressure. The same

emotion, in another individual, may evoke the response of cerebral vasodilation, manifesting a migraine headache.

b. ***Personality Traits:*** Various studies have suggested that individuals with specific personality traits are predisposed to certain disease processes. Although personality cannot account totally for the development of psychophysiological disorders, the literature alluded to the following possible relationships:

Asthma	Dependent personality characteristics
Ulcers, hypertension	Repressed anger
Cancer	Depressive personality
Rheumatoid arthritis, ulcerative colitis	Self-sacrificing and inhibited
Migraine headaches	Compulsive and perfectionistic
Coronary heart disease	Aggressive and competitive

c. ***Learning Theory:*** A third psychosocial theory considers the role of learning in the psychophysiological response to stress (Pasquali et al., 1989). If a child grows up observing the attention, increased dependency, or other secondary gain an individual receives because of the illness, such behaviors may be viewed as desirable responses and subsequently imitated by the child.

d. ***Theory of Family Dynamics:*** Minuchin and coworkers (1978) have suggested the predisposition of those individuals who are members of dysfunctional family systems that use psychophysiological problems to cover up interpersonal conflicts. The anxiety in a dysfunctional family situation is shifted from the conflict to the ailing individual. Anxiety decreases, the conflict is avoided, and the person receives positive reinforcement for his or her symptoms. The situation appears more comfortable, but the real problem remains unresolved.

Symptomatology *(Subjective and Objective Data)*

1. Complaints of physical illness that can be substantiated by objective evidence of physical pathology or known pathophysiological process.
2. Moderate to severe level of anxiety.
3. Denial of emotional problems; client is unable to see a relationship between physical problems and response to stress.

4. Use of physical illness as excuse for noncompliance with psychiatric treatment plan.
5. Repressed anger or anger expressed inappropriately.
6. Verbal hostility.
7. Depressed mood.
8. Low self-esteem.
9. Dependent behaviors.
10. Attention-seeking behaviors.
11. Report (or other evidence) of numerous stressors occurring in person's life.

Common Nursing Diagnoses and Interventions*

(Interventions are applicable to various health-care settings, such as inpatient and partial hospitalization, community outpatient clinic, home health, and private practice.)

INEFFECTIVE INDIVIDUAL COPING

Definition: Inability to form a valid appraisal of the stressors, inadequate choices of practiced responses, and/or inability to use available resources.

Possible Etiologies ("related to")

[Repressed anxiety]
[Inadequate support systems]
[Inadequate coping methods]
[Low self-esteem]
[Unmet dependency needs]
[Negative role modeling]
[Dysfunctional family system]

Defining Characteristics ("evidenced by")

[Initiation or exacerbation of physical illness (specify)]
[Denial of relationship between physical symptoms and emotional problems]
[Use of sick role for secondary gains]

---

*A number of nursing diagnoses common to specific physical disorders or symptoms could be used (e.g., pain, activity intolerance, impaired tissue integrity, diarrhea). For purposes of this chapter, only nursing diagnoses common to the general category are presented.

Inability to meet role expectations
Inability to problem solve

Goals/Objectives

Short-Term Goal

Within 1 week, client will verbalize adaptive ways of coping with stressful situations.

Long-Term Goal

Client will achieve physical wellness and demonstrate the ability to prevent exacerbation of physical symptoms as a coping mechanism in response to stress.

Interventions with *Selected Rationales*

1. Perform thorough physical assessment ***to determine specific care required for client's physical condition.*** Monitor laboratory values, vital signs, intake and output, and other assessments necessary ***to maintain accurate, ongoing appraisal.***
2. Together with the client, identify goals of care and ways in which client believes he or she can best achieve those goals. Client may need assistance with problem solving. ***Personal involvement in his or her care provides a feeling of control and increases chances for positive outcomes.***
3. Encourage client to discuss current life situations that he or she perceives as stressful and the feelings associated with each. ***Verbalization of true feelings in a nonthreatening environment may help client come to terms with unresolved issues.***
4. During client's discussion, note times during which a sense of powerlessness or loss of control over life situations emerges. Focus on these times and discuss ways in which the client may maintain a feeling of control. ***A sense of self-worth develops and is maintained when an individual feels power over his or her own life situations.***
5. As client becomes able to discuss feelings more openly, assist him or her, in a nonthreatening manner, to relate certain feelings to the appearance of physical symptoms. ***Client may be unaware of the relationship between physical symptoms and emotional problems.***
6. Discuss stressful times when physical symptoms did not appear and the adaptive coping strategies that were used during those situations. ***Therapy is facilitated by considering areas of strength and using them to the client's benefit.***

7. Provide positive reinforcement for adaptive coping mechanisms identified or used. Suggest alternative coping strategies but allow client to determine which ones can most appropriately be incorporated into his or her lifestyle. ***Positive reinforcement enhances self-esteem and encourages repetition of desirable behaviors. Client may require assistance with problem solving but must be allowed and encouraged to make decisions independently.***
8. Help client to identify a resource within the community (friend, significant other, group) to use as a support system for the expression of feelings ***in an effort to prevent maladaptive coping through physical illness.***

Outcome Criteria

1. Client is able to demonstrate techniques that may be used in response to stress to prevent the occurrence or exacerbation of physical symptoms.
2. Client verbalizes an understanding of the relationship between emotional problems and physical symptoms.

SELF-ESTEEM DISTURBANCE

Definition: Negative self-evaluation and feelings about self or self-capabilities, which may be directly or indirectly expressed.

Possible Etiologies ("related to")

[Lack of positive feedback]
[Unmet dependency needs]
[Retarded ego development]
[Repeated negative feedback, resulting in diminished self-worth]
[Dysfunctional family system]

Defining Characteristics ("evidenced by")

[Difficulty accepting positive reinforcement]
[Nonparticipation in therapy]
Self-negating verbalizations
Evaluation of self as unable to deal with events
Hesitant to try new things or situations [because of fear of failure]
Hypersensitive to slight or criticism
[Lack of eye contact]
[Inability to form close, personal relationships]

[Degradation of others in an attempt to increase own feelings of self-worth]

Goals/Objectives

Short-Term Goals

1. Client will discuss fear of failure with nurse within 3 days.
2. Client will verbalize aspects he or she likes about self within 5 days.

Long-Term Goals

1. Client will exhibit increased feelings of self-worth as evidenced by verbal expression of positive aspects about self, past accomplishments, and future prospects.
2. Client will exhibit increased feelings of self-worth by setting realistic goals and trying to reach them, thereby demonstrating a decrease in fear of failure.

Interventions with *Selected Rationales*

1. Ensure that goals are realistic. It is important for client to achieve something, so plan activities in which success is likely. ***Success increases self-esteem.***
2. Minimize amount of attention given to physical symptoms. Client must perceive self as a worthwhile person, separate and apart from the role of client. ***Lack of attention may discourage use of undesirable behaviors.***
3. Promote your acceptance of client as a worthwhile person by spending time with him or her. Develop trust through one-to-one interactions, then encourage client to participate in group activities. Support group attendance with your presence until client feels comfortable attending alone. ***The feeling of acceptance by others increases self-esteem.***
4. Ask client to make a written list of positive and negative aspects about self. Discuss each item on the list with client. Develop plans of change for the characteristics viewed as negative. Assist client in implementing the plans. Provide positive feedback for successful change. ***Individuals with low self-esteem often have difficulty recognizing their positive attributes. They may also lack problem-solving skills and require assistance to formulate a plan for implementing the desired changes. Positive feedback enhances self-esteem and encourages repetition of desired behaviors.***
5. Avoid fostering dependence by "doing for" the client. Allow client to perform as independently as physical condition will permit. Offer recognition and praise for accomplishments. ***The ability to perform self-care activities***

independently provides a feeling of self-control and enhances self-esteem. Positive reinforcement encourages repetition of the desirable behavior.

6. Allow client to be an active participant in his or her therapy. Promote feelings of control or power by encouraging input into the decision making regarding treatment, as well as the planning for discharge from treatment. Provide positive feedback for adaptive responses. *Control over own life experiences promotes feelings of self-worth.*

Outcome Criteria

1. Client verbalizes positive perception of self.
2. Client demonstrates ability to manage own self-care, make independent decisions, and use problem-solving skills.
3. Client sets goals that are realistic and works to achieve those goals without evidence of fear of failure.

ALTERED ROLE PERFORMANCE

Definition: The patterns of behavior and self-expression do not match the environmental context, norms, and expectations.

Possible Etiologies ("related to")

[Physical illness accompanied by real or perceived disabling symptoms]
[Unmet dependency needs]
[Dysfunctional family system]

Defining Characteristics ("evidenced by")

Change in self-perception of role
[Change in physical capacity to resume role]
[Assumption of dependent role]
Changes in usual patterns of responsibility [because of conflict within dysfunctional family system]

Goals/Objectives

Short-Term Goal

Client will verbalize understanding that physical symptoms interfere with role performance in order to fill an unmet need.

Long-Term Goal

Client will be able to assume role-related responsibilities by discharge from treatment.

Interventions with *Selected Rationales*

1. Determine client's usual role within the family system. Identify roles of other family members. ***An accurate database is required to formulate appropriate plan of care for the client.***
2. Assess specific disabilities related to role expectations. Assess relationship of disability to physical condition. ***It is important to determine the realism of the client's role expectations.***
3. Encourage client to discuss conflicts evident within the family system. Identify ways in which client and other family members have responded to this conflict. ***It is necessary to identify specific stressors, as well as adaptive and maladaptive responses within the system, before assistance can be provided in an effort to create change.***
4. Help client identify feelings associated with family conflict, the subsequent exacerbation of physical symptoms, and the accompanying disabilities. ***Client may be unaware of the relationship between physical symptoms and emotional problems. An awareness of the correlation is the first step toward creating change.***
5. Help client identify changes he or she would like to occur within the family system.
6. Encourage family participation in the development of plans to effect positive change, and work to resolve the conflict for which the client's sick role provides relief. ***Input from the individuals who will be directly involved in the change will increase the likelihood of a positive outcome.***
7. Allow all family members input into the plan for change: knowledge of benefits and consequences for each alternative, selection of appropriate alternatives, methods for implementation of alternatives, alternate plan in the event initial change is unsuccessful. ***Family may require assistance with this problem-solving process.***
8. Ensure that client has accurate perception of role expectations within the family system. Use role playing to practice areas associated with his or her role that client perceives as painful. ***Repetition through practice may help to desensitize client to the anticipated distress.***
9. As client is able to see the relationship between exacerbation of physical symptoms and existing conflict, discuss more adaptive coping strategies that may be used to prevent interference with role performance during times of stress.

Outcome Criteria

1. Client is able to verbalize realistic perception of role expectations.
2. Client is physically able to assume role-related responsibilities.
3. Client and family are able to verbalize plan for attempt at conflict resolution.

KNOWLEDGE DEFICIT (Psychological Factors Affecting Medical Condition)

Definition: Absence or deficiency of cognitive information related to specific topic.

Possible Etiologies ("related to")

[Lack of interest in learning]
[Severe level of anxiety]
[Low self-esteem]
[Regression to earlier level of development]

Defining Characteristics ("evidenced by")

[Denial of emotional problems]
[Statements such as "I don't know why the doctor put me on the psychiatric unit. I have a physical problem."]
[History of numerous exacerbations of physical illness]
[Noncompliance with psychiatric treatment]
Inappropriate or exaggerated behaviors, for example, hysterical, hostile, agitated, apathetic

Goals/Objectives

Short-Term Goal

Client will cooperate with plan for teaching provided by primary nurse.

Long-Term Goal

By discharge from treatment, client will be able to verbalize psychological factors affecting his or her medical condition.

Interventions with *Selected Rationales*

1. Assess client's level of knowledge regarding effects of psychological problems on the body. *An adequate database is necessary for the development of an effective teaching plan.*

2. Assess client's level of anxiety and readiness to learn. ***Learning does not occur beyond the moderate level of anxiety.***
3. Discuss physical examinations and laboratory tests that have been conducted. Explain purpose and results of each. ***Fear of the unknown may contribute to elevated level of anxiety. "The client has the right to obtain complete current information concerning his diagnosis, treatment, and prognosis . . . " (AHA, 1975).***
4. Explore client's feelings and fears. Go slowly. These feelings may have been suppressed or repressed for so long that their disclosure may be a very painful experience. Be supportive. ***Verbalization of feelings in a nonthreatening environment and with a trusting individual may help the client come to terms with unresolved issues.***
5. Have client keep a diary of appearance, duration, and intensity of physical symptoms. A separate record of situations that the client finds especially stressful should also be kept. ***Comparison of these records may provide objective data from which to observe the relationship between physical symptoms and stress.***
6. Help client identify needs that are being met through the sick role. Together, formulate more adaptive means for fulfilling these needs. Practice by role playing. ***Repetition through practice serves to reduce discomfort in the actual situation.***
7. Provide instruction in assertiveness techniques, especially the ability to recognize the differences among passive, assertive, and aggressive behaviors and the importance of respecting the human rights of others while protecting one's own basic human rights. ***These skills will preserve client's self-esteem while also improving his or her ability to form satisfactory interpersonal relationships.***
8. Discuss adaptive methods of stress management such as relaxation techniques, physical exercise, meditation, breathing exercises, and autogenics. ***Use of these adaptive techniques may decrease appearance of physical symptoms in response to stress.***

Outcome Criteria

1. Client verbalizes an understanding of the relationship between psychological stress and exacerbation of physical illness.
2. Client demonstrates the ability to use adaptive coping strategies in the management of stress.

■ INTERNET REFERENCES

Additional information about Psychophysiological Disorders discussed in this chapter may be located at the following Websites:

- http://www.nci.nih.gov
- http://www.cancer.org
- http://www.amhrt.org/
- http://www.headaches.org/
- http://www.pslgroup.com/ASTHMA.HTM
- http://www.pharminfo.com/disease/immun/asthma/asthma_info.html
- http://www.gastro.org/adhf/ulcers.html
- http://www.pslgroup.com/HYPERTENSION.HTM
- http://pharminfo.com/disease/ra/ra-site.html
- http://www.mediconsult.com/ibd/shareware/colitis/contents.html

CHAPTER 16

*Personality Disorders**

■ BACKGROUND ASSESSMENT DATA

The *DSM-IV* (APA, 1994) describes personality *traits* as "enduring patterns of perceiving, relating to, and thinking about the environment and oneself that are exhibited in a wide range of social and personal contexts." A personality *disorder* is said to exist only when these traits become inflexible and maladaptive and cause either significant functional impairment or subjective distress.

The *DSM-IV* groups the personality disorders into three clusters. They are coded on Axis II in the *DSM-IV* classification. These clusters, and the disorders classified under each, are described as follows:

1. **Cluster A:** Behaviors described as odd or eccentric
   a. 301.0 Paranoid personality disorder
   b. 301.20 Schizoid personality disorder
   c. 301.22 Schizotypal personality disorder
2. **Cluster B:** Behaviors described as dramatic, emotional, or erratic
   a. 301.7 Antisocial personality disorder
   b. 301.83 Borderline personality disorder
   c. 301.50 Histrionic personality disorder
   d. 301.81 Narcissistic personality disorder
3. **Cluster C:** Behaviors described as anxious or fearful
   a. 301.82 Avoidant personality disorder
   b. 301.6 Dependent personality disorder

---

*Reprinted with permission from the *Diagnostic and Statistical Manual of Mental Disorders, Fourth Edition.* Copyright 1994 American Psychiatric Association, 1994.

c. 301.4 Obsessive-compulsive personality disorder
d. Passive-aggressive personality disorder

NOTE: Passive-aggressive personality disorder was included in the *DSM-III-R* (APA, 1987) with the cluster C disorders. In the *DSM-IV,* it is included in the section on *Criteria Provided for Further Study.* For purposes of this text, passive-aggressive personality disorder is described with the cluster C disorders.

Categories of personality disorders described by the *DSM-IV* include the following:

1. **Cluster A**
   a. ***Paranoid Personality Disorder:*** The essential feature is a pervasive and unwarranted suspiciousness and mistrust of people. There is a general expectation of being exploited or harmed by others in some way. Symptoms include guardedness in relationships with others, pathological jealousy, hypersensitivity, inability to relax, unemotionality, and lack of a sense of humor. These individuals are very critical of others but have much difficulty accepting criticism themselves.
   b. ***Schizoid Personality Disorder:*** This disorder is characterized by an inability to form close personal relationships. Symptoms include social isolation; absence of warm, tender feelings for others; indifference to praise, criticism, or the feelings of others; flat, dull affect (appears cold and aloof).
   c. ***Schizotypal Personality Disorder:*** This disorder is characterized by peculiarities of ideation, appearance, and behavior, and deficits in interpersonal relatedness that are not severe enough to meet the criteria for schizophrenia. Symptoms include magical thinking; ideas of reference; social isolation; illusions; odd speech patterns; aloof, cold, suspicious behavior; and undue social anxiety.
2. **Cluster B**
   a. ***Antisocial Personality Disorder:*** This disorder is characterized by a pattern of socially irresponsible, exploitative, and guiltless behavior, as evidenced by the tendency to fail to conform to the law, to sustain consistent employment, to exploit and manipulate others for personal gain, to deceive, and to fail to develop stable relationships. The individual must be at least 18 years of age and have a history of conduct disorder before the age of 15. (Symptoms of this dis-

order are identified later in this chapter, along with predisposing factors and nursing care of the individual with antisocial personality).

b. ***Borderline Personality Disorder:*** The features of this disorder are described as marked instability in interpersonal relationships, mood, and self-image. The instability is significant to the extent that the individual seems to "hover just across the line from psychosis" (Kaplan and Sadock, 1985). (Symptoms of this disorder are identified later in this chapter, along with predisposing factors and nursing care of the individual with borderline personality).

c. ***Histrionic Personality Disorder:*** The essential feature of this disorder is described by the *DSM-IV* as a pervasive pattern of excessive emotionality and attention-seeking behavior. Symptoms include exaggerated expression of emotions, incessant drawing of attention to oneself, overreaction to minor events, constantly seeking approval from others, egocentricity, vain and demanding behavior, extreme concern with physical appearance, and inappropriately sexually seductive appearance or behavior.

d. ***Narcissistic Personality Disorder:*** This disorder is characterized by a grandiose sense of self-importance; preoccupation with fantasies of success, power, brilliance, beauty, or ideal love; a constant need for admiration and attention; exploitation of others for fulfillment of own desires; lack of empathy; response to criticism or failure with indifference or humiliation and rage; and preoccupation with feelings of envy.

3. **Cluster C**

a. ***Avoidant Personality Disorder:*** This disorder is characterized by social withdrawal brought about by extreme sensitivity to rejection. Symptoms include unwillingness to enter into relationships unless given unusually strong guarantees of uncritical acceptance; low self-esteem; social withdrawal in spite of a desire for affection and acceptance. Depression and anxiety are common. Social phobia may be a complication of this disorder.

b. ***Dependent Personality Disorder:*** Individuals with this disorder passively allow others to assume responsibility for major areas of life because of their inability to function independently. They lack self-confidence, are unable to make decisions, perceive self as helpless and stupid, possess fear of being alone or abandoned, and seek constant reassurance and approval from others.

c. ***Obsessive-Compulsive Personality Disorder:*** This disorder is characterized by a pervasive pattern of perfectionism and inflexibility. Interpersonal relationships have a formal and serious quality, and others often perceive these individuals as stilted or "stiff." Other symptoms include difficulty expressing tender feelings, insistence that others submit to his or her way of doing things, excessive devotion to work and productivity to the exclusion of pleasure, indecisiveness, perfectionism, preoccupation with details, depressed mood, and being judgmental of self and others.
d. ***Passive-Aggressive Personality Disorder:*** Characteristic of this disorder is a passive resistance to demands for adequate performance in both occupational and social functioning. Symptoms include obstructionism, procrastination, stubbornness, intentional inefficiency, dawdling, "forgetfulness," criticism of persons in authority, dependency, and low self-esteem. Oppositional defiant disorder in childhood or adolescence is a predisposing factor.

Many of the behaviors associated with the various personality disorders may be manifested by clients with virtually every psychiatric diagnosis, as well as by those individuals described as "healthy." It is only when personality traits or styles repetitively "limit the attempts and potential for mastery; disrupt interpersonal relationships; fail to balance dependence and autonomy; or create insufficient moral parameters in human interactions that a diagnosis of personality disorder is assigned" (Burgess, 1990).

Individuals with personality disorders may be encountered in all types of treatment settings. They are not often treated in acute care settings, but because of the instability of the borderline client, hospitalization is necessary from time to time. The individual with antisocial personality disorder also may be hospitalized as an alternative to imprisonment when a legal determination is made that psychiatric intervention may be helpful. Because of these reasons, suggestions for inpatient care of individuals with these disorders are included in this chapter; however, these interventions may be used in other types of treatment settings as well. Undoubtedly, these clients represent the ultimate challenge for the psychiatric nurse.

Borderline Personality Disorder

Defined

This personality disorder is characterized by instability of affect, behavior, object relationships, and self-image. The term "borderline" came into being because a group of clients seemed to fall on the border between neurosis and psychosis (Platt-Koch, 1983). Transient psychotic symptoms appear during periods of extreme stress. The disorder is more commonly diagnosed in women than in men.

Predisposing Factors

1. **Theory of Object Relations:** This theory suggests that the basis for borderline personality lies in the ways the child relates to the mother and does *not* separate from her. Mahler and associates (1975) define this process in a series of phases described as follows:
   a. **Phase 1 (birth to 1 month), Autistic Phase:** Most of the infant's time is spent in a half-waking, half-sleeping state.
   b. **Phase 2 (1 to 5 months), Symbiotic Phase:** A type of psychic fusion of mother and child. Child views self as extension of mother.
   c. **Phase 3 (5 to 10 months), Differentiation Phase:** Child begins to become aware of separateness between self and mother.
   d. **Phase 4 (10 to 16 months), Practicing Phase:** The child displays increased independence in terms of ability to ambulate and explore on his or her own.
   e. **Phase 5 (16 to 24 months), Rapprochement Phase:** Awareness of separateness from mother increases. This is frightening to the child, who wants to regain some lost closeness but not return to symbiosis. The child just wants mother there as needed for "emotional refueling."
   f. **Phase 6 (24 to 36 months), On the Way to Object Constancy Phase:** In this phase the child completes the individuation process and learns to relate to objects in an effective, constant manner.

The theory of object relations suggests that the individual with borderline personality is fixed in the rapprochement phase of development. This fixation occurs when the mother begins to feel threatened by the increasing autonomy of her child and so withdraws her emotional support during those times *or* she may instead reward clinging, dependent behaviors. In this way, the child comes to believe that

> "To grow up and be independent = a 'bad' child."
> "To stay immature and dependent = a 'good' child."
> "Mom withholds nurturing from 'bad' child."

Consequently, the child develops a deep fear of abandonment that persists into adulthood.

Also, because object constancy is never achieved, the child continues to view objects (people) as parts—either good or bad. This is called *splitting,* the primary defense mechanism of borderline personality.

Symptomatology *(Subjective and Objective Data)*

At least five of the following criteria are required by the *DSM-IV* (APA, 1994) for a diagnosis of borderline personality disorder:

1. Frantic efforts to avoid real or imagined abandonment (does not include suicidal or self-mutilating behavior covered in criterion 5).
2. A pattern of unstable and intense interpersonal relationships characterized by alternating between extremes of idealization and devaluation.
3. Identity disturbance: Markedly and persistently unstable self-image or sense of self.
4. Impulsivity in at least two areas that are potentially self-damaging, such as spending, sex, substance abuse, reckless driving, binge eating (not to include behavior covered in criterion 5).
5. Recurrent suicidal behavior, gestures, or threats, or self-mutilating behavior.
6. Affective instability caused by marked reactivity of mood (e.g., intense episodic dysphoria, irritability, or anxiety, usually lasting a few hours and only rarely more than a few days.)
7. Chronic feelings of emptiness.
8. Inappropriate, intense anger or difficulty controlling anger (e.g., frequent displays of temper, constant anger, recurrent physical fights).

9. Transient, stress-related paranoid ideation or severe dissociative symptoms.

   Other symptoms include the following:

10. Alternating clinging and distancing behaviors.
11. Projection—seeing in others those attitudes they fail to see in themselves.
12. Poor reality testing—misinterpretations of the environment and relationships, resulting from poor ego development.

Common Nursing Diagnoses and Interventions

(Interventions are applicable to various health-care settings, such as inpatient and partial hospitalization, community outpatient clinic, home health, and private practice.)

RISK FOR SELF-MUTILATION/RISK FOR VIOLENCE TO SELF OR OTHERS

Definition: Risk for self-mutilation is a state in which an individual is at risk to perform an act on the self to injure, not kill, which produces tissue damage and tension relief. Risk for violence is defined as: Behaviors in which an individual demonstrates that he/she can be physically, emotionally, and/or sexually harmful either to self or to others.

Related/Risk Factors ("related to")

[Extreme fears of abandonment]
[Feelings of unreality]
[Depressed mood]
[Use of suicidal gestures for manipulation of others]
[Unmet dependency needs]
[Low self-esteem]
[Unresolved grief]
[Rage reactions]
[Physically self-damaging acts (cutting, burning, drug overdose, etc.)]
Body language—rigid posture, clenching of fists and jaw, hyperactivity, pacing, breathlessness, and threatening stances
[History or threats of violence toward self or others or of destruction to the property of others]

Impulsivity
Suicidal ideation, plan, available means
[History of suicide attempts]

Goals/Objectives

Short-Term Goal

Client will seek out staff member if feelings of harming self or others emerge.

Long-Term Goal

Client will not harm self or others.

Interventions with *Selected Rationales*

1. Observe client's behavior frequently. Do this through routine activities and interactions; avoid appearing watchful and suspicious. ***Close observation is required so that intervention can occur if required to ensure client's (and others') safety.***
2. Secure a verbal contract from client that he or she will seek out staff member when urge for self-mutilation is experienced. ***Discussing feelings of self-harm with a trusted individual provides a degree of relief to the client. A contract gets the subject out in the open and places some of the responsibility for his or her safety with the client. An attitude of acceptance of the client as a worthwhile individual is conveyed.***
3. If self-mutilation occurs, care for the client's wounds in a matter-of-fact manner. Do not give positive reinforcement to this behavior by offering sympathy or additional attention. ***Lack of attention to the maladaptive behavior may decrease repetition of its use.***
4. Encourage client to talk about feelings he or she was having just prior to this behavior. ***To problem-solve the situation with the client, knowledge of the precipitating factors is important.***
5. Act as a role model for appropriate expression of angry feelings and give positive reinforcement to the client when attempts to conform are made. ***It is vital that the client express angry feelings, because suicide and other self-destructive behaviors are often viewed as a result of anger turned inward on the self.***
6. Remove all dangerous objects from the client's environment. ***Client safety is a nursing priority.***
7. Try to redirect violent behavior with physical outlets for the client's anxiety (e.g., punching bag, jogging). ***Physi-***

cal exercise is a safe and effective way of relieving pent-up tension.

8. Have sufficient staff available to indicate a show of strength to the client if necessary. ***This conveys to the client evidence of control over the situation and provides some physical security for staff.***
9. Administer tranquilizing medications as ordered by physician or obtain an order if necessary. Monitor the client for effectiveness of the medication and for the appearance of adverse side effects. ***Tranquilizing medications such as anxiolytics or antipsychotics may have a calming effect on the client and may prevent aggressive behaviors.***
10. Use of mechanical restraints or isolation room may be required if less restrictive interventions are unsuccessful. Follow policy and procedure prescribed by the institution in executing this intervention. Most states require that the physician re-evaluate and issue a new order for restraints every 3 hours, except between the hours of midnight and 8:00 AM. If the client has previously refused medication, administer after restraints have been applied. Most states consider this intervention appropriate in emergency situations or in the event that a client would likely harm self or others.
11. Observe the client in restraints every 15 minutes (or according to institutional policy). Ensure that circulation to extremities is not compromised (check temperature, color, pulses). Assist the client with needs related to nutrition, hydration, and elimination. Position the client so that comfort is facilitated and aspiration can be prevented. ***Client safety is a nursing priority.***
12. May need to assign staff on a one-to-one basis if warranted by acuity of the situation. ***Because of their extreme fear of abandonment, leaving clients with borderline personality disorder alone at such a time may cause an acute rise in level of anxiety and agitation.***

Outcome Criteria

1. Client has not harmed self or others.
2. Anxiety is maintained at a level in which client feels no need for aggression.
3. Client denies any ideas of self-harm.
4. Client verbalizes community support systems from which assistance may be requested when personal coping strategies are unsuccessful.

ANXIETY (Severe to Panic)

Definition: A vague uneasy feeling of discomfort or dread accompanied by an autonomic response; the source is often nonspecific or unknown to the individual; a feeling of apprehension caused by anticipation of danger. It is an altering signal that warns of impending danger and enables the individual to take measures to deal with threat.

Possible Etiologies ("related to")

Threat to self-concept
Unmet needs
[Extreme fear of abandonment]
Unconscious conflicts [associated with fixation in earlier level of development]

Defining Characteristics ("evidenced by")

[Transient psychotic symptoms in response to severe stress, manifested by disorganized thinking, confusion, altered communication patterns, disorientation, misinterpretation of the environment]
[Excessive use of projection (attributing own thoughts and feelings to others)]
[Depersonalization (feelings of unreality)]
[Derealization (a feeling that the environment is unreal)]
[Acts of self-mutilation in an effort to find relief from feelings of unreality]

Goals/Objectives

Short-Term Goal

Client will demonstrate use of relaxation techniques to maintain anxiety at manageable level.

Long-Term Goal

Client will be able to recognize events that precipitate anxiety and intervene to prevent disabling behaviors.

Interventions with *Selected Rationales*

1. Symptoms of depersonalization often occur at the panic level of anxiety. Clients with borderline personality disorder often resort to cutting or other self-mutilating acts in an effort to relieve the anxiety. Being able to feel pain or see blood is a reassurance of existence to the person. If injury occurs, care for the wounds in a matter-of-fact manner

without providing reinforcement for this behavior. ***Lack of reinforcement may discourage repetition of the maladaptive behavior.***

2. During periods of panic anxiety, stay with the client and provide reassurance of safety and security. Orient the client to the reality of the situation. ***Client comfort and safety are nursing priorities.***
3. Administer tranquilizing medications as ordered by physician, or obtain order if necessary. Monitor client for effectiveness of the medication as well as for adverse side effects. ***Antianxiety medications (e.g., diazepam, chlordiazepoxide, alprazolam) provide relief from the immobilizing effects of anxiety and may facilitate client's cooperation with therapy.***
4. Correct misinterpretations of the environment as expressed by client. ***Confronting misinterpretations honestly, with a caring and accepting attitude, provides a therapeutic orientation to reality and preserves the client's feelings of dignity and self-worth.***
5. Encourage the client to talk about true feelings. Help him or her recognize ownership of these feelings rather than projecting them onto others in the environment. ***Exploration of feelings with a trusted individual may help the client perceive the situation more realistically and come to terms with unresolved issues.***
6. Assist the client in working toward achievement of object constancy. Client may feel totally abandoned when nurse or therapist leaves at shift change or at end of therapy session. There may even be feelings that the therapist ceases to exist. Leaving a signed note or card with the client for reassurance may help. It is extremely important for more than one nurse to develop a therapeutic relationship with the borderline client. It is also necessary that staff maintain open communication and consistency in the provision of care for these individuals. ***Individuals with borderline personality disorder have a tendency to cling to one staff member, if allowed, transferring their maladaptive dependency to that individual. This dependency can be avoided if the client is able to establish therapeutic relationships with two or more staff members who encourage independent self-care activities.***

Outcome Criteria

1. Client is able to verbalize events that precipitate anxiety and demonstrate techniques for its reduction.
2. Client manifests no symptoms of depersonalization.
3. Client interprets the environment realistically.

DYSFUNCTIONAL GRIEVING

Definition: Extended, unsuccessful use of intellectual and emotional responses by which individuals (families, communities) attempt to work through the process of modifying self-concept based upon the perception of loss.

Possible Etiologies ("related to")

[Maternal deprivation during rapprochement phase of development (internalized as a loss, with fixation in the anger stage of the grieving process)]

Defining Characteristics ("evidenced by")

Anger
[Internalized rage]
[Depressed mood]
Labile affect
[Extreme fear of being alone (fear of abandonment)]
[Acting-out behaviors, such as sexual promiscuity, suicidal gestures, temper tantrums, substance abuse]
[Difficulty expressing feelings]
Alterations in eating habits, sleep patterns, dream patterns, activity level, libido
Repetitive use of ineffectual behaviors associated with attempts to reinvest in relationships
Reliving of past experiences with little or no reduction of intensity of the grief
Prolonged interference with life functioning, with onset or exacerbation of somatic or psychosomatic responses

Goals/Objectives

Short-Term Goal

Client will discuss with nurse or therapist maladaptive patterns of expressing anger.

Long-Term Goal

Client will be able to identify the true source of angry feelings, accept ownership of these feelings, and express them in a socially acceptable manner, in an effort to satisfactorily progress through the grieving process.

Interventions with *Selected Rationales*

1. Convey an accepting attitude—one that creates a nonthreatening environment for the client to express feelings. Be honest and keep all promises. *An accepting attitude*

conveys to the client that you believe he or she is a worthwhile person. Trust is enhanced.

2. Identify the function that anger, frustration, and rage serve for the client. Allow the client to express these feelings within reason. ***Verbalization of feelings in a nonthreatening environment may help the client come to terms with unresolved issues.***
3. Encourage the client to discharge pent-up anger through participation in large motor activities (e.g., brisk walks, jogging, physical exercises, volleyball, punching bag, exercise bike). ***Physical exercise provides a safe and effective method for discharging pent-up tension.***
4. Explore with client the true source of the anger. This is painful therapy that often leads to regression as the client deals with the feelings of early abandonment. It seems that sometimes the client must "get worse before he or she can get better." ***Reconciliation of the feelings associated with this stage is necessary before progression through the grieving process can continue.***
5. As anger is displaced onto the nurse or therapist, caution must be taken to guard against the negative effects of countertransference. These are very difficult clients who have the capacity for eliciting a whole array of negative feelings from the therapist. These feelings must be acknowledged but not allowed to interfere with the therapeutic process.
6. Explain the behaviors associated with the normal, grieving process. Help the client to recognize his or her position in this process. ***Knowledge of the acceptability of the feelings associated with normal grieving may help to relieve some of the guilt that these responses generate.***
7. Help the client to understand appropriate ways to express anger. Give positive reinforcement for behaviors used to express anger appropriately. Act as a role model. ***Positive reinforcement enhances self-esteem and encourages repetition of desirable behaviors. It is appropriate to let the client know when he or she has done something that has generated angry feelings in you. Role modeling ways to express anger in an appropriate manner is a powerful learning tool.***
8. Set limits on acting-out behaviors and explain consequences of violation of those limits. Be supportive, yet consistent and firm in caring for this client. ***Client lacks sufficient self-control to limit maladaptive behaviors, so assistance is required from staff. Without consistency on the part of all staff members working with this client, however, a positive outcome will not be achieved.***

Outcome Criteria

1. Client is able to verbalize ways in which anger and acting-out behaviors are associated with maladaptive grieving.
2. Client is able to discuss the original source of the anger and demonstrates socially acceptable ways of expressing the emotion.

■ IMPAIRED SOCIAL INTERACTION

Definition: The state in which an individual participates in an insufficient or excessive quantity or ineffective quality of social exchange.

Possible Etiologies ("related to")

[Fixation in rapprochement phase of development]
[Extreme fears of abandonment and engulfment]
[Lack of personal identity]

Defining Characteristics ("evidenced by")

[Alternating clinging and distancing behaviors]
[Inability to form satisfactory intimate relationship with another person]
Observed use of unsuccessful social interaction behaviors
[Use of primitive dissociation (splitting) in their relationships (viewing others as all good or all bad)]

Goals/Objectives

Short-Term Goal

Client will discuss with nurse or therapist behaviors that impede the development of satisfactory interpersonal relationships.

Long-Term Goals

1. Client will interact with others in the therapy setting in both social and therapeutic activities without difficulty by discharge from treatment.
2. Client will display no evidence of splitting or clinging and distancing behaviors in relationships by discharge from treatment.

Interventions with *Selected Rationales*

1. Encourage client to examine these behaviors (to recognize that they are occurring). *Client may be unaware of splitting or of clinging and distancing pattern of interaction with others.*

2. Help client realize that you will be available, without reinforcing dependent behaviors. ***Knowledge of your availability may provide needed security for the client.***
3. Give positive reinforcement for independent behaviors. ***Positive reinforcement enhances self-esteem and encourages repetition of desirable behaviors.***
4. Rotate staff who work with client in order to avoid client's developing dependence on particular staff members. ***Client must learn to relate to more than one staff member in an effort to decrease use of splitting and to diminish fears of abandonment.***
5. Explore feelings that relate to fears of abandonment and engulfment with the client. Help client understand that clinging and distancing behaviors are engendered by these fears. ***Exploration of feelings with a trusted individual may help client come to terms with unresolved issues.***
6. Help client understand how these behaviors interfere with satisfactory relationships. ***Client may be unaware of others' perception of him or her and why these behaviors are not acceptable to others.***
7. Assist the client in working toward achievement of object constancy. Be available, without promoting dependency ***so that client may resolve fears of abandonment and develop the ability to establish satisfactory intimate relationships.***

Outcome Criteria

1. Client is able to interact with others in both social and therapeutic activities in a socially acceptable manner.
2. Client does not use splitting or clinging and distancing behaviors in relationships and is able to relate the use of these behaviors to failure of past relationships.

PERSONAL IDENTITY DISTURBANCE

Definition: Inability to distinguish between self and nonself.

Possible Etiologies ("related to")

[Failure to complete tasks of separation/individuation stage of development]
[Underdeveloped ego]
[Unmet dependency needs]
[Absence of, or rejection by, parental sex-role model]

Defining Characteristics ("evidenced by")

[Excessive use of projection]
[Uncertainties regarding gender identity]
[Uncertainties about long-term goals or career choice]
[Ambiguous value system]
[Vague self-image]
[Unable to tolerate being alone]
[Feelings of depersonalization and derealization]
[Self-mutilation (cutting, burning) to validate existence of self]

Goals/Objectives

Short-Term Goal

Client will describe characteristics that make him or her a unique individual.

Long-Term Goal

Client will be able to distinguish own thoughts, feelings, behaviors, and image from those of others, as the initial step in the development of a healthy personal identity.

Interventions with *Selected Rationales*

1. Help client recognize the reality of his or her separateness. Do not attempt to translate client's thoughts and feelings into words. ***Because of the blurred ego boundaries, client may believe you can read his or her mind.*** For this reason, caution should be taken in the use of empathetic understanding. For example, avoid statements such as "I know how you must feel about that."
2. Help client to recognize separateness from nurse by clarifying which behaviors and feelings belong to whom. If deemed appropriate, allow client to touch your hand or arm. ***Touch and physical presence provide reality for the client and serve to strengthen weak ego boundaries.***
3. Encourage client to discuss thoughts and feelings. Help client recognize ownership of these feelings rather than project them onto others in the environment. ***Verbalization of feelings in a nonthreatening environment may help client come to terms with unresolved issues.***
4. Confront statements that project client's feelings onto others. Ask client to validate that others possess those feelings. The expression of ***reasonable doubt*** as a therapeutic technique may be helpful ("I find that hard to believe").
5. If the problem is with gender identity, ask the client to describe his or her perception of appropriate male and female

behaviors. Provide information about role behaviors and sex education, if necessary. Client may require clarification of distorted ideas or misinformation. Convey acceptance of the person regardless of preferred identity. ***An attitude of acceptance reinforces client's feelings of self-worth.***

6. Always call client by his or her name. If client experiences feelings of depersonalization or derealization, orientation to the environment and correction of misperceptions may be helpful. ***These interventions help to preserve client's feelings of dignity and self-worth.***
7. Help client understand that there are more adaptive ways of validating his or her existence than self-mutilation. Contract with the client to seek out staff member when these feelings occur. ***A contract gets the subject out in the open and places some of the responsibility for his or her safety with the client. Client safety is a nursing priority.***
8. Work with client to clarify values. Discuss beliefs, attitudes, and feelings underlying his or her behaviors. Help client to identify those values that have been (or are intended to be) incorporated as his or her own. Care must be taken by the nurse to avoid imposing his or her own value system upon the client. ***Because of underdeveloped ego and fixation in early developmental level, client may not have established own value system. To accomplish this, ownership of beliefs and attitudes must be identified and clarified.***
9. Use of photographs of the client may help to establish or clarify ego boundaries. ***Photographs may help to increase client's awareness of self as separate from others.***
10. Alleviate anxiety by providing assurance to client that he or she will not be left alone. ***Early childhood traumas may predispose borderline clients to extreme fears of abandonment.***
11. Use of touch is sometimes therapeutic in identity confirmation. Before this technique is used, however, assess cultural influences and degree of trust. ***Touch and physical presence provide reality for the client and serve to strengthen weak ego boundaries.***

Outcome Criteria

1. Client is able to distinguish between own thoughts and feelings and those of others.
2. Client claims ownership of those thoughts and feelings and does not use projection in relationships with others.
3. Client has clarified own feelings regarding sexual identity.

SELF-ESTEEM DISTURBANCE

Definition: Negative self-evaluation and feelings about self or self-capabilities, which may be directly or indirectly expressed.

Possible Etiologies ("related to")

[Lack of positive feedback]
[Unmet dependency needs]
[Retarded ego development]
[Repeated negative feedback, resulting in diminished self-worth]
[Dysfunctional family system]
[Fixation in earlier level of development]

Defining Characteristics ("evidenced by")

[Difficulty accepting positive reinforcement]
[Self-destructive behavior]
[Frequent use of derogatory and critical remarks against the self]
[Lack of eye contact]
[Manipulation of one staff member against another in an attempt to gain special privileges]
[Inability to form close, personal relationships]
[Inability to tolerate being alone]
[Degradation of others in an attempt to increase own feelings of self-worth]
Hesitancy to try new things or situations [because of fear of failure]

Goals/Objectives

Short-Term Goals

1. Client will discuss fear of failure with nurse or therapist.
2. Client will verbalize things he or she likes about self.

Long-Term Goals

1. Client will exhibit increased feelings of self-worth as evidenced by verbal expression of positive aspects about self, past accomplishments, and future prospects.
2. Client will exhibit increased feelings of self-worth by setting realistic goals and trying to reach them, thereby demonstrating a decrease in fear of failure.

Interventions with *Selected Rationales*

1. Ensure that goals are realistic. It is important for client to

achieve something, so plan for activities in which success is likely. ***Success increases self-esteem.***

2. Convey unconditional positive regard for client. Promote understanding of your acceptance for him or her as a worthwhile human being. ***Acceptance by others increases feelings of self-worth.***
3. Set limits on manipulative behavior. Identify the consequences for violation of those limits. Minimize negative feedback to the client. Enforce the limits and impose the consequences for violations in a matter-of-fact manner. Consistency among all staff members is essential. ***Negative feedback can be extremely threatening to a person with low self-esteem and possibly aggravate the problem. Consequences should convey unacceptability of the* BEHAVIOR *but not the* PERSON.**
4. Recognize when client is playing one staff member against another. Remember that splitting is the primary defense mechanism of these individuals, and the impressions they have of others as either "good" or "bad" are a manifestation of this defense. Do not listen as client tries to degrade other staff members. Suggest that client discuss the problem directly with staff person involved. ***Lack of reinforcement for these maladaptive behaviors may discourage their repetition.***
5. Encourage independence in the performance of personal responsibilities, as well as in decision making related to client's self-care. Offer recognition and praise for accomplishments. ***Positive reinforcement enhances self-esteem and encourages repetition of desirable behaviors.***
6. Help client increase level of self-awareness through critical examination of feelings, attitudes, and behaviors. ***Self-exploration in the presence of a trusted individual may help the client come to terms with unresolved issues.***
7. Help client identify positive self-attributes, as well as those aspects of the self he or she finds undesirable. Discuss ways to effect change in these areas. ***Individuals with low self-esteem often have difficulty recognizing their positive attributes. They may also lack problem-solving ability and require assistance to formulate a plan for implementing the desired changes.***
8. Discuss client's future. Assist client in the establishment of short-term and long-term goals. What are his or her strengths? How can he or she best use those strengths to achieve those goals? Encourage client to perform at a level realistic to his or her ability. Offer positive reinforcement for decisions made.

Outcome Criteria

1. Client verbalizes positive aspects about self.
2. Client demonstrates ability to make independent decisions regarding management of own self-care.
3. Client expresses some optimism and hope for the future.
4. Client sets realistic goals for self and demonstrates willingness to reach them.

Antisocial Personality Disorder

Defined

This personality disorder is characterized by a pattern of antisocial behavior that began before the age of 15. These behaviors violate the rights of others, and individuals with this disorder display no evidence of guilt feelings at having done so. There is often a long history of involvement with law-enforcement agencies. Substance abuse is not uncommon. The disorder is more frequently diagnosed in men than in women. Individuals with antisocial personalities are often labeled *sociopathic* or *psychopathic* in the lay literature.

Predisposing Factors

1. **Physiological**
   a. ***Genetics:*** The *DSM-IV* reports that antisocial personality is more common among first-degree biological relatives of those with the disorder than among the general population (APA, 1994). Cadoret (1994) reports on studies that implicate the role of genetics in antisocial personality disorder. These studies of families of individuals with antisocial personality show higher numbers of relatives with antisocial personality or alcoholism than are found in the general population. Additional studies have shown that children of parents with antisocial behavior are more likely to be diagnosed as antisocial personality, even when separated at birth from biological parents.
2. **Psychosocial**
   a. ***Psychodynamic Theory:*** Freud (1959) implicated the unmet need for satisfaction and security from significant others in the development of antisocial personality. Because of this rejection or indifference, development of the ego is interrupted, and id behavior is maintained. The child also lacks satisfactory role models at the crucial time when he or

she would be internalizing standards, values, and morals in the development of a superego. This development is impaired, and the individual becomes an adult who nurtures the need for immediate gratification and lacks feelings of guilt.

b. ***Theories of Family Dynamics:*** Several sources have implicated family functioning as an important factor in determining whether or not an individual develops antisocial personality (Cadoret, 1994; APA, 1987; Robinson, 1983). They suggest that the following circumstances may predispose to the disorder:
   (1) Absence of parental discipline.
   (2) Extreme poverty.
   (3) Removal from the home.
   (4) Growing up without parental figures of both sexes.
   (5) Erratic and inconsistent methods of discipline.
   (6) Being "rescued" each time they are in trouble (never having to suffer the consequences of their own behavior).
   (7) Maternal deprivation.

Symptomatology *(Subjective and Objective Data)*

1. Extremely low self-esteem (abuses other people in an attempt to validate his or her own superiority).
2. Inability to sustain satisfactory job performance.
3. Inability to function as a responsible parent.
4. Failure to follow social and legal norms; repeated performance of antisocial acts that are grounds for arrest (whether arrested or not).
5. Inability to develop satisfactory, enduring, intimate relationship with a sexual partner.
6. Aggressive behaviors; repeated physical fights; spouse or child abuse.
7. Extreme impulsivity.
8. Repeated lying for personal benefit.
9. Reckless driving; driving while intoxicated.
10. Inability to learn from punishment.
11. Lack of guilt or remorse felt in response to exploitation of others.
12. Difficulty with interpersonal relationships.
13. Social extroversion; stimulation through interaction with and abuse of others.
14. Repeated failure to honor financial obligations.

Common Nursing Diagnoses and Interventions

(Interventions are applicable to various health-care settings, such as inpatient and partial hospitalization, community outpatient clinic, home health, and private practice.)

RISK FOR VIOLENCE: DIRECTED AT OTHERS

Definition: Behaviors in which an individual demonstrates that he/she can be physically, emotionally, and/or sexually harmful to others.

Related/Risk Factors ("related to")

[Rage reactions]
[Suspiciousness of others]
[Interruption of client's attempt to fulfill own desires]
[Inability to tolerate frustration]
[Learned behavior within client's subculture]
[Vulnerable self-esteem]
Body language—rigid posture, clenching of fists and jaw, hyperactivity, pacing, breathlessness, and threatening stances
[History or threats of violence toward self or others or of destruction to the property of others]
Impulsivity
Availability and/or possession of weapon(s)
[Substance abuse or withdrawal]
[Provocative behavior: argumentative, dissatisfied, overreactive, hypersensitive]
History of witnessing family violence
Neurological impairment (e.g., positive EEG)
History of violence against others

Goals/Objectives

Short-Term Goal

Client will discuss angry feelings and situations that precipitate hostility.

Long-Term Goal

Client will not harm others.

Intervention with *Selected Rationales*

1. Convey an accepting attitude toward this client. Feelings

of rejection are undoubtedly familiar to him or her. Work on development of trust. Be honest, keep all promises, and convey the message to the client that it is not *him* or *her,* but the *behavior* that is unacceptable. ***An attitude of acceptance promotes feelings of self-worth. Trust is the basis of a therapeutic relationship.***

2. Maintain low level of stimuli in client's environment (low lighting, few people, simple decor, low noise level). ***A stimulating environment may increase agitation and promote aggressive behavior.***
3. Observe client's behavior frequently. Do this through routine activities and interactions; avoid appearing watchful and suspicious. ***Close observation is required so that intervention can occur if needed to ensure client's (and others') safety.***
4. Remove all dangerous objects from client's environment. ***Client safety is a nursing priority.***
5. Help client identify the true object of his or her hostility (e.g., "You seem to be upset with . . .") ***Because of weak ego development, client may be misusing the defense mechanism of displacement. Helping him or her recognize this in a nonthreatening manner may help reveal unresolved issues so that they may be confronted.***
6. Encourage client to gradually verbalize hostile feelings. ***Verbalization of feelings in a nonthreatening environment may help client come to terms with unresolved issues.***
7. Explore with client alternative ways of handling frustration (e.g., large motor skills that channel hostile energy into socially acceptable behavior). ***Physically demanding activities help to relieve pent-up tension.***
8. Staff should maintain and convey a calm attitude toward client. ***Anxiety is contagious and can be transferred from staff to client. A calm attitude provides client with a feeling of safety and security.***
9. Have sufficient staff available to present a show of strength to client if necessary. ***This conveys to the client evidence of control over the situation and provides some physical security for staff.***
10. Administer tranquilizing medications as ordered by physician or obtain an order if necessary. Monitor client for effectiveness of the medication as well as for appearance of adverse side effects. ***Antianxiety agents (e.g., diazepam, chlordiazepoxide, oxazepam) produce a calming effect and may help to allay hostile behaviors.*** (NOTE: Medications are often not prescribed for

clients with antisocial personality disorder because of these individuals' strong susceptibility to addictions.)

11. If client is not calmed by "talking down" or by medication, use of mechanical restraints may be necessary. Be sure to have sufficient staff available to assist. Follow protocol established by the institution in executing this intervention. Most states require that the physician re-evaluate and issue a new order for restraints every 3 hours, except between the hours of midnight and 8:00 AM. If client has refused medication, administer after restraints have been applied. Most states consider this intervention appropriate in emergency situations or in the event that a client would likely harm self or others. Never use restraints as a punitive measure but rather as a protective measure for a client who is out of control.
12. Observe the client in restraints every 15 minutes (or according to institutional policy). Ensure that circulation to extremities is not compromised (check temperature, color, pulses). Assist client with needs related to nutrition, hydration, and elimination. Position client so that comfort is facilitated and aspiration can be prevented. *Client safety is a nursing priority.*

Outcome Criteria

1. Client is able to rechannel hostility into socially acceptable behaviors.
2. Client is able to discuss angry feelings and verbalize ways to tolerate frustration appropriately.

INEFFECTIVE INDIVIDUAL COPING

Definition: Inability to form a valid appraisal of the stressors, inadequate choices of practiced responses, and/or inability to use available resources.

Possible Etiologies ("related to")

[Inadequate support systems]
[Inadequate coping method]
[Underdeveloped ego]
[Underdeveloped superego]
[Dysfunctional family system]
[Negative role modeling]
[Absent, erratic, or inconsistent methods of discipline]
[Extreme poverty]

Defining Characteristics ("evidenced by")

[Disregard for societal norms and laws]
[Absence of guilt feelings]
[Inability to delay gratification]
[Extreme impulsivity]
[Inability to learn from punishment]

Goals/Objectives

Short-Term Goal

Client will verbalize understanding of unit rules and regulations and the consequences for violation of those rules and regulations within 24 hours after admission.

Long-Term Goal

Client will be able to cope more adaptively by delaying gratification of own desires and following rules and regulations of the unit by discharge.

Interventions with *Selected Rationales*

1. From the onset, client should be made aware of which behaviors will not be accepted on the unit. Explain consequences of violation of the limits. Consequences must involve something of value to the client. All staff must be consistent in enforcing these limits. Consequences should be administered in a matter-of-fact manner immediately after the infraction. ***Because client cannot (or will not) impose own limits on maladaptive behaviors, these behaviors must be delineated and enforced by staff. Undesirable consequences may help to decrease repetition of these behaviors.***
2. Do not attempt to coax or convince client to do the "right thing." Do not use the words "You should (or shouldn't) . . ."; instead, use "You will be expected to . . ." The ideal would be for this client to eventually internalize societal norms, beginning with this step-by-step, "either/or" approach on the unit (*either* you do [don't do] this, *or* this will occur). ***Explanations must be concise, concrete, and clear, with little or no capacity for misinterpretation.***
3. Provide positive feedback or reward for acceptable behaviors. ***Positive reinforcement enhances self-esteem and encourages repetition of desirable behaviors.***
4. In an attempt to assist client to delay gratification, begin to increase the length of time requirement for acceptable behavior in order to achieve the reward. For example, 2 hours of acceptable behavior may be exchanged for a phone call;

4 hours of acceptable behavior for 2 hours of television; 1 day of acceptable behavior for a recreational therapy bowling activity; 5 days of acceptable behavior for a weekend pass.

5. A milieu unit provides the appropriate environment for the client with antisocial personality. ***The democratic approach, with specific rules and regulations, community meetings, and group therapy sessions emulates the type of societal situation in which the client must learn to live. Feedback from peers is often more effective than confrontation from an authority figure. The client learns to follow the rules of the group as a positive step in the progression toward internalizing the rules of society.***
6. Help client to gain insight into his or her own behaviors. Often these individuals rationalize to such an extent that they deny that their behavior is wrong. (For example, "The owner of this store has so much money, he'll never miss the little bit I take. He has everything, and I have nothing. It's not fair! I deserve to have some of what he has.") ***Client must come to understand that certain behaviors will not be tolerated within the society and that severe consequences will be imposed on those individuals who refuse to comply. Client must want to become a productive member of society before he or she can be helped.***
7. Talk about past behaviors with client. Discuss which behaviors are acceptable by societal norms and which are not. Help client identity ways in which he or she has exploited others. Encourage client to explore how he or she would feel if the circumstances were reversed. ***An attempt may be made to enlighten the client to the sensitivity of others by promoting self-awareness in an effort to assist the client gain insight into his or her own behavior.***
8. Throughout relationship with client, maintain attitude of "It is not *you,* but your *behavior,* that is unacceptable." ***An attitude of acceptance promotes feelings of dignity and self-worth.***

Outcome Criteria

1. Client follows rules and regulations of the milieu environment.
2. Client is able to verbalize which of his or her behaviors are not acceptable.
3. Client shows regard for the rights of others by delaying gratification of own desires when appropriate.

DEFENSIVE COPING

Definition: The state in which an individual repeatedly projects falsely positive self-evaluation based on a self-protective pattern that defends against underlying perceived threats to positive self-regard.

Possible Etiologies ("related to")

[Low self-esteem]
[Retarded ego development]
[Underdeveloped superego]
[Negative role models]
[Lack of positive feedback]
[Absent, erratic, or inconsistent methods of discipline]
[Dysfunctional family system]

Defining Characteristics ("evidenced by")

Denial of obvious problems or weaknesses
Projection of blame or responsibility
Rationalization of failures
Hypersensitivity to criticism
Grandiosity
Superior attitude toward others
Difficulty establishing or maintaining relationships
Hostile laughter or ridicule of others
Difficulty in reality testing of perceptions
Lack of follow-through or participation in treatment or therapy

Goals/Objectives

Short-Term Goal

Client will verbalize personal responsibility for difficulties experienced in interpersonal relationships within (time period reasonable for client).

Long-Term Goal

Client will demonstrate ability to interact with others without becoming defensive, rationalizing behaviors, or expressing grandiose ideas.

Interventions with *Selected Rationales*

1. Recognize and support basic ego strengths. *Focusing on positive aspects of the personality may help to improve self-concept.*
2. Encourage client to recognize and verbalize feelings of inadequacy and need for acceptance from others, and how

these feelings provoke defensive behaviors, such as blaming others for own behaviors. ***Recognition of the problem is the first step in the change process toward resolution.***

3. Provide immediate, matter-of-fact, nonthreatening feedback for unacceptable behaviors. ***Client may lack knowledge about how he or she is being perceived by others. Providing this information in a nonthreatening manner may help to eliminate these undesirable behaviors.***
4. Help client identify situations that provoke defensiveness and practice through role playing more appropriate responses. ***Role playing provides confidence to deal with difficult situations when they actually occur.***
5. Provide immediate positive feedback for acceptable behaviors. ***Positive feedback enhances self-esteem and encourages repetition of desirable behaviors.***
6. Help client set realistic, concrete goals and determine appropriate actions to meet those goals. ***Success increases self-esteem.***
7. Evaluate with client the effectiveness of the new behaviors and discuss any modifications for improvement. ***Because of limited problem-solving ability, assistance may be required to reassess and develop new strategies, in the event that certain of the new coping methods prove ineffective.***

Outcome Criteria

1. Client verbalizes and accepts responsibility for own behavior.
2. Client verbalizes correlation between feelings of inadequacy and the need to defend the ego through rationalization and grandiosity.
3. Client does not ridicule or criticize others.
4. Client interacts with others in group situations without taking a defensive stance.

SELF-ESTEEM DISTURBANCE

Definition: Negative self-evaluation and feelings about self or self-capabilities, which may be directly or indirectly expressed.

Possible Etiologies ("related to")

[Lack of positive feedback]
[Unmet dependency needs]

[Retarded ego development]
[Repeated negative feedback, resulting in diminished self-worth]
[Dysfunctional family system]
[Absent, erratic, or inconsistent parental discipline]
[Extreme poverty]

Defining Characteristics ("evidenced by")

Denial of problems obvious to others
Projection of blame or responsibility for problems
Grandiosity
[Aggressive behavior]
[Frequent use of derogatory and critical remarks against others]
[Manipulation of one staff member against another in an attempt to gain special privileges]
[Inability to form close, personal relationships]

Goals/Objectives

Short-Term Goal

Client will verbalize an understanding that derogatory and critical remarks against others reflect feelings of self-contempt.

Long-Term Goal

Client will experience an increase in self-esteem, as evidenced by verbalizations of positive aspects of self and the lack of manipulative behaviors toward others.

Interventions with *Selected Rationales*

1. Ensure that goals are realistic. It is important for client to achieve something, so plan for activities in which success is likely. ***Success increases self-esteem.***
2. Identify ways in which client is manipulating others. Set limits on manipulative behavior. ***Because client is unable (or unwilling) to limit own maladaptive behaviors, assistance is required from staff.***
3. Explain consequences of manipulative behavior. All staff must be consistent and follow through with consequences in a matter-of-fact manner. ***From the onset, client must be aware of the outcomes his or her maladaptive behaviors will effect. Without consistency of follow-through from all staff, a positive outcome cannot be achieved.***
4. Encourage client to talk about his or her behavior, the limits, and the consequences for violation of those limits. ***Discussion of feelings regarding these circumstances***

may assist the client in achieving a degree of insight into his or her situation.

5. Discuss how manipulative behavior interferes with formation of close personal relationships. ***Client may be unaware of others' perception of him or her and of why these behaviors are not acceptable to others.***
6. Help client identify more adaptive interpersonal strategies. Provide positive feedback for nonmanipulative behaviors. ***Client may require assistance with solving problems. Positive reinforcement enhances self-esteem and encourages repetition of desirable behaviors.***
7. Encourage client to confront the fear of failure by attending therapy activities and undertaking new tasks. Offer recognition of successful endeavors.
8. Assist client in identifying positive aspects of the self and in developing ways to change the characteristics that are socially unacceptable. ***Individuals with low self-esteem often have difficulty recognizing their positive attributes. They may also lack problem-solving ability and require assistance to formulate a plan for implementing the desired changes.***
9. Minimize negative feedback to client. Enforce limit setting in a matter-of-fact manner, imposing previously established consequences for violations. ***Negative feedback can be extremely threatening to a person with low self-esteem, possibly aggravating the problem. Consequences should convey unacceptability of the behavior but not the person.***
10. Encourage independence in the performance of personal responsibilities and in decision making related to own self-care. Offer recognition and praise for accomplishments. ***Positive reinforcement enhances self-esteem and encourages repetition of desirable behaviors.***
11. Help client increase level of self-awareness through critical examination of feelings, attitudes, and behaviors. Help client to understand that it is perfectly acceptable for attitudes and behaviors to differ from those of others, as long as they do not become intrusive. ***As the client becomes more aware and accepting of himself or herself, the need for judging the behavior of others will diminish.***
12. Teach client assertiveness techniques, especially the ability to recognize the differences among passive, assertive, and aggressive behaviors and the importance of respecting the human rights of others while protecting one's own basic human rights. ***These techniques increase***

self-esteem while enhancing the ability to form satisfactory interpersonal relationships.

Outcome Criteria

1. Client verbalizes positive aspects about self.
2. Client does not manipulate others in an attempt to increase feelings of self-worth.
3. Client considers the rights of others in interpersonal interactions.

IMPAIRED SOCIAL INTERACTION

Definition: The state in which an individual participates in an insufficient or excessive quantity or ineffective quality of social exchange.

Possible Etiologies ("related to")

[Low self-esteem]
[Unmet dependency needs]
[Retarded ego development]
[Retarded superego development]
[Negative role modeling]
Knowledge deficit about ways to enhance mutuality

Defining Characteristics ("evidenced by")

Verbalized or observed discomfort in social situations
Verbalized or observed inability to receive or communicate a satisfying sense of belonging, caring, interest, or shared history
Observed use of unsuccessful social interaction behaviors
Dysfunctional interaction with peers, family, or others
[Exploitation of others for the fulfillment of own desires]
[Inability to develop satisfactory, enduring, intimate relationship with a sexual partner]
[Physical and verbal hostility toward others when fulfillment of own desires is thwarted]

Goals/Objectives

Short-Term Goal

Client will develop satisfactory relationship (no evidence of manipulation or exploitation) with nurse or therapist within 1 week.

Long-Term Goal

Client will interact appropriately with others, demonstrating concern for the needs of others as well as his or her own, by discharge from therapy.

Interventions with *Selected Rationales*

1. Develop therapeutic rapport with client. Establish trust by always being honest; keep all promises; convey acceptance of person, separate from unacceptable behaviors ("It is not *you,* but *your behavior,* that is unacceptable.") ***An attitude of acceptance promotes feelings of self-worth. Trust is the basis of a therapeutic relationship.***
2. Offer to remain with client during initial interactions with others on the unit. ***Presence of a trusted individual increases feelings of security during uncomfortable situations.***
3. Provide constructive criticism and positive reinforcement for efforts. ***Positive feedback enhances self-esteem and encourages repetition of desirable behaviors.***
4. Confront client as soon as possible when interactions with others are manipulative or exploitative. Establish consequences for unacceptable behavior, and always follow through. ***Because of the strong id influence on client's behavior, he or she should receive immediate feedback when behavior is unacceptable. Consistency in enforcing the consequences is essential if positive outcomes are to be achieved. Inconsistency creates confusion and encourages testing of limits.***
5. Act as a role model for client through appropriate interactions with him or her and with others. ***Role modeling is a powerful and effective form of learning.***
6. Provide group situations for client. ***It is through these group interactions with positive and negative feedback from his or her peers that client will learn socially acceptable behavior.***

Outcome Criteria

1. Client willingly and appropriately participates in group activities.
2. Client has satisfactorily established and maintained one interpersonal relationship with nurse or therapist, without evidence of manipulation or exploitation.
3. Client demonstrates ability to interact appropriately with others, showing respect for self and others.
4. Client is able to verbalize reasons for inability to form close interpersonal relationships with others in the past.

KNOWLEDGE DEFICIT (Self-Care Activities to Achieve and Maintain Optimal Wellness)

Definition: Absence or deficiency of cognitive information related to a specific topic.

Possible Etiologies ("related to")

Lack of interest in learning
[Low self-esteem]
[Denial of need for information]
[Denial of risks involved with maladaptive lifestyle]
[Unfamiliarity with sources for acquiring information]

Defining Characteristics ("evidenced by")

[History of substance abuse]
[Statement of lack of knowledge]
[Statement of misconception]
[Request for information]
[Demonstrated lack of knowledge regarding basic health practices]
[Reported or observed inability to take the responsibility for meeting basic health practices in any or all functional pattern areas]
[History of lack of health-seeking behavior]
Inappropriate or exaggerated behaviors (e.g., hysterical, hostile, agitated, apathetic)

Goals/Objectives

Short-Term Goal

Client will verbalize understanding of knowledge required to fulfill basic health needs following implementation of teaching plan.

Long-Term Goal

Client will be able to demonstrate skills learned for fulfillment of basic health needs by discharge from therapy.

Interventions with *Selected Rationales*

1. Assess client's level of knowledge regarding positive self-care practices. *An adequate database is necessary for the development of an effective teaching plan.*
2. Assess client's level of anxiety and readiness to learn. *Learning does not occur beyond the moderate level of anxiety.*

3. Determine method of learning most appropriate for client (e.g., discussion, question and answer, use of audio or visual aids, oral, written). Be sure to consider level of education and development. ***Teaching will be ineffective if presented at a level or by a method inappropriate to the client's ability to learn.***
4. Develop teaching plan, including measurable objectives for the learner. Provide information regarding healthful strategies for ADLs, as well as harmful effects of substance abuse on the body. Include suggestions for community resources to assist client when adaptability is impaired.
5. Include significant others in the learning activity, if possible. ***Input from individuals who are directly involved in the potential change increases the likelihood of a positive outcome.***
6. Implement teaching plan at a time that facilitates, and in a place that is conducive to, optimal learning (e.g., in the evening when family members visit; in an empty, quiet classroom or group therapy room). ***Learning is enhanced by an environment with few distractions.***
7. Begin with simple concepts and progress to the more complex. ***Retention is increased if presented introductory material is easy to understand.***
8. Provide activities for client and significant others in which to actively participate during the learning exercise. ***Active participation increases retention.***
9. Ask client and significant others to demonstrate knowledge gained by verbalizing information regarding positive self-care practices. ***Verbalization of knowledge gained is a measurable method of evaluating the teaching experience.***
10. Provide positive feedback for participation, as well as for accurate demonstration of knowledge gained. ***Positive feedback enhances self-esteem and encourages repetition of desirable behaviors.***
11. Evaluate the teaching plan. Identify strengths and weaknesses and any changes that may enhance the effectiveness of the plan.

Outcome Criteria

1. Client is able to verbalize information regarding positive self-care practices.
2. Client is able to verbalize available community resources for obtaining knowledge regarding, and assistance with, deficits related to health care.

■ INTERNET REFERENCES

Additional information about Personality Disorders may be located at the following Websites:

- http://www.mental-health-matters.com/borderline.html
- http://www.cmhc.com/guide/person.htm
- http://www.usd.edu/~pwyss/person.dis.html
- http://www.mentalhealth.com/dis/p20-pe04.html
- http://www.mentalhealth.com/dis/p20-pe08.html
- http://www.mentalhealth.com/dis/p20-pe05.html
- http://www.mentalhealth.com/dis/p20-pe09.html
- http://www.mentalhealth.com/dis/p20-pe06.html
- http://www.mentalhealth.com/dis/p20-pe07.html
- http://www.mentalhealth.com/dis/p20-pe10.html
- http://www.mentalhealth.com/dis/p20-pe01.html
- http://www.mentalhealth.com/dis/p20-pe02.html
- http://www.mentalhealth.com/dis/p20-pe03.html
- http://www.mentalhealth.com/p13.html#Per

UNIT THREE

SPECIAL TOPICS IN PSYCHIATRIC AND MENTAL HEALTH NURSING

CHAPTER 17

Problems Related to Abuse or Neglect

■ BACKGROUND ASSESSMENT DATA

The *DSM-IV* (APA, 1994) lists the following categories for this classification:

1. V61.21 **Physical Abuse of Child:** Physical injury to a child includes any *nonaccidental* physical injury caused by the parent or caretaker. The most obvious way to detect it is by outward physical signs. However, behavioral indicators may also be evident (Townsend, 2000).
2. V61.21 **Sexual Abuse of Child:** This category is defined as engaging in, or assisting any other person to engage in, any sexually explicit conduct or any simulation of such conduct for the purpose of producing any visual depiction of such conduct; or rape, molestation, prostitution, or other form of sexual exploitation of children, or incest with children (NCCAN, 1998). **Incest** is the occurrence of sexual contacts or interaction between, or sexual exploitation of, close relatives, or between participants who are related to each other by a kinship bond that is regarded as a prohibition to sexual relations (e.g., caretakers, stepparents, stepsiblings) (Kaplan and Sadock, 1998).
3. V61.21 **Neglect of Child:** Physical neglect of a child includes refusal of or delay in seeking health care, abandonment, expulsion from the home or refusal to allow a runaway to return home, and inadequate supervision (NCCAN, 1998). Emotional neglect refers to a chronic failure by the parent or caretaker to provide the child with the hope, love, and support necessary

for the development of a sound, healthy personality (KCAPC, 1992).

4. V61.1 **Physical Abuse of Adult:** Physical abuse of an adult may be defined as "the infliction of physical pain or injury with the intent to cause harm which may include slaps, punches, biting, and hair pulling, but in frequency or occurrence generally involves more serious assaults including choking, kicking, breaking bones, stabbing, or shooting; or forcible restraint which may include locking in homes or closets, being tied or handcuffed" (Martin, 1988).
5. V61.1 **Sexual Abuse of Adult:** Sexual abuse of an adult may be defined as the expression of power and dominance by means of sexual violence, most commonly by men over women, although men may also be victims of sexual assault. Sexual assault is identified by the use of force and executed against the person's will.

Predisposing Factors (That Contribute to Patterns of Abuse)

1. **Physiological**
   a. ***Neurophysiological Influences:*** Components of the neurological system in both humans and animals have been implicated in both the facilitation and inhibition of aggressive impulses. Areas of the brain that may be involved include the temporal lobe, the limbic system, and the amygdaloid nucleus (Tardiff, 1994).
   b. ***Biochemical Influences:*** Studies show that various neurotransmitters, in particular norepinephrine, dopamine, and serotonin, may play a role in the facilitation and inhibition of aggressive impulses (Silver and Yudofsky, 1992).
   c. **Genetic Influences:** Some studies have implicated heredity as a component in the predisposition to aggressive behavior. Both direct genetic links and the genetic karyotype XYY have been investigated as possibilities. Evidence remains inconclusive.
   d. ***Disorders of the Brain:*** Various disorders of the brain including tumors, trauma, and certain disease (e.g., encephalitis and epilepsy) have been implicated in the predisposition to aggressive behavior (Silver and Yudofsky, 1992).

2. **Psychosocial**
   a. ***Psychodynamic Theory:*** The psychodynamic theorists have hypothesized that aggression and violence are the overt expressions of powerlessness and low self-esteem, which result when childhood needs for satisfaction and security go unmet (Townsend, 2000).
   b. ***Learning Theory:*** This theory postulates that aggressive and violent behaviors are learned from prestigious and influential role models. Individuals who were abused as children or whose parents disciplined with physical punishment are more likely to behave in a violent manner as adults (Tardiff, 1994).
   c. ***Societal Influences:*** Social scientists believe that aggressive behavior is primarily a product of one's culture and social structure (West, 1983). Societal influences may contribute to violence when individuals come to realize that their needs and desires cannot be met through conventional means, and they resort to delinquent behaviors in an effort to obtain desired ends.

Symptomatology (Subjective and Objective Data)

1. Signs of physical abuse may include the following:
   a. Bruises over various areas of the body. They may present with different colors of bluish purple to yellowish green (indicating various stages of healing).
   b. Bite marks, skin welts, burns.
   c. Fractures, scars, serious internal injuries, even brain damage.
   d. Lacerations, abrasions, or unusual bleeding.
   e. Bald spots indicative of severe hair pulling.
   f. In a child, regressive behaviors (such as thumb sucking and enuresis) are common.
   g. Extreme anxiety and mistrust of others.
2. Signs of neglect of a child may include the following:
   a. Soiled clothing that does not fit and may be inappropriate for the weather.
   b. Poor hygiene.
   c. Always hungry, with possible signs of malnutrition (e.g., emaciated, with swollen belly).
   d. Listless and tired much of the time.
   e. Unattended medical problems.

   f. Social isolation; unsatisfactory peer relationships.
   g. Poor school performance and attendance record.
3. Signs of sexual abuse of a child include the following:
   a. Frequent urinary infections.
   b. Difficulty or pain in walking or sitting.
   c. Rashes or itching in the genital area; scratching the area a great deal or fidgeting when seated.
   d. Frequent vomiting.
   e. Seductive behavior; compulsive masturbation; precocious sex play.
   f. Excessive anxiety and mistrust of others.
   g. Sexually abusing another child.
4. Signs of sexual abuse of an adult include (Burgess, 1984) the following:
   a. Contusions and abrasions about various parts of the body.
   b. Headaches, fatigue, sleep pattern disturbances.
   c. Stomach pains, nausea, and vomiting.
   d. Vaginal discharge and itching, burning on urination, rectal bleeding and pain.
   e. Rage, humiliation, embarrassment, desire for revenge, self-blame.
   f. Fear of physical violence and death.
   g. Overwhelming sense of helplessness and personal violation.

Common Nursing Diagnoses and Interventions

(Interventions are applicable to various health-care settings, such as inpatient and partial hospitalization, community outpatient clinic, home health, and private practice.)

RAPE-TRAUMA SYNDROME

Definition: Forced, violent sexual penetration against the victim's will and consent. The trauma syndrome that develops from this attack or attempted attack includes an acute phase of disorganization of the victim's lifestyle and a long-term process of reorganization of lifestyle.

Possible Etiologies ("related to")

[Having been the victim of sexual violence executed with the use of force and against one's personal will and consent]

Defining Characteristics ("evidenced by")

Disorganization
Change in relationships
Confusion
Physical trauma (e.g., bruising, tissue irritation)
Suicide attempts
Denial; guilt
Paranoia; humiliation, embarrassment
Aggression; muscle tension and/or spasms
Mood swings
Dependence
Powerlessness; helplessness
Nightmare and sleep disturbances
Sexual dysfunction
Revenge; phobias
Loss of self-esteem
Inability to make decisions
Substance abuse; depression
Anger; anxiety; agitation
Shame; shock; fear

Goals/Objectives

Short-Term Goal

The client's physical wounds will heal without complication.

Long-Term Goal

The client will begin a healthy grief resolution, initiating the process of psychological healing (time dimension to be individually determined).

Interventions with *Selected Rationales*

1. Smith (1987a) related the importance of communicating the following four phrases to the rape victim:
   a. I am very sorry this happened to you.
   b. You are safe here.
   c. I am very glad you are alive.
   d. You are not to blame. You are a victim. It was not your fault. Whatever decisions you made at the time of the victimization were the right ones because you are alive. ***The woman who has been sexually assaulted fears for her life and must be reassured of her safety. She may also be overwhelmed with self-doubt and self-blame, and these statements instill trust and validate self-worth.***
2. Explain every assessment procedure that will be conducted

and why. Ensure that data collection is conducted in a caring, nonjudgmental manner *to decrease fear and anxiety and increase trust.*

3. Ensure that the client has adequate privacy for all immediate postcrisis interventions. Try to have as few people as possible providing the immediate care or collecting immediate evidence. *The posttrauma client is extremely vulnerable. Additional people in the environment increase this feeling of vulnerability and escalate anxiety.*
4. Encourage the client to give an account of the assault. Listen, but do not probe. *Nonjudgmental listening provides an avenue for catharsis that the client needs to begin healing. A detailed account may be required for legal follow-up, and a caring nurse, as client advocate, may help to lessen the trauma of evidence collection.*
5. Discuss with the client whom to call for support or assistance. Provide information about referrals for aftercare. *Because of severe anxiety and fear, client may need assistance from others during this immediate postcrisis period. Provide referral information in writing for later reference (e.g., psychotherapist, mental health clinic, community advocacy group).*

Outcome Criteria

1. The client is no longer experiencing panic anxiety.
2. The client demonstrates a degree of trust in the primary nurse.
3. The client has received immediate attention to physical injuries.
4. The client has initiated behaviors consistent with the grief response.

POWERLESSNESS

Definition: The perception that one's own action will not significantly affect an outcome; a perceived lack of control over a current situation or immediate happening.

Possible Etiologies ("related to")

Lifestyle of helplessness
[Low self-esteem]
[Living with, or in a long-term relationship with, an individual who victimizes by inflicting physical pain or injury with the

intent to cause harm, and continues to do so over a long period of time]
[Lack of support network of caring others]
[Lack of financial independence]

Defining Characteristics ("evidenced by")

Verbal expressions of having no control or influence over situation or outcome
Reluctance to express true feelings
Passivity
[Verbalizations of abuse]
[Lacerations over areas of body]
[Fear for personal and children's safety]
[Verbalizations of no way to get out of relationship]

Goals/Objectives

Short-Term Goal

Client will recognize and verbalize choices that are available, thereby perceiving some control over life situation (time dimension to be individually determined).

Long-Term Goal

Client will exhibit control over life situation by making decision about what to do regarding living with cycle of abuse (time dimension to be individually determined).

Interventions with *Selected Rationales*

1. In collaboration with physician, ensure that all physical wounds, fractures, and burns receive immediate attention. It is a good idea to take photographs, if the victim will permit (Smith, 1987b; Burgess, 1990). *Client safety is a nursing priority. Photographs may be called in as evidence if charges are filed.*
2. Take the woman to a private area to do the interview. *If the client is accompanied by the man who did the battering, she is not likely to be truthful about her injuries.*
3. If she has come alone or with her children, assure her of her safety. Encourage her to discuss the battering incident. Ask questions about whether this has happened before; whether the abuser takes drugs; whether the woman has a safe place to go; and whether she is interested in pressing charges. *Some women will attempt to keep secret how their injuries occurred in an effort to protect the partner or because they are fearful that the partner will kill them if they tell.*

4. Ensure that "rescue" efforts are not attempted by the nurse. Offer support, but remember that the final decision must be made by the client. ***Making her own decision gives the client a sense of control over her life situation. Imposing judgments and giving advice are nontherapeutic.***
5. Stress the importance of safety. Smith (1987b) suggests a statement such as, "Yes, it has happened. Now where do you want to go from here?" Burgess (1990) states, "The victim needs to be made aware of the variety of resources that are available to her. These may include crisis hotlines, community groups for women who have been abused, shelters, a variety of counseling opportunities (i.e., couples, individual, or group), and information regarding the victim's rights in the civil and criminal justice system." After a discussion of these available resources, the woman may choose for herself. If her decision is to return to the marriage and home, this choice, too, must be respected. ***Knowledge of available choices can serve to decrease the victim's sense of powerlessness, but true empowerment comes only when she chooses to use that knowledge for her own benefit.***

Outcome Criteria

1. The client has received immediate attention to physical injuries.
2. The client verbalizes assurance of her immediate safety.
3. The client discusses life situation with primary nurse.
4. The client is able to verbalize choices available to her from which she may receive assistance.

ALTERED GROWTH AND DEVELOPMENT

Definition: The state in which an individual demonstrates deviations in norms from his or her age group.

Possible Etiologies ("related to")

Inadequate caretaking

[The infliction by caretakers of physical pain or injury with the intent to cause harm, usually occurring over an extended period of time]

[Ignoring the child's basic physiological needs]

[Indifference to the child]

[Ignoring the child's presence]

[Ignoring the child's social, educational, recreational, and developmental needs]

Defining Characteristics ("evidenced by")

Delay or difficulty in performing skills (motor, social, or expressive) typical of age group
Altered physical growth
Inability to perform self-care or self-control activities appropriate for age
Flat affect
Listlessness
Decreased responses
[Evidence of bruises, burns, lacerations, or other types of physical injury not consistent with performance of everyday activities]
[Expression of fear of parent or caretaker]
[Social isolation]
[Regressive behaviors (e.g., rocking, thumb sucking, enuresis)]
[Wearing clothing inappropriate to weather to cover up the injuries]

Goals/Objectives

Short-Term Goal

Client will develop trusting relationship with nurse and report how evident injuries were sustained (time dimension to be individually determined).

Long-Term Goal

Client will demonstrate behaviors consistent with age-appropriate growth and development.

Interventions with *Selected Rationales*

1. Perform complete physical assessment of the child. Take particular note of bruises (in various stages of healing), lacerations, and client complaints of pain in specific areas. Do not overlook or discount the possibility of sexual abuse. Assess for nonverbal signs of abuse: aggressive conduct, excessive fears, extreme hyperactivity, apathy, withdrawal, age-inappropriate behaviors. ***An accurate and thorough physical assessment is required to provide appropriate care for the client.***
2. Conduct an in-depth interview with the parent or adult who accompanies the child. Consider: If the injury is being reported as an accident, is the explanation reasonable? Is the injury consistent with the child's explanation? Is the injury consistent with the child's developmental capabilities?

Fear of imprisonment or loss of child custody may place the abusive parent on the defensive. Discrepancies may be evident in the description of the incident, and lying to cover up involvement is a common defense that may be detectable in an in-depth interview.

3. Use games or play therapy to gain child's trust. Use these techniques to assist in describing his or her side of the story. *Establishing a trusting relationship with an abused child is extremely difficult. The child may not even want to be touched. These types of play activities can provide a nonthreatening environment that may enhance the child's attempt to discuss these painful issues (Celano, 1990).*
4. Determine whether nature of the injuries warrant reporting to authorities. Specific state statutes must enter into the decision of whether to report suspected child abuse. *A report [is commonly made] if there is reason to suspect that a child has been injured as a result of physical, mental, emotional, or sexual abuse (KCAPC, 1992). "Reason to suspect" exists when there is evidence of a discrepancy or inconsistency in explaining a child's injury. Most states require that the following individuals report cases of suspected child abuse: all health-care workers, all mental health therapists, teachers, child care providers, firefighters, emergency medical personnel, and law enforcement personnel. Reports are made to the Department of Social and Rehabilitative Services (SRS), Department of Human Services (DHS), or a law enforcement agency.*

Outcome Criteria

1. The client has received immediate attention to physical injuries.
2. The client demonstrates trust in primary nurse by discussing abuse through the use of play therapy.
3. The client is demonstrating a decrease in regressive behaviors.

■ INTERNET REFERENCES

Additional information related to Child Abuse may be located at the following Websites:

- http://www.endabuse.com/index.htm
- http://www.childabuse.org/
- http://www.cmhcsys.com/factsfam/sexabuse.htm

Additional information related to Sexual Assault may be located at the following Websites:

- http://www.cs.utk.edu/~bartley/saInfoPage.html
- http://www.ncweb.com/org/rapecrisis

Additional information related to Domestic Violence may be located at the following Websites:

- http://www.ndvh.org/
- http://www.cpsdv.org/
- http://www.cybergrrl.com/dv/book/toc.html
- http://software2.bu.edu/cohis/violence/helpvctm.htm
- http://www.domestic-violence.org/

CHAPTER 18

*Premenstrual Dysphoric Disorder**

BACKGROUND ASSESSMENT DATA

Defined

Premenstrual dysphoric disorder[†] is identified by a variety of physical and emotional symptoms that occur during the last week of the luteal phase of the menstrual cycle and that remit within a few days after the onset of the follicular phase. In most women, these symptoms occur in the week before, and remit within a few days after, the onset of menses. The disorder has also been reported in nonmenstruating women who have had a hysterectomy but retain ovarian function. The diagnosis is given only when the symptoms are sufficiently severe to cause marked impairment in social or occupational functioning, and have occurred during a majority of menstrual cycles in the past year (APA, 1994).

Predisposing Factors

1. **Physiological**
   a. ***Biochemical:*** An imbalance of the hormones estrogen and progesterone have been implicated in the predisposition to premenstrual dysphoric dis-

*Reprinted with permission from the *Diagnostic and Statistical Manual of Mental Disorders, Fourth Edition.* Copyright 1994 American Psychiatric Association, 1994.

[†]Text and criteria are provided in the *DSM-IV* to facilitate systematic clinical research (APA, 1994).

order. It is postulated that excess estrogen or a high estrogen-to-progesterone ratio during the luteal phase causes water retention and that this hormonal imbalance has other effects as well, resulting in the symptoms associated with premenstrual syndrome (Casey and Dwyer, 1987).

b. ***Nutritional:*** A number of nutritional alterations have been implicated in the etiology of premenstrual dysphoric disorder (Casey and Dwyer, 1987). They include vitamin B_6 deficiency, glucose tolerance fluctuations, abnormal fatty acid metabolism, magnesium deficiency, vitamin E deficiency, and caffeine sensitivity. No definitive evidence exists to support any specific nutritional alteration in the etiology of these symptoms.

2. **Psychosocial**
   a. ***Family Dynamics:*** It is possible that the behaviors associated with premenstrual dysphoric disorder are learned through role modeling during the socialization process (Doenges, Townsend, and Moorhouse, 1998). Children may observe and identify with this behavior in significant adults and incorporate it into their own responses as they mature. Positive reinforcement in the form of primary or secondary gains for these behaviors may serve to perpetuate the learned patterns of disability.

Symptomatology (Subjective and Objective Data)

The American Psychiatric Association (1994) has identified the following symptoms as diagnostic for premenstrual (late luteal phase) dysphoric disorder:

1. Markedly depressed mood, feelings of hopelessness, or self-deprecating thoughts.
2. Marked anxiety, tension, feelings of being "keyed up" or "on edge."
3. Marked affective lability (e.g., feeling suddenly sad or tearful or increased sensitivity to rejection).
4. Persistent and marked anger or irritability or increased interpersonal conflicts.
5. Decreased interest in usual activities (e.g., work, school, friends, hobbies).
6. Subjective sense of difficulty in concentrating.
7. Lethargy, easy fatigability, or marked lack of energy.

8. Marked change in appetite, overeating, or specific food cravings.
9. Hypersomnia or insomnia.
10. A subjective sense of being overwhelmed or out of control.
11. Other physical symptoms, such as breast tenderness or swelling, headaches, joint or muscle pain, a sensation of "bloating," or weight gain.

Other subjective symptoms that have been reported include (Doenges, Townsend, and Moorhouse, 1998):

12. Cramps.
13. Alcohol intolerance.
14. Acne.
15. Cystitis.
16. Oliguria.
17. Altered sexual drive.
18. Forgetfulness.
19. Suicidal ideations or attempts.

Common Nursing Diagnoses and Interventions

(Interventions are applicable to various health-care settings, such as inpatient and partial hospitalization, community outpatient clinic, home health, and private practice.)

ACUTE PAIN

Definition: Sudden or slow onset of any intensity from mild to severe with an anticipated or predictable end and a duration of less than 6 months.

Possible Etiologies ("related to")

[Imbalance in estrogen and progesterone levels]
[Possible nutritional alterations, including the following:
- Vitamin B_6 deficiency
- Glucose tolerance fluctuations
- Abnormal fatty acid metabolism, which may contribute to alterations in prostaglandin synthesis
- Magnesium deficiency
- Vitamin E deficiency
- Caffeine sensitivity
- Alcohol intolerance]

[Fluid retention]

Defining Characteristics ("evidenced by")

[Subjective communication of:
- Headache
- Backache
- Joint or muscle pain
- A sensation of "bloating"
- Abdominal cramping
- Breast tenderness and swelling]

Facial mask [of pain]
Sleep disturbance
Self-focus
Changes in appetite and eating

Goals/Objectives

Short-Term Goal

Client cooperates with efforts to manage symptoms of premenstrual syndrome (PMS) and minimize feelings of discomfort.

Long-Term Goal

Client verbalizes relief from discomfort associated with symptoms of PMS.

Interventions with *Selected Rationales*

1. Assess and record location, duration, and intensity of pain. ***Background assessment data are necessary to formulate an accurate plan of care for the client.***
2. Provide nursing comfort measures with a matter-of-fact approach that does not give positive reinforcement to the pain behavior (e.g., back rub, warm bath, heating pad). Give additional attention at times when client is not focusing on physical symptoms. ***These measures may serve to provide some temporary relief from pain. Absence of secondary gains in the form of positive reinforcement may discourage client's use of the pain as attention-seeking behavior.***
3. Encourage the client to get adequate rest and sleep and avoid stressful activity during the premenstrual period. ***Fatigue exaggerates symptoms associated with PMS. Stress elicits heightened symptoms of anxiety, which may contribute to exacerbation of symptoms and altered perception of pain.***
4. Assist client with activities that distract from focus on self and pain. Demonstrate techniques such as visual or auditory distractions, guided imagery, breathing exercises, mas-

sage, application of heat or cold, and relaxation techniques that may provide symptomatic relief. ***These techniques may help to maintain anxiety at manageable level and prevent the discomfort from becoming disabling.***

5. ***In an effort to correct the possible nutritional alterations that may be contributing to PMS,*** the following guidelines may be suggested (Doenges, Townsend, and Moorhouse, 1998):
   a. Reduce intake of fats in the diet, particularly saturated fats.
   b. Limit intake of dairy products to two servings a day (excessive dairy products block the absorption of magnesium).
   c. Increase intake of complex carbohydrates (vegetables, legumes, cereals, and whole grains) and *cis*-linoleic acid–containing foods (e.g., safflower oil).
   d. Decrease refined and simple sugars. (Excess sugar is thought to cause nervous tension, palpitations, headache, dizziness, drowsiness, and excretion of magnesium in the urine, thus preventing the body from breaking down sugar for energy.)
   e. Decrease salt intake to 3 g per day but not less than 0.5 g per day. (Salt restriction prevents edema; too little salt stimulates norepinephrine and causes sleep disturbances.)
   f. Limit intake of caffeine (coffee, tea, colas, and chocolate) and alcohol (one to two drinks a week). Caffeine increases breast tenderness and pain. Alcohol can cause reactive hypoglycemia and fluid retention.
   g. Because some women crave junk food during the premenstrual period, it is important to take a multiple vitamin or mineral tablet to ensure that adequate nutrients are consumed.
6. Administer medications as prescribed. Monitor client response for effectiveness of the medication, as well as for appearance of adverse side effects. ***When other measures are insufficient to bring about relief,*** physician may prescribe symptomatic drug therapy. Provide client with information about the medication to be administered. ***Client has the right to know about the treatment she is receiving.*** Some medications commonly used for symptomatic treatment of PMS are presented in Table 18–1.

Outcome Criteria

1. Client demonstrates ability to manage premenstrual symptoms with minimal discomfort.
2. Client verbalized relief of painful symptoms.

TABLE 18–1 **Medications for Symptomatic Relief of Premenstrual Syndrome**

Medication	Indication
Hydrochlorothiazide (Esidrix, HydroDIURIL), furosemide (Lasix)	Diuretics may provide relief from edema when diet and sodium restriction are not sufficient.
Ibuprofen (Advil, Motrin, Nuprin), naproxen (Naprosyn)	Nonsteroidal antiinflammatory agents may provide relief from joint, muscle, and lower abdominal pain related to increased prostaglandins.
Propranolol (Inderal), verapamil (Isoptin)	β-Blockers and calcium channel blockers are often given for prophylactic treatment of migraine headaches.
Sumatriptan (Imitrex), naratriptan (Amerge), rizatriptan (Maxalt), zolmitriptan (Zomig)	These serotonin 5-HT_1 receptor agonists are highly effective in the treatment of acute migraine attack.
Carisoprodol (Soma), chlorzoxazone (Parafon Forte)	Muscle relaxants may provide relief of muscular tension.
Bromocriptine (Parlodel)	This drug may be prescribed to relieve breast pain and other symptoms of PMS that may be caused by elevated prolactin.

INEFFECTIVE INDIVIDUAL COPING

Definition: Inability to form a valid appraisal of the stressors, inadequate choices of practiced responses, and/or inability to use available resources.

Possible Etiologies ("related to")

[Imbalance in estrogen and progesterone levels]
[Possible nutritional alterations, including the following:
- Vitamin B_6 deficiency
- Glucose tolerance fluctuations
- Abnormal fatty acid metabolism, which may contribute to alterations in prostaglandin synthesis
- Magnesium deficiency

Vitamin E deficiency
Caffeine sensitivity
Alcohol intolerance]
[Learned coping patterns through early role modeling]

Defining Characteristics ("evidenced by")

[Affective liability (sad one minute, angry the next)]
[Marked anger or irritability]
[Feelings of elevated anxiety, tension, being "keyed up" or "on edge"]
[Depressed mood, feelings of hopelessness, or self-deprecating thoughts]
[Decreased interest in usual activities]
[Easy fatigability or marked lack of energy]
[Difficulty concentrating; forgetfulness]
[Changes in appetite]
[Hypersomnia or insomnia]
[Altered sexual drive]
[Suicidal ideations or attempts]
Inability to problem-solve
Inability to meet role expectations

Goals/Objectives

Short-Term Goals

1. Client will seek out support person when having thoughts of suicide.
2. Client will verbalize ways to express anger in an appropriate manner and maintain anxiety at a manageable level.

Long-Term Goals

1. Client will not harm self while experiencing symptoms associated with PMS.
2. Client will demonstrate adaptive coping strategies to use in an effort to minimize disabling behaviors during the premenstrual and perimenstrual period.

Interventions with *Selected Rationales*

1. Assess client's potential for suicide. Has she expressed feelings of not wanting to live? Does she have a plan? A means? ***Depression is the most prevalent disorder that precedes suicide. The risk of suicide is greatly increased if the client has developed a plan and particularly if means exist for the client to execute the plan.***
2. Formulate a short-term verbal contract with the client that she will not harm herself during specific time period. When that contract expires, make another, an so forth.

Discussion of suicidal feelings with a trusted individual provides a degree of relief to the client. A contract gets the subject out in the open and places some of the responsibility for the client's safety with the client. An attitude of acceptance of the client as a worthwhile individual is conveyed.

3. Secure a promise from client that she will seek out a staff member if thoughts of suicide emerge. ***Suicidal clients are often very ambivalent about their feelings. Discussion of feelings with a trusted individual may provide assistance before the client experiences a crisis situation.***
4. Encourage client to express angry feelings within appropriate limits. Provide safe method of hostility release. Help client to identify source of anger, if possible. Work on adaptive coping skills for use outside the health-care system. ***Depression and suicidal behaviors are sometimes viewed as anger turned inward on the self. If this anger can be verbalized in a nonthreatening environment, the client may be able to resolve these feelings, regardless of the discomfort involved.***
5. Encourage client to discharge pent-up anger through participation in large motor activities (e.g., brisk walks, jogging, physical exercises, volleyball, punching bag, exercise bike). ***Physical exercise provides a safe and effective method for discharging pent-up tension.***
6. Assist client in identifying stressors that precipitate anxiety and irritability and in learning new methods of coping with these situations (e.g., stress reduction techniques, relaxation, and visualization skills). ***Knowing stress factors and ways of handling them reduces anxiety and allows client to feel a greater measure of control over the situation.***
7. Identify extent of feelings and situations when loss of control occurs. Assist with problem solving to identify behaviors for protection of self and others (e.g., call support person, remove self from situation). ***Recognition of potential for harm to self or others and development of a plan enables client to take effective actions to meet safety needs.***
8. Encourage client to reduce or shift workload and social activities during the premenstrual period as part of a total stress management program. ***By coping realistically with life stresses, the decreased responsibility should relieve stress and therefore help relieve symptoms.***
9. At each visit, evaluate symptoms and discuss those that

may be most troublesome and continue to persist well after initiation of therapy. ***If traditional measures are inadequate, pharmacological intervention may be required to enhance coping abilities. For example, antidepressants may be administered for depression that remains unresolved after other symptoms have been relieved.***

10. Encourage participation in support group, psychotherapy, marital counseling, or other type of therapy as deemed necessary. ***Professional assistance may be required to help the client and family members learn effective coping strategies and support lifestyle changes that may be needed.***

Outcome Criteria

1. Client participates willingly in treatment regimen, and initiates necessary lifestyle changes.
2. Client demonstrates adaptive coping strategies to deal with episodes of depression and anxiety.
3. Client verbalizes that she has no suicidal thoughts or intentions.

■ INTERNET REFERENCES

- http://www.encyclopedia.com/articles/10485.html
- http://www.womens-health.com/health_center/gynecology/gyn_md_pms.html
- http://www.healthlinkusa.com/254feata.htm

CHAPTER 19

HIV Disease

BACKGROUND ASSESSMENT DATA

The Immune Response to HIV

The cells responsible for nonspecific immune reactions include neutrophils, monocytes, and macrophages. In the normal immune response, they work to destroy an invasive organism and initiate and facilitate repair to damaged tissue. If these cells are not effective in accomplishing a satisfactory healing response, specific immune mechanisms take over.

The elements of the cellular response include the T4 lymphocytes (also called helper T cells). When the body is invaded by a foreign antigen, these T4 cells divide many times, producing antigen-specific T4 cells with other functions. One of these is the T4 killer cell, which serves to help destroy the antigen.

The most conspicuous immunologic abnormality associated with HIV infection is a striking depletion of T4 lymphocytes. The HIV infects the T4 lymphocyte, thereby destroying the very cell the body needs to direct an attack on the virus. An individual with a healthy immune system may present with a T4 cell count between 600 and 1200 mm^3.

Stages and Symptoms of HIV Disease

1. **Early Stage (T4 Cells 1000–500 mm^3)**
   a. ***Acute HIV Infection:*** The acute HIV infection is identified by a characteristic syndrome of symptoms that occurs from 6 days to 6 weeks after exposure to the virus. The symptoms have an abrupt onset, are somewhat vague, and are similar to those sometimes seen in mononucleosis. Symp-

toms of acute HIV infection include fever, myalgia, malaise, lymphadenopathy, sore throat, anorexia, nausea and vomiting, headaches, skin rash, and diarrhea. Most symptoms resolve themselves in 1 to 3 weeks, with the exception of fever, myalgia, lymphadenopathy, and malaise, which may continue for several months.

b. ***Seroconversion:*** Seroconversion, the detectability of HIV antibodies in the blood, most often is detected between 6 and 12 weeks, but can occur anytime between 1 week and (in rare instances) 1 year. The time between infection and seroconversion is called the *window period.*

c. ***Asymptomatic Infection.*** During this stage, there are no manifestations of illness. Blood tests may reveal immunologic and hematologic abnormalities, such as leukopenia, anemia, or thrombocytopenia. This period may last 5 to 10 years or longer.

2. **Middle Stage (T4 Cells 500–200 mm^3)**
   a. ***Persistent Generalized Lymphadenopathy:*** Lymph nodes in at least two different locations in the body (usually the neck, armpit, and groin) swell and remain swollen for months, with no other signs of a related infectious disease.
   b. ***Systemic Complaints:*** Fever, night sweats, chronic diarrhea, fatigue, minor oral infections, headaches, and weight loss.
3. **Late Stage (T4 Cells ≤200 mm^3)**
   a. ***HIV Wasting Syndrome:*** Severe weight loss, large-volume diarrhea, fever and weakness.
   b. ***Opportunistic Infections:*** Opportunistic infections are those that occur because of the altered immune state of the host. These infections, which include protozoan, fungal, viral, and bacterial, have long been a defining characteristic of AIDS. The most common, life-threatening opportunistic infection seen in clients with AIDS is *pneumocystis pneumonia.*
   c. ***AIDS-Related Malignancies:*** HIV-positive individuals are at risk for developing certain types of malignancies. These include Kaposi's sarcoma, non-Hodgkin's lymphoma, Hodgkin's disease, malignant melanoma, testicular cancers, primary hepatocellular carcinoma, and invasive cervical cancer.
   d. ***Altered Mental States:*** The most common alterations in mental states observed in AIDS clients in-

clude delirium (fluctuating consciousness, abnormal vital signs, and psychotic phenomena) and dementia (called HIV-Associated Dementia [HAD]; symptoms include cognitive, motor, and behavioral changes similar to those seen in individuals with other cognitive disorders [see Chap. 4]).

NOTE: Depression is common in HIV disease but can occur at any time during the disease process.

Predisposing Factors

1. **Sexual Transmission**
   a. ***Heterosexual Transmission:*** Because the virus is found in greater concentration in semen than in vaginal secretions, it is more readily transmitted from men to women than from women to men. However, female-to-male transmission is possible, as HIV has been isolated in vaginal secretions.
   b. ***Homosexual Transmission:*** The most significant risk factors for homosexual transmission of HIV are receptive anal intercourse and the number of male sexual partners. The lining of the anal canal is delicate and prone to tearing and bleeding, making anal intercourse an easy way for infections to be passed from one person to another.
2. **Bloodborne Transmission**
   a. ***Transfusion with Blood Products:*** Although laboratory tests are more than 99 percent sensitive, screening problems may occur when donations are received from recently HIV-infected individuals who have not yet developed antibody or from persistently antibody-negative HIV-infected donors.
   b. ***Transmission by Needles Infected with HIV:*** The highest number of cases occurring via this route are among intravenous drug users who share needles and other equipment contaminated with HIV-infected blood. Another bloodborne mode of transmission with contaminated needles is through accidental needle sticks by health-care workers, as well as by other means and with other contaminated equipment used for therapeutic purposes.
3. **Perinatal Transmission**
   a. Modes of transmission include transplacental, exposure to maternal blood and vaginal secretions during delivery, and breast milk. The risk of peri-

natal transmission has been significantly reduced in recent years with the advent of free or low-cost prenatal care, provision of access to anti-HIV medication during pregnancy, and education about the dangers of breastfeeding.

4. **Other Possible Modes of Transmission**
   a. To date, HIV has been isolated from blood, semen, vaginal secretions, saliva, tears, breast milk, cerebrospinal fluid, and amniotic fluid. However, only blood, semen, vaginal secretions, and breast milk have been epidemiologically linked to transmission of the virus.

Common Nursing Diagnoses and Interventions

(Interventions are applicable to various health-care settings, such as inpatient and partial hospitalization, community outpatient clinic, home health, and private practice.)

ALTERED PROTECTION

Definition: A state in which an individual experiences a decrease in the ability to guard self from internal or external threats such as illness or injury.

Possible Etiologies ("related to")

[Compromised immune status secondary to diagnosis of HIV disease]

Defining Characteristics ("evidenced by")

[Laboratory values indicating decreased numbers of T4 cells]
[Presence of opportunistic infections]
[Manifestations of
Fever, night sweats, diarrhea
Anorexia, weight loss
Fatigue, malaise
Swollen lymph glands
Cough, dyspnea
Rash, skin lesions, white patches in mouth
Headache
Ataxia
Bleeding, bruising
Neurological defects]

Goals/Objectives

Short-Term Goal

Client will exhibit no new signs or symptoms of infection.

Long-Term Goal

Client safety and comfort will be maximized.

Interventions with *Selected Rationales*

1. *To prevent infection in an immunocompromised individual:*
   a. Implement universal blood and body fluid precautions.
   b. Wash hands with antibacterial soap before entering and upon leaving client's room.
   c. Monitor vital signs at regular intervals.
   d. Monitor complete blood counts (CBCs) for leukopenia/neutropenia.
   e. Monitor for signs and symptoms of specific opportunistic infections.
   f. Protect client from individuals with infections.
   g. Maintain meticulous sterile technique for dressing changes and any invasive procedure.
   h. Administer antibiotics as ordered.
2. ***To restore nutritional status and decrease nausea, vomiting, and diarrhea:***
   a. Provide low-residue, high-protein, high-calorie, soft, bland diet. Maintain hydration with adequate fluid intake.
   b. Obtain daily weight and record intake and output.
   c. Monitor serum electrolytes and CBCs.
   d. If client is unable to eat, provide isotonic tube feedings as tolerated. Check for gastric residual frequently.
   e. If client is unable to tolerate oral intake or tube feedings, consult physician regarding possibility of parenteral hyperalimentation. Observe hyperalimentation administration site for signs of infection.
   f. Administer antidiarrheals and antiemetics as ordered.
   g. Perform frequent oral care. Promote prevention and healing of lesions in the mouth.
   h. Have the client eat small, frequent meals with high-calorie snacks rather than three large meals per day.
3. ***To promote improvement of skin and mucous membrane integrity:***
   a. Monitor skin condition for signs of redness and breakdown.

b. Reposition client every 1 to 2 hours.
c. Encourage ambulation and chair activity as tolerated.
d. Use "egg crate" mattress or air mattress on bed.
e. Wash skin daily with soap and rinse well with water.
f. Apply lotion to skin to maintain skin softness.
g. Provide wound care as ordered for existing pressure sores or lesions.
h. Cleanse skin exposed to diarrhea thoroughly and protect rectal area with ointment.
i. Apply artificial tears to eyes as appropriate.
j. Perform frequent oral care; apply ointment to lips.

4. *To maximize oxygen consumption and minimize respiratory distress:*
   a. Assess respiratory status frequently:
      (1) Monitor depth, rate, and rhythm of respirations.
      (2) Auscultate lung fields every 2 hours and prn.
      (3) Monitor arterial blood gases.
      (4) Check color of skin, nailbeds, and sclerae.
      (5) Assess sputum for color, odor, and viscosity.
   b. Encourage coughing and deep-breathing exercises.
   c. Provide humidified oxygen as ordered.
   d. Suction as needed using sterile technique.
   e. Space nursing care to allow client adequate rest periods between procedures.
   f. Administer analgesics or sedatives judiciously to prevent respiratory depression.
   g. Administer bronchodilators and antibiotics as ordered.
5. *To minimize the potential for easy bleeding caused by HIV-induced thrombocytopenia:*
   a. Follow protocol for maintenance of skin integrity.
   b. Provide safe environment to minimize falling or bumping into objects.
   c. Provide soft toothbrush or "toothette" swabs for cleaning teeth and gums.
   d. Ensure that client does not take aspirin or other medications that increase the potential for bleeding.
   e. Clean up areas contaminated by client's blood with household bleach (5.25 percent sodium hypochlorite) diluted 1:10 with water (Bartlett & Finkbeiner, 1996).
6. *To maintain near normal body temperature:*
   a. Provide frequent tepid water sponge baths.
   b. Provide antipyretic as ordered by physician (avoid aspirin).
   c. Place client in cool room, with minimal clothing and bedcovers.
   d. Encourage intake of cool liquids (if not contraindicated).

Outcome Criteria

1. Client does not experience respiratory distress.
2. Client maintains optimal nutrition and hydration.
3. Client has experienced no further weight loss.
4. Client maintains integrity of skin and mucus membranes.

ALTERED FAMILY PROCESSES

Definition: A change in family relationships and/or functioning.

Possible Etiologies ("related to")

[Crisis associated with having a family member diagnosed with HIV disease]

Defining Characteristics ("evidenced by")

Changes in availability for affective responsiveness and intimacy
Changes in participation in problem solving and decision making
Changes in communication patterns
Changes in availability for emotional support
Changes in satisfaction with family
Changes in expression of conflict within family

Goals/Objectives

Short-Term Goal

Family members will express feelings regarding loved one's diagnosis and prognosis.

Long-Term Goal

Family will verbalize areas of dysfunction and demonstrate ability to cope more effectively.

Interventions with *Selected Rationales*

1. Create an environment that is comfortable, supportive, private, and promotes trust. ***Basic needs of the family must be met before crisis resolution can be attempted.***
2. Encourage each individual member to express feelings regarding loved one's diagnosis and prognosis. ***Each individual is unique and must feel that his or her private needs can be met within the family constellation.***

3. If the client is homosexual, and this is the family's first awareness, help them deal with guilt and shame they may experience. Help parents to understand they are not responsible and their child is still the same individual they have always loved. ***Resolving guilt and shame enables family members to respond adaptively to the crisis. Their response can affect the client's remaining future and the family's future as well (Christ, Siegel, and Moynihan, 1988).***
4. Serve as facilitator between client's family and homosexual lover. The family may have difficulty accepting the lover as a person who is as significant as a spouse. Clarify roles and responsibilities of family and lover. Do this by bringing both parties together to define and distribute the tasks involved in the client's care. ***By minimizing the lack of legally defined roles, and by focusing on the need for making realistic decisions about the client's care, communication and resolution of conflict are enhanced (Christ, Siegel and Moynihan, 1988).***
5. Encourage use of stress management techniques (e.g., relaxation exercises, guided imagery, attendance at support group meetings for significant others of AIDS clients). ***Reduction of stress and support from others who share similar experiences enable individuals to begin to think more clearly and develop new behaviors to cope with this situational crisis.***
6. Provide educational information about AIDS and opportunity to ask questions and express concerns. ***Many misconceptions about the disease abound within the public domain. Clarification may calm some of the family's fears and facilitate interaction with the client.***
7. Make family referrals to community organizations that provide supportive help or financial assistance to AIDS clients. ***Extended care can place a financial burden on client and family members. Respite care may provide family members with occasional much-needed relief away from the stress of physical and emotional caregiving responsibilities.***

Outcome Criteria

1. Family members are able to discuss feelings regarding client's diagnosis and prognosis.
2. Family members are able to make rational decisions regarding care of their loved one and the effect on family functioning.

KNOWLEDGE DEFICIT (Prevention of Transmission and Protection of the Client)

Definition: Absence or deficiency of cognitive information related to a specific topic.

Possible Etiologies ("related to")

Cognitive limitation
Information misinterpretation
Lack of exposure [to accurate information]

Defining Characteristics ("evidenced by")

Verbalization of the problem
Inappropriate or exaggerated behaviors
Inaccurate follow-through of instruction
[Inaccurate statements by client and family]

Goals/Objectives

Short-Term Goal

Client and family verbalize understanding about disease process, modes of transmission, and prevention of infection.

Long-Term Goals

1. Client and family demonstrate ability to execute precautions for preventing transmission of HIV and infection of the client.
2. Transmission of HIV and infection of the client are prevented.

Interventions with *Selected Rationales**

1. Present the following information *in an effort to clarify misconceptions, calm fears, and support an environment of appropriate interventions for care of the client with AIDS.* Teach that HIV cannot be contracted from:
   a. Casual or household contact with an AIDS client.
   b. Shaking hands, hugging, social (dry) kissing, holding hands, or other nonsexual physical contact.

---

*The nursing interventions for this care plan have been adapted from "Nursing Care Plan for the AIDS Patient," written by the nursing staff of Hospice, Inc., Wichita, KS, with permission.

c. Touching unsoiled linens or clothing, money, furniture, or other inanimate objects.
d. Being near someone who has AIDS at work, school, restaurants, or elevators.
e. Toilet seats, bathtubs, towels, showers, or swimming pools.
f. Dishes, silverware, or food handled by a person with AIDS.
g. Animals (pets may transmit opportunistic organisms).
h. (Very unlikely spread by) coughing, sneezing, spitting, kissing, tears, or saliva.

2. AIDS virus dies quickly outside the body because it requires living tissue to survive. It is readily killed by soap, cleansers, hot water, and disinfectants.
3. Teach client to protect self from infections by taking the following precautions:
   a. Avoid unpasteurized milk or milk products.
   b. Cook all raw vegetables and fruits before eating them. ***Raw or improperly washed foods may transmit microbes.***
   c. Cook all meals well before eating.
   d. Avoid direct contact with persons with known contagious illnesses.
   e. Consult physician before getting a pet. ***Pets require extra infection control precautions owing to the opportunistic organisms carried by animals.***
   f. Avoid touching animal feces, urine, emesis, litter boxes, aquariums, or bird cages. Always wear mask and gloves when cleaning up after a pet.
   g. Avoid traveling in countries with poor sanitation.
   h. Avoid vaccines or vaccinations that contain live organisms. ***Vaccination with live organisms may be fatal to severely immunosuppressed persons.***
   i. Exercise regularly.
   j. Control stress factors. A counselor or support group may be helpful.
   k. Stop smoking. ***Smoking predisposes to respiratory infections.***
   l. Maintain good personal hygiene.
4. Teach client and significant others about prevention of transmission:
   a. Do not donate blood, plasma, body organs, tissues, or semen.
   b. Inform physician, dentist, and anyone providing care that client has AIDS.
   c. Do not share needles or syringes.
   d. Do not share personal items, such as toothbrushes, ra-

zors, or other implements that may be contaminated with blood or body fluids.

e. Do not eat or drink from the same dinnerware and utensils without washing them between use.
f. Avoid becoming pregnant if at risk for HIV infection.
g. Engage in only "safer" sexual practices (those ***not*** involving exchange of body fluids).
h. Avoid sexual practices medically classified as "unsafe," such as anal or vaginal intercourse and oral sex.
i. Avoid the use of recreational drugs because of their immunosuppressive effects.

5. Teach the home caregiver(s) to protect self from HIV infection by taking the following precautions:
   a. Wash hands thoroughly with liquid antibiotic soap before and after each client contact. Use moisturizing lotion afterward to prevent dry, cracking skin.
   b. Wear gloves when in contact with blood or body fluids (e.g., open wounds, suctioning, feces). Gown or aprons may be worn if soiling is likely.
   c. Wear a mask:
      (1) When client has a productive cough and tuberculosis has not been ruled out.
      (2) To protect client if caregiver has a cold.
      (3) During suctioning.
   d. Bag disposable gloves and masks with client's trash.
   e. Dispose of the following in the toilet:
      (1) Organic material on clothes or linen before laundering.
      (2) Blood or body fluids.
      (3) Soiled tissue or toilet paper.
      (4) Cleaners or disinfectants used to clean contaminated articles.
      (5) Solutions contaminated with blood or body fluids.
   f. Double-bag client's trash and soiled dressings in an impenetrable, plastic bag. ***Tie*** the bag shut and discard with household trash.
   g. Do not recap needles, syringes, and other sharp items. Use puncture-proof covered containers for disposal (e.g., coffee cans, jars).
   h. Place soiled linen and clothing in a plastic bag and tie shut until washed. Launder these separately from other laundry. Use bleach or other disinfectant in hot water.
   i. When house cleaning, all equipment used in care of the client, as well as bathroom and kitchen surfaces, should be cleaned with a 1:10 dilute bleach solution
   j. Mops, sponges, and other items used for cleaning should be reserved specifically for that purpose.

Outcome Criteria

1. Client and family as well as significant other(s) are able to verbalize information presented regarding ways in which HIV can and cannot be transmitted, ways to protect the client from infections, and ways to prevent transmission to caregivers and others.
2. Transmission to others and infection of the client have been avoided.

■ INTERNET REFERENCES

Additional information about HIV/AIDS may be located at the following Websites:

- http://www.avert.org/
- http://www.kc-reach.org/
- http://www.infoweb.org/
- http://www.aegis.com/main/
- http://www.aidsnews/index.html
- http://www.critpath.org/
- http://www.healthcg.com/hiv/
- http://www.medscape.com/Home/Topics/AIDS/AIDS.htm
- http://www.HIVpositive.com/
- http://www.guides4living.com/links.html
- http://research.med.umkc.edu/teams/cml/AIDS.html
- http://www.alzheimer-europe.org/aids.html

CHAPTER 20

Homelessness

BACKGROUND ASSESSMENT DATA

It is difficult to determine how many individuals are homeless in the United States. Estimates have been between 250,000 and 4 million.

Who are the homeless?

1. **Age:** Studies have produced a variety of statistics related to age of the homeless: 25 percent are younger than 18 years of age, individuals between 31 and 50 comprise 51 percent, and the range of persons aged 55 to 60 has been estimated at 2.5 to 19.4 percent.
2. **Gender:** More men than women are homeless. The U.S. Conference of Mayors (1998) study found that single men comprised 45 percent of the urban homeless population and single women 14 percent.
3. **Families:** Families with children are among the fastest growing segments of the homeless population. Families comprise 38 percent of the urban homeless population, but research indicates that this number is likely higher in rural areas, where families, single mothers, and children make up the largest group of homeless people.
4. **Ethnicity:** The study by the U.S. Conference of Mayors (1998) found that the homeless population was 53 percent African-American, 35 percent Caucasian, 12 percent Hispanic, 4 percent Native American, and 3 percent Asian. The ethnic makeup of homeless populations varies according to geographic location.

Mental Illness and Homelessness

It is thought that approximately 20 to 25 percent of the single adult homeless population suffers from some form of severe and persistent mental illness (Koegel, Burnam, and Baumohl, 1996). Frequently described as the most common diagnosis is schizophrenia. Other prevalent disorders include bipolar affective disorder, substance abuse and dependence, depression, personality disorders, and organic mental disorders.

Predisposing Factors to Homelessness Among the Mentally Ill

1. **Deinstitutionalization:** Between 1955 and 1981, the population of state and county mental hospitals dropped nationally from 559,000 to 125,000 clients (Dato and Rafferty, 1985). Deinstitutionalization began out of expressed concern by mental health professionals and others who described the "deplorable conditions" under which mentally ill individuals were housed. Some individuals believed that institutionalization deprived the mentally ill of their civil rights. Not the least of the motivating factors for deinstitutionalization was the financial burden these clients placed on state governments.
2. **Poverty:** Cuts in various government entitlement programs have depleted the allotments available for chronically mentally ill individuals living in the community. Even when the unemployment rate in general is low, the job market remains prohibitive for individuals whose behavior is incomprehensible or even frightening to many. The stigma and discrimination associated with mental illness may be diminishing slowly, but it is highly visible to those who suffer from its effects.
3. **Scarcity of Affordable Housing:** Wallsten (1992) states:

   > Economic policies and issues have contributed to the growing numbers and different profiles of the homeless. Urban redevelopment projects eliminated a considerable amount of low-cost housing options for poor people. A growing number of impoverished families have been doubling and tripling up in single housing units as affordable housing becomes more scarce. A sizable proportion of residents in these renewal areas were poor elderly renting rooms in houses, residential hotels, and missions. (p. 21)

   In addition, the number of single-room-occupancy (SRO) hotels has diminished drastically. These SRO hotels provided a means of relatively inexpensive housing for chronic psychiatric clients. Although some people believe that these facilities nurtured isolation, they provided adequate shelter from the elements for their occupants. So many individuals currently frequent the shelters of our cities that there is concern that the shelters are becoming mini-institutions for the chronically mentally ill.

4. **Lack of Affordable Health Care:** For families barely able to scrape together enough money to pay for day-to-day living, a catastrophic illness can create the level of poverty that starts the downward spiral to homelessness.
5. **Domestic Violence:** The study by the U.S. Conference of Mayors (1998) revealed that 46 percent identified domestic violence as a primary cause of homelessness. Battered women are often forced to choose between an abusive relationship and homelessness.
6. **Addiction Disorders:** For individuals with alcohol or drug addictions, in the absence of appropriate treatment, the chances increase for being forced into life on the street. The National Coalition for the Homeless (NCH) (1999) cites the following as obstacles to addiction treatment for homeless persons: lack of health insurance, lack of documentation, waiting lists, scheduling difficulties, daily contact requirements, lack of transportation, ineffective treatment methods, lack of supportive services, and cultural insensitivity.

Symptomatology (Commonly Associated with Homelessness)

1. Mobility and migration (the penchant for frequent movement to various geographic locations).
2. Substance abuse.
3. Nutritional deficiencies.
4. Difficulty with thermoregulation.
5. Increased incidence of tuberculosis.
6. Increased incidence of sexually transmitted diseases.
7. Increased incidence of gastrointestinal and respiratory disorders.
8. In homeless children (compared with control samples), increased incidence of:
   a. Ear disorders.
   b. Gastrointestinal disorders.
   c. Infestational ailments.
   d. Developmental delays.
   e. Psychological problems.

Common Nursing Diagnoses and Interventions

(Interventions are applicable to various health-care settings, such as inpatient and partial hospitalization, community health clinic, "street clinic," and homeless shelters.)

ALTERED HEALTH MAINTENANCE

Definition: Inability to identify, manage and/or seek out help to maintain health.

Possible Etiologies ("related to")

Perceptual/cognitive impairment
Lack of, or significant alteration in, communication skills
Unachieved developmental tasks
Lack of material resources
Lack of ability to make deliberate and thoughtful judgments
Ineffective individual coping

Defining Characteristics ("evidenced by")

History of lack of health-seeking behavior
Reported or observed lack of equipment, financial and/or other resources
Reported or observed impairment of personal support systems
Demonstrated lack of knowledge regarding basic health practices
Demonstrated lack of adaptive behaviors to internal/external environmental changes
Reported or observed inability to take responsibility for meeting basic health practices in any or all functional pattern areas

Goals/Objectives

Short-Term Goal

Client will seek and receive assistance with current health matters.

Long-Term Goals

1. Client will assume responsibility for own health-care needs within level of ability.
2. Client will adopt lifestyle changes that support individual health-care needs.

Interventions with *Selected Rationales*

1. The triage nurse in the emergency department, street clinic, or shelter will begin the biopsychosocial assessment of the

homeless client. ***An adequate assessment is required to ensure that appropriate nursing care is provided.***

2. Assess developmental level of functioning and ability to communicate. Use language that the client can comprehend. ***This information is essential to ensure that client achieves an accurate understanding of presented information and that the nurse correctly interprets what the client is attempting to convey.***
3. Assess client's use of substances, including use of tobacco. Discuss eating and sleeping habits. ***These actions may be contributing to current health problems.***
4. Assess sexual practices ***to determine level of personal risk.***
5. Assess oral hygiene practices ***to determine specific self-care needs.***
6. Assess client's ability to make decisions. ***Client may need assistance in determining the type of care that is required and how to determine the most appropriate time to seek that care.***
7. Hunter (1992) suggests that three basic questions must be asked of the homeless client:
   a. Do you understand what your problem is?
   b. How will you get your prescriptions filled?
   c. Where are you going when you leave here or where will you sleep tonight?

   Answers to these questions at admission will initiate discharge planning for the client.
8. Teach client the basics of self-care (e.g., proper hygiene, facts about nutrition). ***The client must have this type of knowledge if he or she is to become more self-sufficient.***
9. Teach client about safe sex practices ***in an effort to avoid sexually transmitted diseases.***
10. Identify immediate problems and assist with crisis intervention. ***Emergency departments, "storefront" clinics, or shelters may be the homeless client's only resource in a crisis situation.***
11. Tend to physical needs immediately. Ensure that client has a thorough physical examination. ***The client cannot deal with psychosocial issues until physical problems have been addressed.***
12. Assess mental health status. ***Many homeless individuals have some form of mental illness.*** Ensure that appropriate psychiatric care is provided. If possible, inquire about possible long-acting medication injections for this client. ***The client may be less likely to discontinue taking the medication if he or she does not have to take pills every day.***

13. Refer client to others who can provide assistance (e.g., case manager, social worker). ***If the client is to be discharged to a shelter, a case manager or social worker may be the best link between the client and the health-care system to ensure that he or she obtains appropriate follow-up care.***

Outcome Criteria

1. Client verbalizes understanding of information presented regarding optimal health maintenance.
2. Client is able to verbalize signs and symptoms that should be reported to a health-care professional.
3. Client verbalizes knowledge of available resources from whom he or she may seek assistance as required.

POWERLESSNESS

Definition: Perception that one's own action will not significantly affect an outcome; a perceived lack of control over a current situation or immediate happening.

Possible Etiologies ("related to")

Lifestyle of helplessness
[Homelessness]

Defining Characteristics ("evidenced by")

Verbal expressions of having no control over self-care
Verbal expressions of having no control or influence over situation
Verbal expressions of having no control or influence over outcome
Apathy

Goals/Objectives

Short-Term Goal

Client will identify areas over which he or she has control.

Long-Term Goal

Client will make decisions that reflect control over present situation and future outcome.

Interventions with *Selected Rationales*

1. Provide opportunities for the client to make choices about his or her present situation. ***Providing client with choices will increase his or her feeling of control.***

2. Avoid arguing or using logic with the client who feels powerless. ***Client will not believe it can make a difference.***
3. Accept expressions of feelings, including anger and hopelessness. ***An attitude of acceptance enhances feelings of trust and self-worth.***
4. Assist the client in identifying personal strengths and establishing realistic life goals. ***Unrealistic goals set the client up for failure and reinforce feelings of powerlessness.***
5. Help client identify areas of life situation that he or she can control. ***Client's emotional condition interferes with his or her ability to solve problems. Assistance is required to perceive the benefits and consequences of available alternatives accurately.***
6. Help client identify areas of life situation that are not within his or her ability to control. Encourage verbalization of feelings related to this inability ***in an effort to deal with unresolved issues and accept what cannot be changed.***
7. Encourage client to seek out support group or shelter resources. ***Social isolation promotes feelings of powerlessness and hopelessness.***

Outcome Criteria

1. Client verbalizes choices made in a plan to maintain control over his or her life situation.
2. Client verbalizes honest feelings about life situations over which he or she has no control.
3. Client is able to verbalize system for problem solving as required to maintain hope for the future.

■ INTERNET REFERENCES

- http://earthsystems.org/ways/
- http://www.absoluteauthority.com/homelessness
- http://www.chn.org/homeless/

CHAPTER 21

Psychiatric Home Nursing Care

■ BACKGROUND ASSESSMENT DATA

Dramatic changes in the health-care delivery system and skyrocketing costs have created a need to find a way to provide quality, cost-effective care to psychiatric clients. Home health care has become one of the fastest growing areas in the health-care system and is now recognized by many reimbursement factions as a preferred method of community-based service. Just what is home health care? The National Association for Home Care (NAHC) (1996) contributes the following definition:

> Home care is a simple phrase that encompasses a wide range of health and social services. These services are delivered at home to recovering, disabled, chronically or terminally ill persons in need of medical, nursing, social, or therapeutic treatment and/or assistance with essential activities of daily living.

Psychiatric home nursing care expounds upon this definition to include the delivery of mental health services to clients in their home setting. Duffey and Miller (1996) state:

> Psychiatric home care nurses must have physical and psychosocial nursing skills to meet the demands of the patient population they serve. Inpatient psychiatric nurses are likely to have some familiarity with physical nursing skills. Psychiatric nurses in home care must adapt their skills to fit within the home care nursing arena. (p. 104)

Predisposing Factors

In 1996, 3.4 percent of all clients receiving home care services had a primary psychiatric diagnosis (NAHC,

1999). Richie and Lusky (1987) cite the following reasons for the continued increase in psychiatric home care:

1. Earlier hospital discharges.
2. Increased demand for home care as an alternative to institutional care.
3. Broader third-party payment coverage.
4. Greater physician acceptance of home care.

Psychiatric home nursing care is provided through private home health agencies, private hospitals, public hospitals, government institutions such as the Department of Veterans Affairs, and community mental health centers. Most often, home care is viewed as follow-up care to inpatient, partial, or outpatient hospitalization.

The majority of home health care is paid for by Medicare. Other sources include Medicaid, private insurance, self-pay, and others. Medicare requires that the following criteria be met to qualify for psychiatric home care:

1. Certification by a physician that the client is homebound.
2. The client has an acute psychiatric diagnosis or an acute exacerbation of such an illness.
3. The client requires the specialized knowledge, skills, and abilities of a psychiatric registered nurse (Pelletier, 1988).

Case (1993) reports:

> Medicare's interpretation of 'homebound' status for psychiatric clients diverges from the medical application with which most have been familiar in the past. Patients don't have to be physically homebound; they can be mentally homebound. In other words, they can be patients physically able to leave their homes but mentally unwilling. It deals more with not wanting to leave the home because of factors such as anxiety, cognitive impairment, and vegetative depression. Agency nurses must be able to document that patients truly are homebound by such factors. (p. 61)

Although Medicare and Medicaid are the largest reimbursement providers, a growing number of health maintenance organizations (HMOs) and preferred provider organizations (PPOs) are beginning to recognize the cost effectiveness of psychiatric home nursing care and are including it as part of their benefit packages. Most managed care agencies require that treatment, or even a specific number of visits, be preauthorized for psychiatric home nursing care. The plan of treatment and subsequent charting must explain why the client's psychiatric disorder keeps him or her at home, as well as justify the need for services.

Symptomatology (Subjective and Objective Data)

Homebound clients most often have diagnoses of schizophrenia, major depression, bipolar disorder, substance abuse, agoraphobia, paranoia, and generalized anxiety (Hellwig, 1993). Many elderly clients are homebound owing to medical conditions that impair mobility and necessitate home care.

Finkelman (1997) states:

> Psychiatric home care is provided to patients with psychiatric diagnoses who may or may not have been hospitalized in the past, to medical patients who do not have a formal psychiatric diagnosis but do have major psychiatric symptoms, and to medical patients with psychological responses to their medical illnesses. (p. xv)

Richie and Lusky (1987) identify three predominant client populations that benefit from psychiatric home health nursing:

1. **The elderly:** These individuals are without a history of chronic mental illness but are experiencing acute psychosocial and developmental problems that have arisen from medical and sociocultural factors. Depression and social isolation are common.
2. **The chronically mentally ill:** These individuals have a history of three or more psychiatric hospitalizations and require long-term medications and supportive care. Common diagnoses include depression, schizoaffective disorders, schizophrenia, and borderline personality disorder.
3. **Those with acute mental health problems:** These individuals are experiencing crisis situations and are in need of crisis intervention and/or short-term psychotherapy.

The following components should be included in the comprehensive assessment of the homebound client (Wheeler, 1998):

1. Client's perception of the problem and need for assistance.
2. Information regarding client's strengths and personal habits.

3. Health history.
4. Recent changes.
5. Support systems.
6. Vital signs.
7. Current medications.
8. Client's understanding and compliance with medications.
9. Nutritional and elimination assessment.
10. Activities of daily living (ADLs) assessment.
11. Substance use assessment.
12. Neurological assessment.
13. Mental status examination (see Appendix M).
14. Comprehension of proverbs.
15. Global Assessment of Functioning (GAF) Scale rating (see Appendix K).

Other important assessments include information about acute or chronic medical conditions, patterns of sleep and rest, solitude and social interaction, use of leisure time, education and work history, issues related to religion or spirituality, and adequacy of the home environment.

Nursing Diagnoses and Interventions Common to Psychiatric Homebound Clients

INEFFECTIVE MANAGEMENT OF THERAPEUTIC REGIMEN: INDIVIDUALS

Definition: A pattern of regulating and integrating into daily living a program for treatment of illness and the sequelae of illness that is unsatisfactory for meeting specific health goals.

Possible Etiologies ("related to")

Perceived barriers
Social support deficits
Powerlessness
Perceived benefits
Mistrust of regimen
Knowledge deficits
Complexity of therapeutic regimen

Defining Characteristics ("evidenced by")

Choices of daily living ineffective for meeting the goals of a treatment or prevention program
Verbalized that did not take action to reduce risk factors for progression of illness and sequelae
Verbalized difficulty with regulation/integration of one or more prescribed regimens for treatment of illness and its effects or prevention of complications
Acceleration of illness symptoms
Verbalized that did not take action to include treatment regimens in daily routines

Goals/Objectives

Short-Term Goals

1. Client will verbalize understanding of barriers to management of therapeutic regimen.
2. Client will participate in problem-solving efforts toward adequate management of therapeutic regimen.

Long-Term Goal

Client will incorporate changes in lifestyle necessary to maintain therapeutic regimen.

Interventions with *Selected Rationales*

1. Assess client's knowledge of condition and treatment needs. ***Client may lack full comprehension of need for treatment regimen.***
2. Identify client's perception of treatment regimen. ***Client may be mistrustful of treatment regimen or of healthcare system in general.***
3. ***Promote a trusting relationship with the client*** by being honest, encouraging client to participate in decision making, and conveying genuine positive regard.
4. Assist client in recognizing strengths and past successes. ***Recognition of strengths and past successes increases self-esteem and indicates to client that he or she can be successful in managing therapeutic regimen.***
5. Provide positive reinforcement for efforts. ***Positive reinforcement increases self-esteem and encourages repetition of desirable behaviors.***
6. Emphasize importance of need for treatment/medication. ***Client must understand that the consequence of lack of follow-through is possible decompensation.***
7. ***In an effort to incorporate lifestyle changes and promote wellness,*** assist client in developing plans for man-

aging therapeutic regimen, such as support groups, social and family systems, and financial assistance.

Outcome Criteria

1. Client verbalizes understanding of information presented regarding management of therapeutic regimen.
2. Client demonstrates desire and ability to perform strategies necessary to maintain adequate management of therapeutic regimen.
3. Client verbalizes knowledge of available resources from whom he or she may seek assistance as required.

IMPAIRED ADJUSTMENT

Definition: Inability to modify lifestyle or behavior in a manner consistent with a change in health status.

Possible Etiologies ("related to")

Low state of optimism
Intense emotional state
Negative attitudes toward health behavior
Failure to intend to change behavior
Multiple stressors
Absence of social support for changed beliefs and practices
Disability or health status change requiring change in lifestyle
Lack of motivation to change behaviors

Defining Characteristics ("evidenced by")

Denial of health status change
Failure to achieve optimal sense of control
Failure to take actions that would prevent further health problems
Demonstration of nonacceptance of health status change

Goals/Objectives

Short-Term Goals

1. Client will discuss with home health nurse the kinds of lifestyle changes that will occur because of the change in health status.
2. With the help of home health nurse, client will formulate a plan of action for incorporating those changes into his or her lifestyle.
3. Client will demonstrate movement toward independence, considering change in health status.

Long-Term Goal

Client will demonstrate competence to function independently to his or her optimal ability, considering change in health status, by discharge from home health care.

Interventions with *Selected Rationales*

1. Encourage client to talk about lifestyle prior to the change in health status. Discuss coping mechanisms that were used at stressful times in the past. ***It is important to identify the client's strengths so that they may be used to facilitate adaptation to the change or loss that has occurred.***
2. Encourage client to discuss the change or loss and particularly to express anger associated with it. ***Some individuals may not realize that anger is a normal stage in the grieving process. If it is not released in an appropriate manner, it may be turned inward on the self, leading to pathological depression.***
3. Encourage client to express fears associated with the change or loss, or alteration in lifestyle that the change or loss has created. ***Change often creates a feeling of disequilibrium and the individual may respond with fears that are irrational or unfounded. He or she may benefit from feedback that corrects misperceptions about how life will be with the change in health status.***
4. Provide assistance with ADLs as required, but encourage independence to the limit that client's ability will allow. Give positive feedback for activities accomplished independently. ***Independent accomplishments and positive feedback enhance self-esteem and encourage repetition of desired behaviors. Successes also provide hope that adaptive functioning is possible and decrease feelings of powerlessness.***
5. Help client with decision making regarding incorporation of change or loss into lifestyle. Identify problems that the change or loss is likely to create. Discuss alternative solutions, weighing potential benefits and consequences of each alternative. Support client's decision in the selection of an alternative. ***The high degree of anxiety that usually accompanies a major lifestyle change often interferes with an individual's ability to solve problems and to make appropriate decisions. Client may need assistance with this process in an effort to progress toward successful adaptation.***
6. Use role playing ***to decrease anxiety*** as client anticipates stressful situations that might occur in relation to the

health status change. ***Role playing decreases anxiety and provides a feeling of security by preparing the client with a plan of action to respond in an appropriate manner when a stressful situation occurs.***

7. Ensure that client and family are fully knowledgeable regarding the physiology of the change in health status and its necessity for optimal wellness. Encourage them to ask questions, and provide printed material explaining the change to which they may refer following discharge.
8. Help client identify resources within the community from which he or she may seek assistance in adapting to the change in health status. Examples include self-help or support groups, counselor, or social worker. Encourage client to keep follow-up appointments with physician or to call physician's office prior to follow-up date if problems or concerns arise.

Outcome Criteria

1. Client is able to perform ADLs independently.
2. Client is able to make independent decisions regarding lifestyle considering change in health status.
3. Client is able to express hope for the future with consideration of change in health status.

SOCIAL ISOLATION

Definition: Aloneness experienced by the individual and perceived as imposed by others and as a negative or threatened state.

Possible Etiologies ("related to")

Alterations in mental status
Inability to engage in satisfying personal relationships
Unaccepted social values
Unaccepted social behavior
Inadequate personal resources
Immature interests
Alterations in physical appearance
Altered state of wellness

Defining Characteristics ("evidenced by")

Expresses feelings of aloneness imposed by others
Expresses feelings of rejection
Inappropriate interests for developmental stage
Inability to meet expectations of others

Insecurity in public
Absence of supportive significant other(s)
Projects hostility in voice and behavior
Withdrawn; uncommunicative
Seeks to be alone
Preoccupation with own thoughts
Sad, dull affect

Goals/Objectives

Short-Term Goal

Client will verbalize willingness to be involved with others.

Long-Term Goal

Client will participate in interactions with others at level of ability or desire.

Interventions with *Selected Rationales*

1. Convey an accepting attitude by making regular visits. ***An accepting attitude increases feelings of self-worth and facilitates trust.***
2. Show unconditional positive regard. ***This conveys your belief in the client as a worthwhile human being.***
3. Be honest and keep all promises. ***Honesty and dependability promote a trusting relationship.***
4. Be cautious with touch until trust has been established. ***A suspicious client may perceive touch as a threatening gesture.***
5. Be with the client to offer support during activities that may be frightening or difficult for him or her. ***The presence of a trusted individual provides emotional security for the client.***
6. Take walks with the client. Help him or her perform simple tasks around the house. ***Increased activity enhances both physical and mental status.***
7. Assess lifelong patterns of relationships. ***Basic personality characteristics will not change. Most individuals keep the same style of relationship development that they had in the past.***
8. Help the client identify present relationships that are satisfying and activities that he or she considers interesting. ***Only the client knows what he or she truly likes, and these personal preferences will facilitate success in reversing social isolation.***
9. Consider the feasibility of a pet. ***There are many documented studies of the benefits of companion pets.***

Outcome Criteria

1. Client demonstrates willingness and desire to socialize with others.
2. Client independently pursues social activities with others.

CAREGIVER ROLE STRAIN

Definition: A caregiver's felt or exhibited difficulty in performing the family caregiver role.

Possible Etiologies ("related to")

Severity of the care receiver's illness
Illness chronicity [of the care receiver]
Lack of respite and recreation for the caregiver
Caregiver's competing role commitments
Inadequate physical environment for providing care
Family or caregiver isolation
Complexity and amount of caregiving tasks
Psychological or cognitive problems in care receiver
Unpredictable illness course or instability in the care receiver's health

Defining Characteristics ("evidenced by")

Apprehension about possible institutionalization of care receiver
Apprehension about future regarding care receiver's health and caregiver's ability to provide care
Difficulty performing required activities
Inability to complete caregiving tasks
Apprehension about care receiver's care when caregiver is ill or deceased

Goals/Objectives

Short-Term Goal

Caregivers will verbalize understanding of ways to facilitate the caregiver role.

Long-Term Goal

Caregivers will demonstrate effective problem-solving skills and develop adaptive coping mechanisms to regain equilibrium.

Interventions with *Selected Rationales*

1. Assess caregiver's ability to anticipate and fulfill client's unmet needs. Provide information to assist caregivers with

this responsibility. Ensure that caregivers encourage client to be as independent as possible. ***Caregivers may be unaware of what the client can realistically accomplish. They may be unaware of the nature of the illness.***

2. Ensure that caregivers are aware of available community support systems from which they can seek assistance when required. Examples include respite care services, day treatment centers, and adult day-care centers. ***Caregivers require relief from the pressures and strain of providing 24-hour care for their loved one. Studies have shown that abuse arises out of caregiving situations that place overwhelming stress on the caregivers.***
3. Encourage caregivers to express feelings, particularly anger. ***Release of these emotions can serve to prevent psychopathology, such as depression or psychophysiological disorders from occurring.***
4. Encourage participation in support groups composed of members with similar life situations. Provide information about support groups that may be helpful:
   a. National Alliance for the Mentally Ill—800-950-NAMI
   b. National Clearinghouse on Family Support—800-628-1696
   c. Association on Mental Retardation—800-424-3688
   d. Association for Retarded Citizens—817-261-6003
   e. Alzheimer's Disease and Related Disorders Association—800-621-0379

   Hearing others who are experiencing the same problems discuss ways in which they have coped may help the caregiver adopt more adaptive strategies. Individuals who are experiencing similar life situations provide empathy and support for each other.

Outcome Criteria

1. Caregivers are able to problem-solve effectively regarding care of the client.
2. Caregivers demonstrate adaptive coping strategies for dealing with stress of caregiver role.
3. Caregivers openly express feelings.
4. Caregivers express desire to join support group of other caregivers.

■ INTERNET REFERENCES

- http://www.hcfa.gov/
- http://www.nahc.org/Consumer/wihc.html
- http://www.nahc.org/Consumer/hcstats.html

CHAPTER 22

Forensic Nursing

■ BACKGROUND ASSESSMENT DATA

The International Association of Forensic Nurses (IAFN) and the American Nurses Association (ANA) (1997) define forensic nursing as "the application of forensic science combined with the bio-psychological education of the registered nurse, in the scientific investigation, evidence collection and preservation, analysis, prevention and treatment of trauma and/or death related medical-legal issues" (p. v).

Hufft and Peternelj-Taylor (1999) offer the following definition: "A nursing specialty that integrates nursing and forensic science to bridge the gap between the health care system and the criminal justice system" (p. 1).

Areas of forensic nursing include the following:

1. Clinical Forensic Nursing
2. The Sexual Assault Nurse Examiner (SANE)
3. Forensic Psychiatric Nursing Specialty
4. Correctional/Institutional Nursing Specialty
5. Nurses in General Practice

Clinical Forensic Nursing in Trauma Care

Assessment

Lynch (1995) states that forensic nurses who work in trauma care settings may

> . . . become the designated clinicians who will evaluate and assess surviving victims of rape, drug and alcohol addiction, domestic violence (including abuse of spouse, children, elderly), assaults, automobile/pedestrian accidents, suicide attempts, occupationally related injuries, incest, medical malpractice and the injuries sustained therefrom, and food and drug tampering.

All traumatic injuries in which liability is suspected are considered within the scope of forensic nursing. Reports to legal agencies are required to ensure follow-up investigation; however, the protection of clients' rights remains a nursing priority.

Several areas of assessment in which the clinical forensic nurse specialist in trauma care may become involved include:

1. **Preservation of Evidence:** Evidence from both crime-related and self-inflicted traumas must be safeguarded in a manner consistent with the investigation. Evidence such as clothing, bullets, blood stains, hairs, fibers, and small pieces of material such as fragments of metal, glass, paint, and wood should be saved and documented in all medical accident instances that have legal implications.
2. **Investigation of Wound Characteristics:** Wounds that the nurse must be able to identify include:
    a. ***Sharp Injuries:*** Sharp-force injuries including stab wounds and other wounds resulting from penetration with a sharp object.
    b. ***Blunt-Force Injuries:*** Includes cuts and bruises resulting from the impact of a blunt object against the body.
    c. ***Dicing Injuries:*** Multiple, minute cuts and abrasions caused by contact with shattered glass (e.g., often occur in motor vehicle accidents).
    d. ***Patterned Injuries:*** Specific injuries that reflect the pattern of the weapon used to inflict the injury.
    e. ***Bite-Mark Injuries:*** A type of patterned injury inflicted by human or animal.
    f. ***Defense Wounds:*** Injuries that reflect the victim's attempt to defend himself or herself from attack.
    g. ***Hesitation Wounds:*** Usually superficial, sharp-force wounds; often found perpendicular to the lower part of the body and may reflect self-inflicted wounds.
    h. ***Fast-Force Injuries:*** Usually gunshot wounds; may reflect various patterns of injury.
3. **Deaths in the Emergency Department:** When deaths occur in the emergency department as a result of abuse or accident, evidence must be retained, the death must be reported to legal authorities, and an investigation is conducted (Lynch, 1995). It is therefore essential that the nurse carefully document the appearance, condi-

tion, and behavior of the victim upon arrival at the hospital. The information gathered from the client and family (or others accompanying the client) may serve to facilitate the postmortem investigation and may be used during criminal justice proceedings.

The critical factor is the ability to determine whether the cause of death is natural or unnatural. In the emergency department, most deaths are sudden and unexpected. Those that are considered natural most commonly involve the cardiovascular, respiratory, and central nervous systems (Lynch, 1995). Deaths that are considered unnatural include those from trauma, from self-inflicted acts, or from injuries inflicted by another. Legal authorities must be notified of all deaths related to unnatural circumstances.

Common Nursing Diagnoses and Interventions *(For forensic nursing in trauma care.)*

POSTTRAUMA SYNDROME

Definition: A sustained maladaptive response to a traumatic, overwhelming event.

Possible Etiologies ("related to")

Physical and psychosocial abuse
Tragic occurrence involving multiple deaths
Sudden destruction of one's home or community
Epidemics
Rape
Natural or man-made disasters
Serious accidents
Witnessing mutilation, violent death, or other horrors
Serious threat or injury to self or loved ones
Industrial and motor vehicle accidents

Defining Characteristics ("evidenced by")

[Physical injuries related to trauma]
Avoidance
Repression
Difficulty concentrating
Grief; guilt
Intrusive thoughts

Neurosensory irritability
Palpitations
Anger and/or rage; aggression
Intrusive dreams; nightmares; flashbacks
Panic attacks; fear
Gastric irritability
Psychogenic amnesia
Substance abuse

Goals/Objectives

Short-Term Goals

1. The client's physical wounds will heal without complication.
2. The client will begin a healthy grief resolution, initiating the process of psychological healing.

Long-Term Goal

The client will demonstrate ability to deal with emotional reactions in an individually appropriate manner.

Interventions with *Selected Rationales*

1. Smith (1987a) relates the importance of communicating the following four phrases to the rape victim:
   a. I am very sorry this happened to you.
   b. You are safe here.
   c. I am very glad you are alive.
   d. You are not to blame. You are a victim. It was not your fault. Whatever decisions you made at the time of the victimization were the right ones because you are alive.

   The woman who has been sexually assaulted fears for her life and must be reassured of her safety. She may also be overwhelmed with self-doubt and self-blame, and these statements instill trust and validate self-worth.
2. Explain every assessment procedure that will be conducted and why. Ensure that data collection is conducted in a caring, nonjudgmental manner ***to decrease fear and anxiety and increase trust.***
3. Ledray and Arndt (1994) suggest the following five essential components of a forensic examination of the sexual assault survivor in the emergency department:
   a. Treatment and documentation of injuries. Samples of blood, semen, hair, and fingernail scrapings should be sealed in paper, not plastic, bags, ***to prevent the possible growth of mildew from accumulation of moisture inside the plastic container and the subsequent contamination of the evidence.***

b. Maintaining the proper chain of evidence. Samples must be properly labeled, sealed, and refrigerated when necessary, and kept under observation or properly locked until rendered to the proper legal authority, ***to ensure the proper chain of evidence and freshness of the samples.***
c. Treatment and evaluation of sexually transmitted diseases (STDs). If conducted within 72 hours of the attack, several tests and interventions are available for prophylactic treatment of certain STDs.
d. Pregnancy risk evaluation and prevention. Prophylactic regimens are 97 to 98 percent effective if started within 24 hours of the sexual attack and are generally recommended within 72 hours only (AMA, 1999).
e. Crisis intervention and arrangements for follow-up counseling. ***Because a survivor is often too ashamed or fearful to seek follow-up counseling,*** it may be important for the nurse to obtain the individual's permission to allow a counselor to call her to make a follow-up appointment.

4. In the case of other types of trauma (e.g., gunshot victims, automobile/pedestrian hit-and-run victims), ***ensure that any possible evidence is not lost.*** Clothing that is removed from a victim should not be shaken, and each separate item of clothing should be placed carefully in a paper bag, sealed, dated, timed, and signed.
5. Ensure that the client has adequate privacy for all immediate postcrisis interventions. Try to have as few people as possible providing the immediate care or collecting immediate evidence. ***The posttrauma client is extremely vulnerable. Additional people in the environment increase this feeling of vulnerability and escalate anxiety.***
6. Encourage the client to give an account of the trauma/assault. Listen, but do not probe. ***Nonjudgmental listening provides an avenue for catharsis that the client needs to begin healing. A detailed account may be required for legal follow-up, and a caring nurse, as client advocate, may help to lessen the trauma of evidence collection.***
7. Discuss with the client whom to call for support or assistance. Provide information about referrals for aftercare. ***Because of severe anxiety and fear, client may need assistance from others during this immediate postcrisis period. Provide referral information in writing for later reference (e.g., psychotherapist, mental health clinic, community advocacy group).***

8. In the event of a sudden and unexpected death in the trauma care setting, the clinical forensic nurse may be called upon to present information associated with an anatomic request to the survivors. ***The clinical forensic nurse specialist is an expert in legal issues and has the knowledge and sensitivity to provide coordination between organ/tissue procurement and the medical examiner/coroner system (Lynch, 1995).***

Outcome Criteria

1. The client is no longer experiencing panic anxiety.
2. The client demonstrates a degree of trust in the primary nurse.
3. The client has received immediate attention to physical injuries.
4. The client has initiated behaviors consistent with the grief response.
5. Necessary evidence has been collected and preserved to proceed appropriately within the legal system.

Forensic Psychiatric Nursing in Correctional Facilities

Assessment

It was believed that deinstitutionalization increased the freedom of mentally ill individuals in accordance with the principle of "least restrictive alternative." However, because of inadequate community-based services, many of these individuals drifted into poverty and homelessness, increasing their vulnerability to criminalization. Because the bizarre behavior of mentally ill individuals living on the street is sometimes offensive to community standards, law enforcement officials have the authority to protect the welfare of the public, as well as the safety of the mentally ill individual, by initiating emergency hospitalization. However, legal criteria for commitment are so stringent in most cases that arrest becomes an easier way of getting the mentally ill person off the street if a criminal statute has been violated. It is estimated that between 10 and 35 percent of all inmates have some form of psychological disorder or mental disability (Wark, 1998). Some of these individuals are incarcerated as a result of the increasingly popular "guilty but mentally ill" verdict. Lego (1995) stated, "prisons are becoming the 1990s' 'state psychiatric hospitals.' "

Psychiatric diagnoses commonly identified at the time of incarceration include schizophrenia, affective psychoses, personality disorders, and substance disorders (Rice, Harris, and Quinsey, 1996). Common psychiatric behaviors include hallucinations, suspiciousness, thought disorders, anger/agitation, impulsivity, and denial of problems. In a study by Rice, Harris, and Quinsey (1996), the behavior "denial of problems" ranked as most significant among this population. Use of substances and medication noncompliance are common obstacles to rehabilitation. Substance abuse has been shown to have a strong correlation with recidivism among the prison population (Rice, Harris, and Quinsey, 1996). Many individuals report that they were under the influence of substances at the time of their criminal actions, and dual diagnoses are common. Detoxification frequently occurs in jails and prisons, and some inmates have died from the withdrawal syndrome because of lack of adequate treatment during this process (Bernier, 1991).

Common Nursing Diagnoses and Interventions *(For forensic psychiatric nursing in correctional facilities.)*

DEFENSIVE COPING

Definition: The state in which an individual repeatedly projects falsely positive self-evaluation based on a self-protective pattern that defends against underlying perceived threats to positive self-regard.

Possible Etiologies ("related to")

[Low self-esteem]
[Retarded ego development]
[Underdeveloped superego]
[Negative role models]
[Lack of positive feedback]
[Absent, erratic, or inconsistent methods of discipline]
[Dysfunctional family system]

Defining Characteristics ("evidenced by")

Denial of obvious problems or weaknesses
Projection of blame or responsibility
Rationalization of failures
Hypersensitivity to criticism
Grandiosity

Superior attitude toward others
Difficulty establishing or maintaining relationships
Hostile laughter or ridicule of others
Difficulty in reality testing of perceptions
Lack of follow-through or participation in treatment or therapy

Goals/Objectives

Short-Term Goal

Client will verbalize personal responsibility for own actions, successes, and failures.

Long-Term Goal

Client will demonstrate ability to interact with others and adapt to lifestyle goals without becoming defensive, rationalizing behaviors, or expressing grandiose ideas.

Interventions with *Selected Rationales*

1. Recognize and support basic ego strengths. ***Focusing on positive aspects of the personality may help to improve self-concept.***
2. Encourage client to recognize and verbalize feelings of inadequacy and need for acceptance from others, as well as ways in which these feelings provoke defensive behaviors, such as blaming others for own behaviors. ***Recognition of the problem is the first step in the change process toward resolution.***
3. Provide immediate, matter-of-fact, nonthreatening feedback for unacceptable behaviors. ***Client may lack knowledge about how he or she is being perceived by others. Direct the behavior in a nonthreatening manner to a more acceptable behavior.***
4. Help client identify situations that provoke defensiveness and practice through role playing more appropriate responses. ***Role playing provides confidence to deal with difficult situations when they actually occur.***
5. Provide immediate positive feedback for acceptable behaviors. ***Positive feedback enhances self-esteem and encourages repetition of desirable behaviors.***
6. Help client set realistic, concrete goals and determine appropriate actions to meet those goals. ***Success increases self-esteem.***
7. Evaluate with client the effectiveness of the new behaviors and discuss any modifications for improvement. ***Because of limited problem-solving ability, assistance may be required in reassessing and developing new strategies, in the event that certain of the new coping methods prove ineffective.***

8. Use confrontation judiciously *to help client begin to identify defense mechanisms (e.g., denial/projection) that are hindering development of satisfying relationships and adaptive behaviors.*

Outcome Criteria

1. Client verbalizes and accepts responsibility for own behavior.
2. Client verbalizes correlation between feelings of inadequacy and the need to defend the ego through rationalization and grandiosity.
3. Client does not ridicule or criticize others.
4. Client interacts with others in group situations without taking a defensive stance.

DYSFUNCTIONAL GRIEVING

Definition: Extended, unsuccessful use of intellectual and emotional responses by which individuals, families, communities attempt to work through the process of modifying self-concept based upon the perception of loss.

Possible Etiologies ("related to")

Loss of freedom

Defining Characteristics ("evidenced by")

Anger
[Internalized rage]
[Depressed mood]
Labile affect
[Extreme fear of being alone (fear of abandonment)]
[Acting-out behaviors, such as sexual promiscuity, suicidal gestures, temper tantrums, substance abuse]
[Difficulty expressing feelings]
Alterations in eating habits, sleep patterns, dream patterns, activity level
Prolonged interference with life functioning with onset or exacerbation of somatic or psychosomatic responses

Goals/Objectives

Short-Term Goal

Client will verbalize feelings of grief related to loss of freedom.

Long-Term Goal

Client will satisfactorily progress through the grieving process.

Interventions with *Selected Rationales*

1. Convey an accepting attitude—one that creates a nonthreatening environment for the client to express feelings. Be honest and keep all promises. ***An accepting attitude conveys to the client that you believe he or she is a worthwhile person. Trust is enhanced.***
2. Identify the function that anger, frustration, and rage serve for the client. Allow the client to express these feelings within reason. ***Verbalization of feelings in a nonthreatening environment may help the client come to terms with unresolved grief.***
3. Encourage the client to discharge pent-up anger through participation in large motor activities (e.g., physical exercises, volleyball, punching bag). ***Physical exercise provides a safe and effective method for discharging pent-up tension.***
4. Anger may be displaced onto the nurse or therapist, and caution must be taken to guard against the negative effects of countertransference. These are very difficult clients who have the capacity for eliciting a whole array of negative feelings from the therapist. These feelings must be acknowledged but not allowed to interfere with the therapeutic process.
5. Explain the behaviors associated with the normal grieving process. Help the client to recognize his or her position in this process. ***This knowledge about normal grieving may help facilitate the client's progression toward resolution of grief.***
6. Help the client understand appropriate ways to express anger. Give positive reinforcement for behaviors used to express anger appropriately. Act as a role model. ***Positive reinforcement enhances self-esteem and encourages repetition of desirable behaviors. It is appropriate to let the client know when he or she has done something that has generated angry feelings in you. Role modeling ways to express anger in an appropriate manner is a powerful learning tool.***
7. Set limits on acting-out behaviors and explain consequences of violation of those limits. Be supportive, yet consistent and firm in working with this client. ***Client lacks sufficient self-control to limit maladaptive behaviors, so assistance is required from staff. Without consistency on the part of all staff members working with this client, a positive outcome will not be achieved.***
8. Provide a safe and protective environment for the client against risk of self-directed violence. ***Depression is the***

emotion that most commonly precedes suicidal attempts.

Outcome Criteria

1. Client is able to verbalize ways in which anger and acting-out behaviors are associated with maladaptive grieving.
2. Client expresses anger and hostility outwardly in a safe and acceptable manner.
3. Client has not harmed self or others.

RISK FOR INJURY

Definition: A state in which the individual is at risk of injury as a result of [internal or external] environmental conditions interacting with the individual's adaptive and defensive resources.

Related/Risk Factors ("related to")

[Substance use/detoxification at time of incarceration, exhibiting any of the following:
Substance intoxication
Substance withdrawal
Disorientation
Seizures
Hallucinations
Psychomotor agitation
Unstable vital signs
Delirium
Flashbacks
Panic level of anxiety]

Goals/Objectives

Short-Term Goal

Client's condition will stabilize within 72 hours.

Long-Term Goal

Client will not experience physical injury.

Interventions with *Selected Rationales*

1. Assess client's level of disorientation to determine specific requirements for safety. *Knowledge of client's level of functioning is necessary to formulate appropriate plan of care.*
2. Obtain a drug history, if possible, to determine

   a. Type of substance(s) used.
   b. Time of last ingestion and amount consumed.
   c. Length and frequency of consumption.
   d. Amount consumed on a daily basis.
3. Obtain urine sample for laboratory analysis of substance content. ***Subjective history is often not accurate. Knowledge regarding substance ingestion is important for accurate assessment of client condition.***
4. Place client in quiet room, if possible. ***Excessive stimuli increase client agitation.***
5. Institute necessary safety precautions:
   a. Observe client behaviors frequently; assign staff on one-to-one basis if condition is warranted; accompany and assist client when ambulating; use wheelchair for transporting long distances.
   b. Be sure that side rails are up when client is in bed.
   c. Pad headboard and side rails of bed with thick towels to protect client in case of seizure.
   d. Use mechanical restraints as necessary to protect client if excessive hyperactivity accompanies the disorientation. ***Client safety is a nursing priority.***
6. Ensure that smoking materials and other potentially harmful objects are stored outside client's access. ***Client may harm self or others in disoriented, confused state.***
7. Monitor vital signs every 15 minutes initially and less frequently as acute symptoms subside. ***Vital signs provide the most reliable information regarding client condition and need for medication during acute detoxification period.***
8. Follow medication regimen, as ordered by physician. Common medical intervention for detoxification from the following substances includes:
   a. ***Alcohol:*** Chlordiazepoxide (Librium) is given orally every 4 to 8 hours in decreasing doses until withdrawal is complete. In clients with liver disease, accumulation of the longer-acting agents, such as chlordiazepoxide (Librium), may be problematic, and the use of the shorter-acting benzodiazepine oxazepam (Serax) is more appropriate. Some physicians may order anticonvulsant medication to be used prophylactically; however, this is not a universal intervention. Multivitamin therapy, in combination with daily thiamine (either by mouth or by injection), is common protocol.
   b. ***Narcotics:*** Narcotic antagonists, such as naloxone (Narcan), nalorphine (Nalline), or levallorphan (Lorfan), are administered intravenously for narcotic overdose. With-

drawal is managed with rest and nutritional therapy. Substitution therapy may be instituted to decrease withdrawal symptoms using propoxyphene (Darvon) for weaker effects or methadone (Dolophine) for longer effects.

c. ***Depressants:*** Substitution therapy may be instituted to decrease withdrawal symptoms using a long-acting barbiturate, such as phenobarbital (Luminal). Some physicians prescribe oxazepam (Serax) as needed for objective symptoms, gradually decreasing the dosage until the drug is discontinued.
d. ***Stimulants:*** Treatment of overdose is geared toward stabilization of vital signs. Intravenous antihypertensives may be used, along with intravenous diazepam (Valium) to control seizures. Chlordiazepoxide may be administered orally for the first few days while the client is "crashing."
e. ***Hallucinogens and Cannabinols:*** Medications are normally not prescribed for withdrawal from these substances. However, in the event of overdose, diazepam (Valium) or chlordiazepoxide (Librium) may be given as needed to decrease agitation.

Outcome Criteria

1. Client is no longer exhibiting any signs or symptoms of substance intoxication or withdrawal.
2. Client shows no evidence of physical injury obtained during substance intoxication or withdrawal.

■ INTERNET REFERENCES

- http://www.forensiceducation.com/eduinternational.htm
- http://www.forensicnurse.org/
- http://www.forensicnurse.org/resource/links.htm

CHAPTER 23

Complementary Therapies

INTRODUCTION

The connection between mind and body, and the influence of each on the other, is well recognized by all clinicians, and particularly by psychiatrists. Currently, traditional medicine as it is practiced in the United States is based on scientific methodology. Traditional medicine is also known as *allopathic* medicine; it is the type historically taught in U.S. medical schools.

The term *alternative medicine* has come to be recognized as practices that differ from the usual traditional practices in the treatment of disease. A recent national survey by the American Medical Association's Council on Scientific Affairs revealed that 33 percent of those polled reported at least one alternative treatment during the previous 12 months (Money World, 1997). More than $15 billion a year is spent on alternative medical therapies in the United States (Kaplan and Sadock, 1998).

In 1991, an Office of Alternative Medicine (OAM) was established by the National Institutes of Health (NIH) to study nontraditional therapies and to evaluate their usefulness and their effectiveness. The mission statement of the OAM states the following: "The NIH Office of Alternative Medicine facilitates research and evaluation of unconventional medical practices and disseminates this information to the public" (Complementary & Alternative Medicine, 1998).

Some health maintenance organizations (HMOs) appear to be bowing to public pressure by including alternative providers in their networks of providers for treatments such as acupuncture and massage therapy.

Chiropractic care has been covered by some third-party payers for many years. Individuals who seek alternative therapy, however, are often reimbursed at lower rates than those who choose traditional practitioners.

Credit, Hartunian, and Nowak (1998) view these treatments not as *alternatives,* but as *complements,* in partnership with traditional medical practice. They acknowledge the superiority of traditional medical intervention in certain medical situations. However, they do not discount "the body's ability to heal itself with the help of natural, noninvasive therapies that are effective and without harmful side effects" (p. 3).

Client education is an important part of complementary care. Positive lifestyle changes are encouraged, and practitioners serve as educators as well as treatment specialists (Credit et al., 1998). Complementary medicine is viewed as *holistic* health care that deals not only with the physical perspective, but also with the emotional and spiritual components of the individual. Dr. Tom Coniglione, former professor of medicine at the Oklahoma University Health Sciences Center states:

> We must look at treating the "total person" in order to be more efficient and balanced within the medical community. Even finding doctors who are well-rounded and balanced has become a criteria in the admitting process for medical students. Medicine has changed from just looking at the "scientist perspective of organ and disease" to the total perspective of lifestyle and real impact/results to the patient. This evolution is a progressive and very positive shift in the right direction (Coniglione, 1998).

Terms such as *harmony* and *balance* are often associated with complementary care. In fact, restoring harmony and balance between body and mind is often the goal of complementary health-care approaches (Credit et al., 1998).

■ TYPES OF COMPLEMENTARY THERAPIES

Herbal Medicine

The use of plants to heal is probably as old as humankind. Virtually every culture in the world has relied on herbs and plants to treat illness. Clay tablets from about 4000 BC reveal that the Sumerians had apothecaries for dispensing medicinal herbs, and the *Pen Tsao,* a Chinese text written around 3000 BC, contained some 1000 herbal formulas that had probably been used as remedies for thousands of years (Guinness, 1993). When the Pilgrims came to America in the 1600s, they brought with them a variety of herbs to be established and used for medicinal purposes, and they soon discovered that the Native Americans also had their own varieties of plants for healing.

Most medicines today are derived from synthetic methods. However, 25 percent of all prescription drugs in the United States are derived from plants (Guinness, 1993). These plant-derived medications can be just as potent and produce just as many adverse effects as synthetic medicines. For this reason, many people are seeking a return to herbal remedies, with about $1.5 billion a year being spent on these substances. Because the Food and Drug Administration (FDA) classifies herbal remedies as dietary supplements or food additives, their labels cannot indicate medicinal uses. They are not subjected to FDA approval and they lack uniform standards of quality control. Several organizations have been established to attempt regulation and control of the herbal industry. They include the Council for Responsible Nutrition, the American Herbal Association, and the American Botanical Council.

The Commission E of the German Federal Health Agency is responsible for researching and regulating the safety and efficacy of herbs and plant medicines in Germany. Recently, all 380 German Commission E monographs of herbal medicines have been translated into English and compiled into one text. This should prove to be an invaluable reference for practitioners of holistic medicine.

Until more extensive testing has been completed on humans and animals, the use of herbal medicines must be approached with caution and responsibility. The notion that because something is "natural," it is therefore completely safe, is a myth. In fact, some of the plants from which prescription drugs are derived are highly toxic in their "natural" state (Guinness, 1993). Also, because of lack of regulation and standardization, ingredients may be adulterated and method of manufacture may alter potency. For example, dried herbs lose potency rapidly because of exposure to air. Guinness (1993) offers the following points for practitioners and individuals contemplating the use of herbal medicines:

1. **Be careful of your sources:** Owing to the lack of government scrutiny, the purity and potency of the herbal medicines cannot be guaranteed. The buyer must be careful to select reputable brands.
2. **Choose the most reliable forms:** Tinctures and freeze-dried products have been prepared to retard spoilage and prevent loss of potency.
3. **More is not better:** Always take the recommended dosages at the suggested intervals. Adverse effects can occur from overdosing with herbal medicines, just as with prescription pharmaceuticals.
4. **Monitor your reactions:** Discontinue the herbal medication at the first sign of allergic or other adverse reacton or, after a reasonable length of time, if there seems to be no significant indication that it is producing the desired effect.
5. **Take no risks:** Do not self-medicate with herbal remedies for serious illnesses or injuries. Do not take herbal medications without a physician's approval if you are pregnant or lactating, very young or very old, or taking other medications.

Table 23–1 lists information about certain herbs with possible implications for psychiatric and mental health nursing, including their botanical name, medicinal uses, and safety profile.

Acupressure and Acupuncture

Acupressure and acupuncture are healing techniques based on the ancient philosophies of traditional Chinese medicine dating back to 3000 BC. The main concept behind Chinese medicine is that healing energy (*chi*) flows through the body along specific pathways called *meridians*. It is believed that these meridians of chi connect various parts of the body in a way similar to that in which lines on a road map link various locations. The pathways link a conglomerate of points, called *acupoints;* therefore, it is possible to treat a part of the body distant to another, because they are linked by a meridian. Credit and associates (1998) state, "The goal of traditional Chinese medicine is to keep the body in balance and harmony through the free flow of chi. Disease is a result of blockages in this energy current."

In acupressure, the fingers, thumbs, palms, or elbows are used to apply pressure to the acupoints. This pressure is thought to dissolve any obstructions in the flow of heal-

TABLE 23–1 **Herbal Remedies**

Common Names (Botanical Name)	Medicinal Uses/ Possible Action	Safety Profile
Black cohosh (*Cimicifuga racemosa*)	May provide relief of menstrual cramps; improved mood; calming effect; extracts from the roots are thought to have action similar to estrogen.	Generally considered safe in low doses; toxic in large doses, causing dizziness, nausea, headaches, stiffness, and trembling; should not take with heart problems, concurrently with antihypertensives, or during pregnancy.
Cascara sagrada (*Rhamnus purshiana*)	Relief of constipation.	Generally recognized as safe; sold as over-the-counter drug in the United States; should not be used during pregnancy.
Chamomile (*Matricaria chamomilla*)	As a tea, is effective as a mild sedative in the relief of insomnia; may also aid digestion, relieve menstrual cramps, and settle upset stomach.	Generally recognized as safe when consumed in reasonable amounts.
Echinacea (*Echinacea angustifolia and Echinacea purpurea*)	Stimulates immune system; may have value in fighting infections and easing the symptoms of colds and flu.	Considered safe in reasonable doses; observe for side effects of allergic reaction.
Fennel (*Foeniculum vulgare*)	Used to ease stomach aches and to aid digestion; taken in a tea or in extracts to stimulate the appetites of anorectics (1–2 tsp seeds steeped in boiling water for making tea).	Generally recognized as safe when consumed in reasonable amounts.

TABLE 23–1 **Herbal Remedies (*Continued*)**

Common Names (Botanical Name)	Medicinal Uses/ Possible Action	Safety Profile
Feverfew (*Tanacetum parthenium*)	Prophylaxis and treatment of migraine headaches; effective in either the fresh leaf or freeze-dried forms (2–3 fresh leaves [or equivalent] per day).	A small percentage of individuals may experience the adverse effect of temporary mouth ulcers; considered safe in reasonable doses.
Ginger (*Zingiber officinale*)	Ginger tea to ease stomach aches and to aid digestion; two powdered gingerroot capsules have been shown to be effective in preventing motion sickness.	Generally recognized as safe.
Ginkgo (*Ginkgo biloba*)	Used to treat senility, short-term memory loss, and peripheral insufficiency; has been shown to dilate blood vessels; usual dosage is 120 mg/day.	Safety has been established at recommended dosages; possible side effects include headache, gastrointestinal problems, and dizziness; contraindicated in pregnancy and lactation and in patients with bleeding disorder.
Ginseng (*Panax ginseng*)	Ancient Chinese saw this herb as one that increased wisdom and longevity; current studies support a possible positive effect on the cardiovascular system; action not known.	Generally considered safe; side effects may include headache, insomnia, anxiety, skin rashes, diarrhea.
Hops (*Humulus lupulus*)	Used in cases of nervousness, mild anxiety, and insomnia; also may relieve the cramp-	Generally recognized as safe when consumed in recommended dosages.

Table continued on following page

TABLE 23–1 **Herbal Remedies (*Continued*)**

Common Names (Botanical Name)	Medicinal Uses/ Possible Action	Safety Profile
	ing associated with diarrhea; may be taken as a tea, in extracts, or capsules.	
Kava-Kava (*Piper methysticum*)	Used to reduce anxiety while promoting mental acuity; dosage range: 70–400/day.	Generally considered safe; may cause scaly skin rash when taken at the higher dosage range for long periods; concurrent use with alcohol may produce additive tranquilizing effects.
Passion flower (*Passiflora incarnata*)	Used in tea, capsules, or extracts to treat nervousness and insomnia; depresses the central nervous system to produce a mild sedative effect.	Generally recognized as safe in recommended doses.
Peppermint (*Mentha piperita*)	Used as a tea to relieve upset stomachs, headaches, and as a mild sedative; pour boiling water over 1 tbsp dried leaves and steep to make a tea.	Considered to be safe when consumed in normal quantities.
Psyllium (*Plantago ovata and Plantago major*)	Psyllium seeds are a popular bulk laxative commonly used for chronic constipation.	Approved as an over-the-counter drug in the United States.
Scullcap (*Scutellaria lateriflora*)	Used as a sedative for mild anxiety and nervousness.	Considered safe in reasonable amounts.
St. John's wort (*Hypericum perforatum*)	• Used in the treatment of mild to moderate depression; may block reuptake of	Generally recognized as safe when taken at recommended dosages; side

TABLE 23–1 **Herbal Remedies (*Continued*)**

Common Names (Botanical Name)	Medicinal Uses/ Possible Action	Safety Profile
	serotonin/norepinephrine and have a mild monoamine oxidase inhibiting effect; effective dose: 900 mg/day • May also have antiviral, antibacterial, and anti-inflammatory properties; currently being tested in high doses as anti-HIV drug	effects include mild gastrointestinal irritation that is lessened with food; photosensitivity when taken in high dosages over long periods; not to be taken with other psychoactive medications.
Valerian (*Valeriana officinalis*)	Used to treat insomnia; produces restful sleep without morning "hangover"; the root may be used to make a tea, or capsules are available at a common dosage of 400 mg; mechanism of action is similar to benzodiazepines but without addicting properties.	Generally recognized as safe when taken at recommended dosages; side effects may include mild headache or upset stomach; taking doses higher than recommended may result in severe headache, nausea, morning grogginess, blurry vision; should not be taken concurrently with other sedatives.

Adapted from Guinness, 1993; Kaplan and Sadock, 1998; Institute for Natural Resources, 1998; Yeager, 1998; and PDR for Herbal Medicines, 1998.

ing energy and to restore the body to a healthier functioning. In acupuncture, hair-thin, sterile, disposable, stainless steel needles are inserted into acupoints to dissolve the obstructions along the meridians. The needles may be left in place for a specified length of time, or they may be rotated or a mild electric current may be applied. An occasional tingling or numbness is experienced, but little to no pain is associated with the treatment (Credit et al., 1998).

The Western medical philosophy regarding acupressure and acupuncture is that they stimulate the body's own painkilling chemicals, the morphine-like substances known as endorphins. The treatment has been found to be effective in the treatment of asthma, headaches, dysmenorrhea, cervical pain, insomnia, anxiety, depression, substance abuse, stroke rehabilitation, nausea of pregnancy, postoperative- and chemotherapy-induced nausea and vomiting, tennis elbow, fibromyalgia, low back pain, and carpal tunnel syndrome (Kaplan and Sadock, 1998; National Institutes of Health, 1997).

Acupuncture is gaining wide acceptance in the United States by both patients and physicians. This treatment can be administered at the same time other techniques, such as conventional Western techniques, are being used, although it is essential that all health-care providers have knowledge of all treatments being received. Acupuncture should be administered by a physician or an acupuncturist who is board certified by the National Commission for the Certification of Acupuncturists (NCCA), which requires more than 1000 hours of acupuncture training. Currently 34 states have set licensure standards for acupuncturists (Institute for Natural Resources, 1998).

Diet and Nutrition

The value of nutrition in the healing process has long been underrated. Lutz and Przytulski (1994) state:

> Today many diseases are linked to lifestyle behaviors such as smoking, lack of adequate physical activity, and poor nutritional habits. Health care providers, in their role as educators, emphasize the relationship between lifestyle and risk of contracting disease. People are increasingly managing their health problems and making personal commitments to lead healthier lives. Nutrition is, in part, a preventive science. How and what one eats is a lifestyle choice. (p. 5)

Individuals select the foods they eat based on a number of factors, not the least of which is enjoyment. Eating must serve social and cultural, as well as nutritional needs. The U.S. Department of Agriculture (USDA) and the U.S. Department of Health and Human Services (USDHHS) (1995) have collaborated on a set of guidelines to help individuals understand what types of foods to eat to promote health and prevent disease. Following is a list of these guidelines.

1. **Eat a Variety of Foods:** No single food can supply all nutrients in the amounts needed for good health. A variety of foods should be selected from the Food Guide Pyramid (Figure 23–1). Most of the daily servings of food should be selected from the food groups that are the largest in the picture and closest to the base of the pyramid. Smaller, sedentary persons should select from the lower range of servings. The higher number of servings is meant for larger, more active individuals. Table 23–2 provides a summary of information about essential vitamins and minerals.
2. **Balance the Food You Eat with Physical Activity—Maintain or Improve Your Weight:** Many individuals gain weight with age, increasing their chance of developing a number of health problems associated with excess weight. These include high blood pressure, heart disease, stroke, diabetes, certain types of cancer, arthritis, breathing problems, and other illnesses. Thirty minutes or more of moderate physical activity such as walking regularly 3–5 days a week can help to increase calorie expenditure and assist in maintaining a healthy weight.

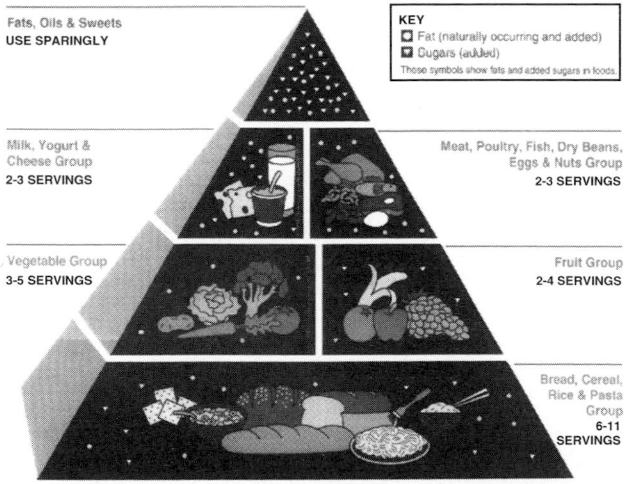

Source U.S. Department of Agriculture, Human Nutrition Information Services

Figure 23–1 The Food Guide Pyramid

TABLE 23–2 **Essential Vitamins and Minerals**

Vitamin/Mineral	Function	RDA*	Food Sources	Comments
Vitamin A	Prevention of night blindness; calcification of growing bones; resistance to infection	MEN: 1000 μg WOMEN: 800 μg	Liver, butter, cheese, whole milk, egg yolk, fish liver oil, green leafy vegetables, carrots	May be of benefit in prevention of cancer because of antioxidant properties associated with control of free radicals that damage DNA and cell membranes.
Vitamin D	Promotes absorption of calcium and phosphorus in the small intestine; prevention of rickets	MEN: 5 μg WOMEN: 5 μg	Fortified milk and dairy products, egg yolk, fish liver oils, liver, oysters; formed in the skin by exposure to sunlight	Without Vitamin D, very little dietary calcium can be absorbed.
Vitamin E	An antioxidant that prevents cell membrane destruction	MEN: 10 mg WOMEN: 8 mg	Vegetable oils, wheat germ, whole grain or fortified cereals, green leafy vegetables	As an antioxidant, may have implications in the prevention of Alzheimer's disease, heart disease, breast cancer.
Vitamin K	Synthesis of prothrombin and other clotting factors; normal	MEN: 80 μg WOMEN: 65 μg	Formed in intestines by bacteria; also found in	

	blood coagulation		green leafy vegetables, meats, dairy products	
Vitamin C	Formation of collagen in connective tissues; a powerful antioxidant; facilitates iron absorption; aids in the release of epinephrine from the adrenal glands during stress	MEN AND WOMEN: 60 mg	Citrus fruits, tomatoes, potatoes, green leafy vegetables, strawberries	As an antioxidant, may have implications in the prevention of cancer, cataracts, heart disease; it may stimulate the immune system to fight various types of infection.
Vitamin B_1 (Thiamine)	Essential for normal functioning of nervous tissue; coenzyme in carbohydrate metabolism	MEN: 1.5 mg WOMEN: 1.1 mg	Whole grains, legumes, nuts, egg yolk, meat, green leafy vegetables	Large doses may improve mental performance in people with Alzheimer's disease.
Vitamin B_2 (Riboflavin)	Coenzyme in the metabolism of protein and carbohydrate	MEN: 1.7 mg WOMEN: 1.3 mg	Meat, dairy products, whole or enriched grains, legumes	May help in the prevention of cataracts; high-dose therapy may be effective in migraine prophylaxis (Schoenen et al., 1998).
Vitamin B_3 (Niacin)	Coenzyme in the metabolism of protein and carbohydrate	MEN: 19 mg WOMEN: 15 mg	Milk, eggs, meats, legumes, whole grain and enriched cereals	High doses of niacin have been successful in decreasing levels of cholesterol in some individuals.

Table continued on following page

TABLE 23–2 **Essential Vitamins and Minerals (*Continued*)**

Vitamin/Mineral	Function	RDA*	Food Sources	Comments
Vitamin B_6 (Pyridoxine)	Coenzyme in the synthesis and catabolism of amino acids; essential for metabolism of tryptophan to niacin	MEN: 2 mg WOMEN: 1.6 mg	Meat, fish, grains, legumes, bananas, figs	May decrease depression in some individuals by increasing levels of serotonin; deficiencies may contribute to memory problems; also used in the treatment of migraines and pre-menstrual discomfort.
Vitamin B_{12}	Necessary in the formation of DNA and the production of red blood cells; associated with folic acid metabolism	MEN AND WOMEN: 2 μg	Animal products (e.g., meats, eggs, dairy products)	Deficiency may contribute to memory problems; vegetarians can get this vitamin from fortified foods; intrinsic factor must be present in the stomach for absorption of Vitamin B_{12}.
Folic Acid (Folate)	Necessary in the formation of DNA and the production of red blood cells	MEN: 200 μg WOMEN: 180 μg	Meat, green leafy vegetables, beans, peas, oranges, cantaloupes	Important in women of childbearing age to prevent fetal neural tube defects; may contribute to

				prevention of heart disease and colon cancer.
Calcium	Necessary in the formation of bones and teeth; neuron and muscle functioning; blood clotting	MEN AND WOMEN: 800 mg	Dairy products, green leafy vegetables, sardines, oysters, salmon	Calcium has been associated with preventing headaches, muscle cramps, osteoporosis, and premenstrual problems; requires vitamin D for absorption.
Phosphorus	Necessary in the formation of bones and teeth; a component of DNA, RNA, ADP† and ATP†, helps control acid-base balance in the blood	MEN AND WOMEN: 800 mg	Milk, cheese, fish, meat	
Magnesium	Protein synthesis and carbohydrate metabolism; muscular relaxation following contraction; and bone formation	MEN: 350 mg WOMEN: 280 mg	Green vegetables, legumes, seafood, milk	May aid in prevention of asthmatic attacks and migraine headaches; deficiencies may contribute to insomnia, premenstrual problems.

Table continued on following page

TABLE 23–2 **Essential Vitamins and Minerals (*Continued*)**

Vitamin/Mineral	Function	RDA*	Food Sources	Comments
Iron	Synthesis of hemoglobin and myoglobin; cellular oxidation	MEN AND WOMEN: 10 mg (lactating women and those of childbearing age: 15 mg)	Meats, egg yolks, shellfish, dark green leafy vegetables, dried fruit	Iron deficiencies can result in headaches and feeling chronically fatigued.
Iodine	Aids in the synthesis of T_3 and T_4	MEN AND WOMEN: 150 μg	Iodized salt, seafood	Exerts strong controlling influence on overall body metabolism.
Selenium	Works with vitamin E to protect cellular compounds from oxidation	MEN: 70 μg WOMEN: 55 μg	Seafood, low-fat meats, whole grains, dairy products, legumes	As an antioxidant combined with Vitamin E, may have some anticancer effect; deficiency has also been associated with depressed mood.

Zinc	Involved in synthesis of DNA and RNA; energy metabolism and protein synthesis; wound healing; increased immune functioning; necessary for normal smell and taste sensation	MEN AND WOMEN: 15 mg	Meat, seafood, grains, legumes	An important source for prevention of infection and improvement in wound healing.

*Recommended Dietary Allowances.
†ADP = adenosine diphosphate; ATP = adenosine triphosphate.
Source: Adapted from Yeager, 1998; Lutz and Przytulski, 1994; Scanlon and Sanders, 1995; and Institute for Natural Resources, 1998.

3. **Choose a Diet with Plenty of Grain Products, Vegetables, and Fruits:** Consumption of these foods is associated with a substantially lower risk for many chronic diseases, including certain types of cancer. These foods are emphasized in this guideline because they are an excellent source of vitamins, minerals, complex carbohydrates (starch and dietary fiber), and, depending upon how they are prepared, they are also low in fat.
4. **Choose a Diet Low in Fat, Saturated Fat, and Cholesterol:** Heart disease and some types of cancer (e.g., breast, colon) have been linked to high-fat diets. Some dietary fat is required for good health. Fats supply energy and essential fatty acids as well as promote absorption of the fat-soluble vitamins A, D, E, and K. However, fats should comprise no more than 30 percent of the total daily calorie intake. Choose foods with monounsaturated and polyunsaturated fat sources, and keep daily cholesterol intake below 300 mg.
5. **Choose a Diet Moderate in Sugars:** Many foods that contain sugars supply unnecessary calories and few nutrients. A significant health problem from eating too much sugar is tooth decay. Scientific evidence indicates that diets high in sugars do not cause hyperactivity or diabetes. A recent study by Dr. W.B. Grant of the Atmospheric Sciences Division of NASA's Langley Research Center reports that sugar may be the highest dietary risk factor for heart disease in women 35 and older (*The Sunday Oklahoman,* 1998). He states that "fructose metabolizes into triglycerides, then is incorporated into very low density lipoprotein cholesterol." Sugars should be used in moderation by most healthy people and sparingly by people with low-calorie needs.
6. **Choose a Diet Moderate in Salt and Sodium:** Sodium and sodium chloride (salt) occur naturally in foods, usually in small amounts. Most foods are prepared with some salt, and some has been added during processing. In studies with many diverse populations, it has been established that a high intake of salt is associated with high blood pressure. It is therefore important for individuals at risk for high blood pressure to consume less salt in their diets (as well as increase physical activity and control weight).
7. **If You Drink Alcoholic Beverages, Do So in Moderation:** High levels of alcohol intake raise the risk for

high blood pressure, stroke, heart disease, certain cancers, accidents, violence, suicides, birth defects, and overall mortality. Too much alcohol may cause cirrhosis of the liver, inflammation of the pancreas, and damage to the brain and heart. Heavy drinkers also are at risk of malnutrition because alcohol contains calories that may substitute for those in more nutritious foods. The USDA/USDHHS report defines "moderation" as ". . . no more than one drink per day for women and no more than two drinks per day for men. Count as a drink:

- 12 ounces of regular beer (150 calories)
- 5 ounces of wine (100 calories)
- 1.5 ounces of 80-proof distilled spirits (100 calories)"

Good nutrition can help with adaptation to the inevitable stresses of life by promoting a healthy body and a feeling of well-being. Knowledge of good nutrition is learned and not necessarily something that comes naturally. Nurses are in an ideal situation for providing individuals with this type of information.

Chiropractic Medicine

Chiropractic is probably the most widely used form of alternative healing in the United States. It was developed in the late 1800s by a self-taught healer named David Palmer. It was later reorganized and expanded by his son, Joshua, a trained practitioner. Palmer's objective was to find a cure for disease and illness that did not rely on drugs, which he considered harmful (Guinness, 1993). Palmer's theory behind chiropractic medicine was that energy flows from the brain to all parts of the body through the spinal cord and spinal nerves. When vertebrae of the spinal column become displaced, they may press on a nerve and interfere with normal nerve transmission. Palmer named the displacement of these vertebrae *subluxations* and alleged that the way to restore normal function was to manipulate the vertebrae back into their normal positions. These manipulations are called *adjustments* (Guinness, 1993).

Adjustments are usually performed by hand, although some chiropractors have special treatment tables equipped to facilitate these manipulations. Other processes used to facilitate the outcome of the spinal adjustment by providing muscle relaxation include massage tables, application of heat or cold, and ultrasound treatments.

The chiropractor takes a medical history and performs a clinical examination, which usually includes x-rays of the spine. Today's chiropractors may practice "straight" therapy; that is, the only therapy provided is that of subluxation adjustments. "Mixer" is a term applied to chiropractors who combine adjustments with adjunct therapies, such as exercise, heat treatments, or massage.

Individuals seek treatment from chiropractors for many types of ailments and illnesses, the most common being back pain. In addition, chiropractors treat clients with headaches, sciatica, shoulder pain, tennis and golfer's elbow, leg and foot pain, hand and wrist pain, allergies, asthma, stomach disorders, and menstrual problems (Guinness, 1993). Some chiropractors are employed by professional sports teams as their team physicians.

Chiropractors are licensed to practice in all 50 states and treatment is covered by government and most private insurance plans. They treat approximately 20 million people in the United States annually (Kaplan and Sadock, 1998).

Therapeutic Touch and Massage

Therapeutic Touch

The technique of therapeutic touch was developed in the 1970s by Dolores Krieger, a nurse associated with the New York University School of Nursing. This therapy is based on the philosophy that the human body projects a field of energy around it. When this field of energy becomes blocked, pain or illness occurs. Practitioners of therapeutic touch use this technique to correct the blockages, thereby relieving the discomfort and improving health.

Based on the premise that the energy field extends beyond the surface of the body, the practitioner need not actually touch the client's skin. The therapist's hands are passed over the client's body, remaining two to four inches from the skin. The goal is to repattern the energy field (Credit et al., 1998). This is done by performing slow, rhythmic, sweeping hand motions over the entire body. Heat should be felt where the energy is blocked. The therapist "massages" the energy field in that area, smoothing it out, and thus correcting the obstruction. Therapeutic touch is thought to reduce pain and anxiety and promote relaxation and health maintenance. It has been useful in the treatment of chronic health conditions.

Massage

Massage is the technique of manipulating the muscles and soft tissues of the body. Ancient Chinese physicians prescribed massage for the treatment of disease more than 5000 years ago. The Eastern style focuses on balancing the body's vital energy (chi) as it flows through pathways called *meridians*. The Western style of massage affects muscles, connective tissues such as tendons and ligaments, and the cardiovascular system. The Swedish massage, which is probably the best known of the Western variety, uses a variety of gliding and kneading strokes, along with deep circular movements and vibrations, to relax the muscles, improve circulation, and increase mobility (Guinness, 1993).

Massage has been shown to be beneficial in the following conditions: anxiety, chronic back and neck pain, arthritis, sciatica, migraine headaches, muscle spasms, insomnia, pain of labor and delivery, stress-related disorders, and whiplash. Massage is contraindicated in certain conditions such as high blood pressure, acute infection, osteoporosis, phlebitis, skin conditions, varicose veins, or the site of a recent injury, bruises, or burns.

Massage therapists require specialized training in a program accredited by the American Massage Therapy Association and must pass the National Certification Examination for Therapeutic Massage and Bodywork.

Yoga

It is thought that yoga was developed in India some 5000 years ago and is attributed to an Indian physician and Sanskrit scholar, Patanjali. The ultimate goal of yoga is to unite the human soul with the universal spirit (Guinness, 1993). Yoga has been found to be especially helpful in relieving stress and in improving overall physical and psychological wellness. Proper breathing is a major component of yoga. It is believed that yoga breathing, a deep, diaphramatic breathing, increases oxygen to brain and body tissues, thereby easing stress and fatigue as well as boosting energy.

Another component of yoga is meditation. Individuals who practice the meditation and deep breathing associated with yoga find that they are able to achieve a profound feeling of relaxation.

The most familiar type of yoga practiced in the Western countries is hatha yoga. Hatha yoga uses body postures, along with meditation and breathing exercises, to achieve a balanced, disciplined workout that releases muscle tension, tones the internal organs, and energizes the mind, body, and spirit so that natural healing can occur (Credit et al., 1998). The complete routine of poses is designed to work all parts of the body, stretching and toning muscles, while also keeping joints flexible. Studies have shown that yoga has provided beneficial effects to some individuals with back pain, stress, migraine, insomnia, high blood pressure, rapid heart rates, and limited mobility (Guiness, 1993).

Pet Therapy

The therapeutic value of pets is no longer just theory. Evidence has shown that animals can directly influence a person's mental and physical well-being. Pet therapy programs have been established across the country and the numbers are increasing regularly.

A number of studies have provided information about the positive results of human interaction with pets. Some of these include the following:

1. One year following heart attack, clients who have pets have one-fifth the death rate as those who do not (Friedmann and Thomas, 1995).
2. Petting a dog or cat has been shown to lower blood pressure (Sobel and Ornstein, 1996).
3. Bringing a pet into a nursing home or hospital has been shown to enhance a client's mood and social interaction (Sobel and Ornstein, 1996).

Some researchers believe that animals actually may retard the aging process among those who live alone. Loneliness often results in premature death, and having a pet mitigates the effects of loneliness and isolation.

It may never be known precisely why animals affect humans the way they do, but for those who have pets to love, it comes as no surprise. Pets provide unconditional, nonjudgmental love and affection, which can be the perfect antidote for a depressed mood or a stressful situation. The role of animals in the human healing process still requires more research, but its validity is now widely accepted in both the medical and lay communities.

■ SUMMARY

Complementary therapies assist the practitioner in viewing the client in a holistic manner. Most complementary therapies consider the mind and body connection and strive to enhance the body's own natural healing powers. The OAM of the NIH has established a list of alternative therapies to be used in practice and for investigative purposes. More than $15 billion a year is spent on alternative medical therapies in the United States.

This chapter has examined herbal medicine, acupressure, acupuncture, diet and nutrition, chiropractic medicine, therapeutic touch, massage, yoga, and pet therapy. Nurses must be familiar with these therapies as more and more clients seek out the healing properties of these complementary strategies to traditional care.

■ INTERNET REFERENCES

- http://www.herbalgram.org/
- http://www.amfoundation.org/herbmed.htm
- http://www.eatright.org/adap0298b.html
- http://www.chiropractic.org/
- http://www.pawssf.org/
- http://www.superdog.com/therapy.htm
- http://www.holisticmed.com/www/acupuncture.html
- http://www.amcricanyogaassociation.org/

UNIT FOUR

PSYCHOTROPIC MEDICATIONS

■ PHARMACOLOGY: ADJUNCT PSYCHOTHERAPY

What sort of behavior warrants the label of "mental illness?" Horwitz (1982) has suggested a strong cultural influence in the application of this label. Behaviors considered indicative of mental illness in one society may not necessarily be considered as such in another. Standards by which behaviors are measured include:

1. The degree to which the behavior conforms to societal norms
2. The ability of an observer to comprehend the behavior (or the motivation behind the behavior)

Historically, reaction to and treatment of the mentally ill ranged from benign involvement to intervention some would consider inhumane. Mentally ill individuals were feared because of common beliefs associating them with demons or the supernatural. They were looked upon as loathsome and often were mistreated.

Beginning in the late 18th century, a type of "moral reform" in the treatment of the mentally ill began to occur. This resulted in the establishment of community and state hospitals concerned with the needs of the mentally ill. Considered a breakthrough in the humanization of care, these institutions, however well-intentioned, fostered the concept of custodial care. Clients were assured of the provision of food and shelter but had little or no hope of change for the future. As they became increasingly dependent on the institution to fill their needs, the likelihood of their return to the family or community diminished.

The early part of the 20th century saw the advent of the somatic therapies in psychiatry. Mentally ill individuals were treated with insulin shock therapy, wet sheet packs, ice baths, electroconvulsive therapy, and psychosurgery. Before 1950, no important chemical agents existed in psychiatric practice except sedatives and amphetamines, which had limited use because of their toxicity and addicting effects (Burgess, 1990). Since the 1950s, the development of psychopharmacology has expanded to include widespread use of antipsychotic, antidepressant, and antianxiety medications. Research into how these drugs work has provided an understanding of the etiology of many psychiatric disorders.

Psychotropic medications are not intended to "cure"

mental illness. Most physicians who prescribe these medications for their clients use them as an adjunct to individual or group psychotherapy. Although the contribution of these drugs to psychiatric care cannot be minimized, it must be emphasized that psychotropic medications relieve physical and/or behavioral symptoms. They do not resolve any underlying condition or emotional problems that may exist.

Nurses must understand the legal implications associated with administration of psychotropic medications. Laws differ from state to state, but most adhere to the client's right to refuse treatment. Exceptions exist in emergency situations when it has been determined that clients are likely to harm themselves or others.

It is important for nurses to be familiar with the psychotropic medications being administered. This unit is designed to provide the information needed to administer medication in a safe manner and to provide a framework of the nursing process for delivery of care. Common psychotropic medications are included, as well as other medications that have implications in psychiatry. Each chemical class of medications includes generic and trade names, controlled substance categories (where appropriate), indications, action, contraindications and precautions, adverse reactions and side effects, half-life, daily adult dosage range, available forms, and therapeutic serum levels (where appropriate). In addition, application of the nursing process as it relates specifically to each classification is discussed. This includes assessment data, as previously described, NANDA-accepted nursing diagnoses with potential or actual relevance to administration of the medication, and nursing actions important in the implementation of drug administration, including a section on client/family education.

This integration of psychopharmacology with nursing process will provide the nurse with a useful, quick, and up-to-date reference for systematic and accurate administration of medications commonly used in psychiatry.

CHAPTER 24

Antianxiety Agents

■ CHEMICAL CLASS: ANTIHISTAMINES

Indications

- Anxiety disorders
- Temporary relief of anxiety symptoms
- Acute alcohol withdrawal
- Allergic reactions producing pruritic or asthmatic conditions
- Antiemetic
- Reduction of narcotic requirement, alleviation of anxiety, and control of emesis in preoperative and postoperative and prepartum and postpartum clients.

Action

- Exert CNS-depressant activity at the subcortical level of the CNS

Contraindications and Precautions

Contraindicated in:

- Hypersensitivity
- Pregnancy and lactation.

Use Cautiously in:

- Elderly or debilitated clients (dosage reduction recommended)
- Hepatic or renal dysfunction
- Concomitant use of other CNS depressants.

Adverse Reactions and Side Effects

- Dry mouth
- Drowsiness
- Pain at intramuscular site.

Examples

Generic (Trade) Name	Half-Life (hr)	Daily Adult Dosage Range (mg)	Available Forms (mg)
Hydroxyzine (Atarax)	3	100–400	**TABS:** 10, 25, 50, 100 **SYRUP:** 10/5mL
(Vistaril)	3	100–400	**CAPS:** 25, 50, 100 **ORAL SUSP:** 25/5mL **INJECT:** 25, 50, 100

■ CHEMICAL CLASS: BENZODIAZEPINES

Indications

- Anxiety disorders
- Anxiety symptoms
- Acute alcohol withdrawal
- Skeletal muscle spasms
- Convulsive disorders and status epilepticus
- Preoperative sedation and relief of anxiety.

Action

Benzodiazepines are thought to potentiate the effects of gamma-aminobutyric acid (GABA), a powerful inhibitory neurotransmitter, thereby producing a calmative effect. The activity may involve the spinal cord, brain stem, cerebellum, limbic system, and cortical areas.

Contraindications and Precautions

Contraindicated in:

- Hypersensitivity
- Narrow-angle glaucoma
- Pre-existing CNS depression
- Pregnancy and lactation
- Shock
- Coma

Use Cautiously in:

- Elderly or debilitated clients (reduced dosage recommended)
- Hepatic and renal impairment

- History of drug abuse/dependence
- Depressed/suicidal clients
- Children

Adverse Reactions and Side Effects

- Drowsiness
- Dizziness
- Ataxia
- Lethargy
- Hypotension (with intravenous use)
- Tolerance
- Physical and psychological dependence.

Examples

Generic (Trade) Name	Controlled Categories	Half-Life (hr)	Daily Adult Dosage Range (mg)	Available Forms (mg)
Alprazolam (Xanax)	C-IV	6–26	0.75–4	**TABS:** 0.25, 0.5, 1.0, 2.0 **ORAL SOLU:** 0.5/5mL
Chlordia-zepoxide (Librium)	C-IV	5–30	15–100	**TABS & CAPS:** 5, 10, 25 **INJECT:** 100
Clonazepam (Klonopin)	C-IV	18–50	1.5–20	**TABS:** 0.5, 1.0, 2.0
Clorazepate (Tranxene)	C-IV	30–100	15–60	**TABS & CAPS:** 3.75, 7.5, 15 **SINGLE DOSE:** 11.25, 22.5
Diazepam (Valium)	C-IV	20–80	4–40	**TABS:** 2, 5, 10 **CAPS (SR):** 15 **ORAL SOLU:** 5/5mL, 5/mL **INJECT:** 5/mL
Lorazepam (Ativan)	C-IV	10–20	2–6	**TABS:** 0.5, 1.0, 2.0 **ORAL SOLU:** 2/mL **INJECT:** 2/mL, 4/mL
Oxazepam (Serax)	C-IV	5–20	30–120	**TABS:** 15 **CAPS:** 10, 15, 30

■ CHEMICAL CLASS: PROPANEDIOLS

Indications

- Anxiety disorders
- Temporary relief of anxiety symptoms.

Actions

- Depress multiple sites in the CNS, including the hypothalamus, thalamus, limbic system, and spinal cord.

Contraindications and Precautions

Contraindicated in:

- Hypersensitivity to the drug
- Combination with other CNS depressants
- Children under 6
- Pregnancy and lactation
- Acute intermittent porphyria.

Use Cautiously in:

- Elderly or debilitated clients
- Hepatic or renal dysfunction
- Individuals with a history of drug abuse/addiction
- Clients with a history of seizure disorders
- Depressed/suicidal clients.

Adverse Reactions and Side Effects

- Drowsiness
- Dizziness
- Ataxia
- Reduced seizure threshold
- Tolerance
- Physical and psychological dependence.

Examples

Generic (Trade) Name	Controlled Categories	Half-Life (hr)	Daily Adult Dosage Range (mg)	Available Forms (mg)
Meprobamate (Equanil)	C-IV	6–17	400–2400	TABS: 200, 400
(Miltown)	C-IV	6–17	400–2400	TABS: 200, 400, 600

■ CHEMICAL CLASS: AZASPIRODECANEDIONES

Indications

- Generalized anxiety states.

UNLABELED USE:

- Symptomatic management of premenstrual syndrome.

Actions

- Unknown
- May produce desired effects through interactions with serotonin, dopamine, and other neurotransmitter receptors
- Delayed onset (a lag time of 10 days to 2 weeks between onset of therapy and subsiding of anxiety symptoms
- Cannot be used on a prn basis.

Contraindications and Precautions

Contraindicated in:

- Hypersensitivity to the drug.

Use Cautiously in:

- Clients using monoamine oxidase inhibitors
- Elderly or debilitated clients
- Clients with hepatic or renal dysfunction
- Pregnancy and lactation
- Children under 18 years of age
- Buspirone will not block the withdrawal syndrome in clients with a history of chronic benzodiazepine or other sedative/hypnotic use. Clients should be withdrawn gradually from these medications before beginning therapy with buspirone.

Adverse Reactions and Side Effects

- Drowsiness
- Dizziness
- Headache
- Nervousness
- Nausea.

Example

Generic (Trade) Name	Half-Life (hr)	Daily Adult Dosage Range (mg)	Available Forms (mg)
Buspirone HCl (BuSpar)	2–11	15–60	TABS: 5, 10

■ NURSING DIAGNOSES RELATED TO ALL ANTIANXIETY AGENTS

1. Risk for injury related to seizures, panic anxiety, acute agitation from alcohol withdrawal (indications); abrupt withdrawal from the medication after long-term use; effects of medication intoxication or overdose.
2. Anxiety (specify) related to threat to physical integrity or self-concept.
3. Risk for activity intolerance related to medication side effects of sedation, confusion, lethargy.
4. Sleep pattern disturbance related to situational crises, physical condition, severe level of anxiety.
5. Knowledge deficit related to medication regimen.

■ NURSING IMPLICATIONS FOR ANTIANXIETY AGENTS

1. Instruct client not to drive or operate dangerous machinery while taking the medication.
2. Advise client receiving long-term therapy not to quit taking the drug abruptly. Abrupt withdrawal can be life-threatening (with exception of buspirone). Symptoms include depression, insomnia, increased anxiety, abdominal and muscle cramps, tremors, vomiting, sweating, convulsions, and delirium.
3. Instruct client not to drink alcohol or take other medications that depress the CNS while taking this medication.
4. Assess mood daily. ***May aggravate symptoms in depressed persons.*** Take necessary precautions for potential suicide.
5. Monitor lying and standing blood pressure and pulse every shift. Instruct client to arise slowly from a lying or sitting position.

6. Withhold drug and notify the physician should paradoxical excitement occur.
7. Have client take frequent sips of water, ice chips, suck on hard candy, or chew sugarless gum to relieve dry mouth.
8. Have client take drug with food or milk to prevent nausea or vomiting.
9. Symptoms of sore throat, fever, malaise, easy bruising, or unusual bleeding should be reported to the physician immediately. They may be indications of blood dyscrasias.
10. Ensure that client taking buspirone (BuSpar) understands there is a lag time of 10 days to 2 weeks between onset of therapy and subsiding of anxiety symptoms. Client should continue to take the medication during this time. (NOTE: This medication is not recommended for prn administration because of this delayed therapeutic onset. There is no evidence that buspirone creates tolerance or physical dependence as do the CNS depressant anxiolytics.)

■ CLIENT AND FAMILY EDUCATION RELATED TO ALL ANTIANXIETY AGENTS

- Do not drive or operate dangerous machinery. Drowsiness and dizziness can occur.
- Do not stop taking the drug abruptly. Can produce serious withdrawal symptoms, such as depression, insomnia, anxiety, abdominal and muscle cramps, tremors, vomiting, sweating, convulsions, and delirium.
- (With buspirone only): Be aware of lag time between start of therapy and subsiding of symptoms. Relief is usually evident within 10 to 14 days. Take the medication regularly, as ordered, so that it has sufficient time to take effect.
- Do not consume other CNS depressants (including alcohol).
- Do not take nonprescription medication without approval from physician.
- Rise slowly from the sitting or lying position to prevent a sudden drop in blood pressure.
- Report to physician immediately symptoms of sore

throat, fever, malaise, easy bruising, unusual bleeding, or motor restlessness.

- Be aware of risks of taking these drugs during pregnancy. (Congenital malformations have been associated with use during the first trimester.) If pregnancy is suspected or planned, notify the physician of the desirability to discontinue the drug.
- Be aware of possible side effects. Refer to written materials furnished by health-care providers regarding the correct method of self-administration.
- Carry card or piece of paper at all times stating names of medications being taken.

INTERNET REFERENCES

- http://www.mentalhealth.com/fr30.html
- http://www.nimh.nih.gov/publicat/medicate.cfm
- http://www.fadavis.com/catalog/Nursing/Psychiatric%20and%20Mental%20Health%20Nursing/0483-monograph.htm

CHAPTER 25

Antidepressants

■ CHEMICAL CLASS: TRICYCLICS

Indications

- Major depression
- Depressive phase of bipolar disorder
- Depression accompanied by anxiety (doxepin)
- Childhood enuresis (imipramine)
- Depression associated with organic disease, alcoholism, schizophrenia, or mental retardation
- Obsessive-compulsive disorder (clomipramine)

INVESTIGATIONAL USES:

- Attention-deficit disorder in children
- Panic disorder
- Chronic pain.

Action

- Inhibit reuptake of norepinephrine or serotonin at the presynaptic neuron.

Contraindications and Precautions

Contraindicated in:

- Hypersensitivity to tricyclics
- Concomitant use with monoamine oxidase inhibitors (MAOIs)
- Acute recovery period following myocardial infarction
- Untreated angle-closure glaucoma
- Pregnancy and lactation (safety not established).

Use Cautiously in:

- Clients with history of seizures
- Urinary retention
- Benign prostatic hypertrophy

- Cardiovascular disorders
- Hepatic or renal insufficiency
- Psychotic clients
- Elderly or debilitated clients

Adverse Reactions and Side Effects

- Drowsiness
- Dry mouth
- Orthostatic hypotension
- Tachycardia
- Constipation
- Urinary retention
- Blood dyscrasias
- Nausea and vomiting
- Photosensitivity.

Examples

Generic (Trade) Name	Half-Life (hr)	Daily Adult Dosage Range (mg)	Therapeutic Plasma Level Range (ng/mL)	Available Forms (mg)
Amitriptyline (Elavil; Endep)	31–46	50–300	110–250 (incl. metabolite)	**TABS:** 10, 25, 50, 75, 100, 150
Amoxapine (Asendin)	8	50–600	200–500	**TABS:** 25, 50, 100, 150
Clomipramine (Anafranil)	19–37	25–250	80–100	**CAPS:** 25, 50, 75
Desipramine (Norpramin)	12–24	25–300	125–300	**TABS:** 10, 25, 50, 75, 100, 150
Doxepin (Sinequan)	8–24	25–300	100–200 (incl. metabolite)	**CAPS:** 10, 25, 50, 75, 100, 150 **ORAL CONC:** 10/mL
Imipramine (Tofranil)	11–25	30–300	200–350 (incl. metabolite)	**TABS:** 10, 25, 50 **CAPS:** 75, 100, 125, 150 **INJECT:** 25/2 mL
Nortriptyline (Aventyl; Pamelor)	18–44	30–100	50–150	**CAPS:** 10, 25, 50, 75 **ORAL SOLU:** 10/5 mL

Generic (Trade) Name	Half-Life (hr)	Daily Adult Dosage Range (mg)	Therapeutic Plasma Level Range (ng/mL)	Available Forms (mg)
Protriptyline (Vivactil)	67–89	15–60	100–200	TABS: 5, 10
Trimipramine (Surmontil)	7–30	50–300	180 (incl. active metabolite)	CAPS: 25, 50, 100

■ CHEMICAL CLASS: HETEROCYCLICS

Indications

- Major depression
- Depressive phase of bipolar disorder
- Dysthymic disorder
- Smoking cessation (bupropion [Zyban]).

UNLABELED USES (trazodone):

- Aggressive behavior
- Panic disorder
- Agoraphobia with panic attacks.

Action

- Block neuronal reuptake of serotonin and norepinephrine, increasing the availability of these neurotransmitters at receptor sites in the brain and other tissues.

Contraindications and Precautions

Contraindicated in:

- Hypersensitivity to the drug
- Concomitant use with, or within 2 weeks' use of, MAOIs
- Known or suspected seizure disorder (maprotiline; bupropion)
- Acute phase of myocardial infarction
- Bulimia or anorexia nervosa (buproprion).

Use Cautiously in:

- Urinary retention
- Hepatic, renal, or cardiovascular disease
- Suicidal clients
- Pregnancy and lactation (safety not established)
- Elderly and debilitated clients.

Adverse Reactions and Side Effects

- Dry mouth
- Sedation

- Tachycardia
- Headache
- Nausea/vomiting
- Priapism (trazodone)
- Seizures (maprotiline; bupropion)
- Hypotension.

Examples

Generic (Trade) Name	Half-Life (hr)	Daily Adult Dosage Range (mg)	Therapeutic Plasma Level Range (ng/mL)	Available Forms (mg)
Bupropion (Wellbutrin; Zyban)	8–24	200–450	Not well established	TABS: 75, 100 TABS (SR): 100, 150
Maprotiline (Ludiomil)	21–25	50–225	200–300 (incl. metabolite)	TABS: 25, 50, 75
Mirtazapine (Remeron)	20–40	15–45	Not well established	TABS: 15, 30
Trazodone (Desyrel)	4–9	150–600	800–1600	TABS: 50, 100, 150, 300

■ CHEMICAL CLASS: SELECTIVE SEROTONIN REUPTAKE INHIBITORS

Indications

- Depression (citalopram, fluoxetine, paroxetine, sertraline)
- Obsessive-compulsive disorder (fluvoxamine, fluoxetine, paroxetine, sertraline)
- Bulimia nervosa (fluoxetine)
- Panic disorder (citalopram, paroxetine, sertraline).

UNLABELED USES:

Fluoxetine:

- Alcoholism
- Anorexia nervosa
- Attention-deficit/hyperactivity disorder
- Premenstrual syndrome
- Migraine headaches
- Obesity.

Sertraline:

- Post-traumatic stress disorder.

Action

- Selectively inhibit the CNS neuronal uptake of serotonin (5-HT), thereby potentiating its activity.

Contraindications and Precautions

Contraindicated in:

- Hypersensitivity to selective serotonin reuptake inhibitors (SSRIs)
- Concomitant use with, or within 2 weeks' use of, MAOIs.

Fluvoxamine:

- Concomitant use with astemizole or cisapride.

Use Cautiously in:

- Clients with history of seizures
- Underweight or anorectic clients
- Hepatic or renal insufficiency
- Elderly or debilitated clients
- Clients with history of drug abuse
- Suicidal clients.

Adverse Reactions and Side Effects

- Headache
- Insomnia
- Nausea
- Sexual dysfunction
- Somnolence
- Dry mouth
- Serotonin syndrome (if taken concurrently with, or within 2 weeks of [5 weeks with fluoxetine], MAOIs or other drugs that increase levels of serotonin). Symptoms of serotonin syndrome include diarrhea, cramping, tachycardia, labile blood pressure, diaphoresis, fever, tremor, shivering, restlessness, confusion, disorientation, mania, myoclonus, hyperreflexia, ataxia, seizures, cardiovascular shock, and death.

Examples

Generic (Trade) Name	Half-Life (hr)	Daily Adult Dosage Range (mg)	Therapeutic Plasma Level Ranges	Available Forms (mg)
Citalopram (Celexa)	24–48	20–40	Not well established	**TABS:** 20, 40
Fluoxetine (Prozac)	2–9 days (incl. metabolite)	20–80	Not well established	**CAPS:** 10, 20 **CONC:** 20/5 mL

Generic (Trade) Name	Half-Life (hr)	Daily Adult Dosage Range (mg)	Therapeutic Plasma Level Ranges	Available Forms (mg)
Fluvoxamine (Luvox)	13.6–15.6	50–300	Not well established	**TABS:** 50, 100
Paroxetine (Paxil)	10–24	10–50	Not well established	**TABS & CAPS:** 10, 20, 30, 40
Sertraline (Zoloft)	1–4 (incl. metabolite)	50–200	Not well established	**TABS:** 25, 50, 100

■ CHEMICAL CLASS: NONSELECTIVE REUPTAKE INHIBITORS

Indications

- Treatment of depression.

Action

- Inhibit neuronal reuptake of serotonin and norepinephrine
- Venlafaxine is also a weak inhibitor of dopamine reuptake.

Contraindications and Precautions

Contraindicated in:

- Hypersensitivity to the drug
- Children and pregnancy (safety not established)
- Concomitant use with MAOIs.

Nefazodone:

- Concomitant use with astemizole.

Use Cautiously in:

- Hepatic and renal insufficiency
- Elderly and debilitated clients
- Clients with history of drug abuse
- Suicidal clients
- Clients with history of or existing cardiovascular disease
- Clients with history of mania
- Clients with history of seizures.

Adverse Reactions and Side Effects

- Headache
- Dry mouth

- Nausea
- Somnolence
- Dizziness
- Insomnia
- Asthenia.

Examples

Generic (Trade) Name	Half-Life (hr)	Daily Adult Dosage Range (mg)	Therapeutic Plasma Level Ranges	Available Forms (mg)
Nafazodonc (Serzone)	2–4	200–600	Not well established	**TABS:** 50, 100, 150, 200, 250
Venlafaxine (Effexor)	5–11 (incl. metabolite)	75–375	Not well established	**TABS:** 25, 37.5, 50, 75, 100 **CAPS (XR):** 37.5, 75, 150

■ CHEMICAL CLASS: MONOAMINE OXIDASE INHIBITORS

Indications

- Treatment of depression

UNLABELED USES:

- Bulimia
- Night terrors
- Posttraumatic stress disorder
- Seasonal affective disorder
- Panic disorder.

Action

- Inhibit the enzyme monoamine oxidase, resulting in an increase in the concentration of endogenous epinephrine, norepinephrine, and serotonin in storage sites throughout the nervous system.

Contraindications and Precautions

Contraindicated in:

- Hypersensitivity
- Pheochromocytoma
- Hepatic or renal insufficiency

- History of or existing cardiovascular disease
- Hypertension
- History of severe or frequent headaches
- Concomitant use with guanethidine
- Concomitant use with tricyclic antidepressants or SSRIs
- Children less than 16 years of age
- Pregnancy and lactation (safety not established).

Use cautiously in:

- Clients with a history of seizures
- Diabetes mellitus
- Suicidal clients
- Schizophrenia
- Agitated or hypomanic clients
- History of angina pectoris or hyperthyroidism.

Adverse Reactions and Side Effects

- Dizziness
- Headache
- Orthostatic hypotension
- Constipation
- Nausea
- Disturbances in cardiac rate and rhythm.

Examples

Generic (Trade) Name	Half-Life (hr)	Daily Adult Dosage Range (mg)	Therapeutic Plasma Level Range	Available Forms (mg)
Isocarboxazid (Marplan)	Not established	30–50	Not well established	TABS: 10
Phenelzine (Nardil)	Not established	45–90	Not well established	TABS: 15
Tranylcypromine (Parnate)	2.4–2.8	30–60	Not well established	TABS: 10

■ NURSING DIAGNOSES RELATED TO ALL ANTIDEPRESSANTS

1. Risk for self-directed violence related to depressed mood.
2. Risk for injury related to side effects of sedation, lowered seizure threshold, orthostatic hypotension, pri-

apism, photosensitivity, arrhythmias, and hypertensive crisis.
3. Social isolation related to depressed mood.
4. Constipation related to side effects of the medication.

Nursing Implications for Antidepressants

The plan of care should include monitoring for the following side effects from antidepressant medications. Nursing implications are designated by an asterisk(*).

1. **May Occur with All Chemical Classes**
   a. ***Dry Mouth***
      * Offer the client sugarless candy, ice, frequent sips of water.
      * Strict oral hygiene is very important.

   b. ***Sedation***
      * Request an order from the physician for the drug to be given at bedtime.
      * Request that the physician decrease the dosage or perhaps order a less sedating drug.
      * Instruct the client not to drive or use dangerous equipment while experiencing sedation.

   c. ***Nausea***
      * Medication may be taken with food to minimize gastrointestinal distress.

2. **Most Commonly Occur with Tricyclics or Heterocyclics**
   a. ***Blurred Vision***
      * Offer reassurance that this symptom should subside after a few weeks.
      * Instruct the client not to drive until vision is clear.
      * Clear small items from routine pathway to prevent falls.

   b. ***Constipation***
      * Order foods high in fiber, increase fluid intake if not contraindicated, and encourage the client to increase physical exercise, if possible.

   c. ***Urinary Retention***
      * Instruct the client to report hesitancy or inability to urinate.
      * Monitor intake and output.
      * Various methods to stimulate urination may be tried, such as running water in the bathroom or pouring water over the perineal area.

   d. ***Orthostatic Hypotension***
      * Instruct the client to rise slowly from a lying or sitting position.

* Monitor blood pressure (lying and standing) frequently, and document and report significant changes.
* Avoid long hot showers or baths.

e. ***Reduction of Seizure Threshold***
* Clients with history of seizures should be observed closely.
* Institute seizure precautions as specified in hospital procedure manual.
* Bupropion (Wellbutrin) should be administered in doses of no more than 150 mg and should be given at least 4 hours apart. Bupropion has been associated with a relatively high incidence of seizure activity in anorectic and cachectic clients.

f. ***Tachycardia, Arrhythmias***
* Carefully monitor blood pressure and pulse rate and rhythm, and report any significant change to the physician.

g. ***Photosensitivity***
* Ensure that client wears protective sunscreens, clothing, and sunglasses while outdoors.

h. ***Weight Gain***
* Provide instructions for reduced-calorie diet.
* Encourage increased level of activity, if appropriate.

3. **Most Commonly Occur with SSRIs**

a. ***Insomnia, Agitation***
* Take dose early in the day.
* Avoid caffeinated food and drinks.
* Teach relaxation techniques to use before bedtime.

b. **Headache**
* Most common with fluoxetine (Prozac).
* Administer analgesics, as prescribed.
* May need to switch to another SSRI or to another class of antidepressants.

c. ***Weight Loss***
* Ensure that client is provided with caloric intake sufficient to maintain desired weight.
* Caution should be taken in prescribing these drugs for anorectic clients.
* Weigh client daily or every other day, at the same time and on the same scale if possible.

d. ***Sexual Dysfunction***
* (Males) May report abnormal ejaculation or impotence.
* (Females) May experience delay or loss of orgasm.

* If side effect becomes intolerable, a switch to another antidepressant may be necessary.

e. ***Serotonin Syndrome***

* Discontinue offending agent immediately.
* The physician will prescribe medications to block serotonin receptors, relieve hyperthermia and muscle rigidity, and prevent seizures. Artificial ventilation may be required.
* Symptomatic measures, such as cooling blankets to decrease fever, may be instituted.

4. **Most Commonly Occur with MAOIs**

a. ***Hypertensive Crisis***

* This occurs if the individual consumes foods or other substances containing tyramine while receiving MAOI therapy. Foods that should be avoided include aged cheeses, raisins, fava beans, red wines, smoked and processed meats, caviar, pickled herring, soy sauce, monosodium glutamate (MSG), beer, chocolate, yogurt, and bananas. Drugs that should be avoided include other antidepressants (tricyclics, heterocyclics, SSRIs), sympathomimetics (including over-the-counter cough and cold preparations), stimulants (including over-the-counter diet drugs), antihypertensives, meperidine and other opioid narcotics, and antiparkinsonian agents such as levodopa.
* Symptoms of hypertensive crisis include severe occipital headache, palpitations, nausea and vomiting, nuchal rigidity, fever, sweating, marked increase in blood pressure, chest pain, and coma.
* Treatment of hypertensive crisis: Discontinue drug immediately; monitor vital signs; administer short-acting antihypertensive medication as ordered by physician; use external cooling measures to control hyperpyrexia.

5. **Miscellaneous Side Effects**

a. ***With Trazodone (Desyrel): Priapism***

* This is a rare side effect, but it has occurred in some men taking trazodone.
* If the client complains of prolonged or inappropriate penile erection, withhold medication dosage and notify the physician immediately.
* This can become very problematic, requiring surgical intervention, and, if not treated successfully, can result in impotence.

■ CLIENT AND FAMILY EDUCATION RELATED TO ALL ANTIDEPRESSANTS

- Continue to take the medication even though the symptoms have not subsided. The therapeutic effect may not be seen for as long as 4 weeks. If after this length of time no improvement is noted, the physician may prescribe a different medication.
- Use caution when driving or operating dangerous machinery. Drowsiness and dizziness can occur. If these side effects become persistent or interfere with ADLs, report them to the physician. Dosage adjustment may be necessary.
- Do not stop taking the drug abruptly. To do so might produce withdrawal symptoms, such as nausea, vertigo, insomnia, headache, malaise, and nightmares
- If taking a tricyclic, use sunscreens and wear protective clothing when spending time outdoors. The skin may be sensitive to sunburn.
- Report occurrence of any of the following symptoms to the physician immediately: sore throat, fever, malaise, unusual bleeding, easy bruising, persistent nausea and vomiting, severe headache, rapid heart rate, difficulty urinating, anorexia or weight loss, seizure activity, stiff or sore neck, and chest pain.
- Rise slowly from a sitting or lying position to prevent a sudden drop in blood pressure.
- Take frequent sips of water, chew sugarless gum, or suck on hard candy if dry mouth is a problem. Good oral care (frequent brushing, flossing) is very important.
- Do not consume the following foods or medications while taking MAOIs: aged cheese, wine (especially chianti), beer, chocolate, colas, coffee, tea, sour cream, beef or chicken livers, canned figs, soy sauce, overripe and fermented foods, pickled herring, preserved sausages, yogurt, yeast products, broad beans, cold remedies, diet pills. To do so could cause a life-threatening hypertensive crisis.
- Avoid smoking while receiving tricyclic therapy. Smoking increases the metabolism of tricyclics, requiring an adjustment in dosage to achieve the therapeutic effect.
- Do not drink alcohol while undergoing antidepres-

sant therapy. These drugs potentiate the effects of each other.

- Do not consume other medications (including over-the-counter medications) without the physician's approval while receiving antidepressant therapy. Many medications contain substances that, in combination with antidepressant medication, could precipitate a life-threatening hypertensive crisis.
- Notify physician immediately if inappropriate or prolonged penile erections occur while taking trazodone (Desyrel). If the erection persists longer than 1 hour, seek emergency department treatment. This condition is rare, but has occurred in some men who have taken trazodone. If measures are not instituted immediately, impotence can result.
- Do not "double up" on medication if a dose of bupropion (Wellbutrin) is missed, unless advised to do so by the physician. Taking bupropion in divided doses will decrease the risk of seizures and other adverse effects.
- Be aware of possible risks of taking antidepressants during pregnancy. Safe use during pregnancy and lactation has not been fully established. These drugs are believed to readily cross the placental barrier; if so, the fetus could experience adverse effects of the drug. Inform the physician immediately if pregnancy occurs, is suspected, or is planned.
- Be aware of the side effects of antidepressants. Refer to written materials furnished by health-care providers for safe self-administration
- Carry a card or other identification at all times describing the medications being taken.

■ INTERNET REFERENCES

- http://www.mentalhealth.com/fr30.html
- http://www.nimh.nih.gov/publicat/medicate.cfm
- http://www.fadavis.com/catalog/Nursing/Psychiatric%20and%20Mental%20Health%20Nursing/0483-monograph.htm

CHAPTER 26

Mood-Stabilizing Drugs

■ CHEMICAL CLASS: ANTIMANICS

Indications

- Manic episodes associated with bipolar disorder
- Maintenance therapy to prevent or diminish intensity of subsequent manic episodes
- Depression associated with bipolar disorder.

INVESTIGATIONAL USES:

- Major depression
- Neutropenia
- Cluster or migraine headaches (prophylaxis)
- Alcohol dependence
- Shizoaffective disorder.

Action

- Not fully understood but may enhance reuptake of norepinephrine and serotonin, decreasing the levels in the body, resulting in decreased hyperactivity (may take 1–3 weeks for symptoms to subside).

Contraindications and Precautions

Contraindicated in:

- Hypersensitivity
- Cardiac or renal disease
- Dehydration
- Sodium depletion
- Brain damage
- Pregnancy and lactation.

Use Cautiously in:

- Elderly clients
- Thyroid disorders
- Diabetes mellitus
- Urinary retention
- History of seizure disorder.

Adverse Reactions and Side Effects

- Drowsiness, dizziness, headache
- Dry mouth, thirst
- Gastrointestinal upset
- Fine hand tremors
- Hypotension, arrhythmias, pulse irregularities
- Polyuria, dehydration
- Weight gain.

Examples

Generic (Trade) Name	Half-Life (hr)	Daily Adult Dosage Range (mg)	Therapeutic Plasma Level Range (mEq/L)	Available Forms (mg)
Lithium carbonate (Eskalith; Lithane; Lithobid)	10–50	ACUTE MANIA: 1800–2400 MAINTENANCE: 300–1200	ACUTE MANIA: 1.0–1.5 MAINTENANCE: 0.6–1.2	CAPS: 150, 300, 600 TABS: 300 TABS (SR): 300, 450
Lithium citrate				SYRUP: 8 mEq (as citrate equivalent to 300 mg lithium)/ 5 mL

■ CHEMICAL CLASS: ANTICONVULSANTS

Indications

- Absence, akinetic, myoclonic, grand mal, and psychomotor seizures.

UNLABELED USES:

- Bipolar disorder.

Carbamazepine:

- Rage reactions
- Resistant schizophrenia.

Valproic acid:
- Migraine headache prophylaxis.

Action

- Action in the treatment of bipolar disorder is unclear.

Contraindications and Precautions

Contraindicated in:
- Hypersensitivity
- Lactation.

Carbamazepine:
- Concomitant use with MAOIs.

Clonazepam:
- Acute angle-closure glaucoma.

Valproic acid:
- Severe liver disease.

Use Cautiously in:
- Elderly and debilitated clients
- Clients with hepatic, renal, or cardiac disease
- Pregnancy.

Clonazepam:
- Clients with history of drug abuse/addiction or depression/suicidal ideation.

Adverse Reactions and Side Effects

- Drowsiness
- Dizziness
- Nausea/vomiting.

Carbamazepine:
- Blood dyscrasias.

Valproic acid:
- Prolonged bleeding time.

Examples

Generic (Trade) Name	Half-Life (hr)	Daily Adult Dosage Range (mg)	Therapeutic Plasma Level Range	Available Forms (mg)
Carbamazepine (Tegretol)	25–65 (initial) 12–17 (repeated doses)	400–1200	4–12 μg/mL	TABS: 100, 200 TABS (XR): 100, 200, 400 CAPS (XR): 200, 300 SUSP: 100/5 mL
Clonazepam (C-IV) (Klonopin)	18–50	1.5–20	20–80 ng/mL	TABS: 0.5, 1, 2

Generic (Trade) Name	Half-Life (hr)	Daily Adult Dosage Range (mg)	Therapeutic Plasma Level Range	Available Forms (mg)
Valproic acid (Depakene; Depakote)	6–16	500–1500	50–100 μg/mL	CAPS: 250 SYRUP: 250/5 mL TABS (DR): 125, 250, 500 CAPS (SPRINKLE): 125 INJECT: 5 mL (single dose vial)

■ CHEMICAL CLASS: CALCIUM CHANNEL BLOCKERS

Indications

- Angina
- Hypertension
- Arrhythmias.

UNLABELED USES:

- Bipolar mania
- Migraine headache prophylaxis.

Action

- Action in the treatment of bipolar disorder is unclear.

Contraindications and Precautions

Contraindicated in:

- Hypersensitivity
- Heart block
- Hypotension
- Cardiogenic shock
- Congestive heart failure
- Pregnancy and lactation.

Use Cautiously in:

- Liver or renal disease
- Cardiomyopathy
- Intracranial pressure
- Elderly clients.

Adverse Reactions and Side Effects

- Drowsiness
- Dizziness
- Hypotension
- Bradycardia
- Nausea
- Constipation.

Examples

Generic (Trade) Name	Half-Life (hr)	Daily Adult Dosage Range (mg)	Therapeutic Plasma Level Range (ng/mL)	Available Forms (mg)
Verapamil (Calan; Isoptin)	3–7 (initially) 4.5–12 (repeated dosing)	240–480	80–300	TABS: 40, 80, 120 TABS (SR): 120, 180, 240 CAPS (SR): 120, 180, 240, 360 INJECT: 5/ 2 mL

■ NURSING DIAGNOSES RELATED TO ALL MOOD-STABILIZING DRUGS

1. Risk for injury related to manic hyperactivity.
2. Risk for violence: self-directed or directed at others related to unresolved anger turned inward on the self or outward on the environment.
3. Risk for injury related to lithium toxicity.
4. Risk for activity intolerance related to side effects of drowsiness and dizziness.

■ NURSING IMPLICATIONS FOR MOOD-STABILIZING DRUGS

1. Assess for changes in mood, particularly mood swings.
2. For the client on lithium therapy, assess for signs of lithium toxicity: ataxia, blurred vision, severe diarrhea, persistent nausea and vomiting, and tinnitus.
3. Instruct client to take medication on a regular basis,

even when feeling well. Discontinuation can result in return of symptoms.

4. Ensure that client does not drive or operate dangerous machinery until response is stabilized. Drowsiness and dizziness can occur.
5. Ensure that the client on lithium therapy receives sufficient dietary sodium intake and 2500 to 3000 mL of water per day.
6. Notify the physician if vomiting or diarrhea occurs. These symptoms in the client on lithium therapy can result in increased risk of toxicity.
7. Some clients may gain weight on this therapy. Assist client in planning appropriate diet from the Food Guide Pyramid to ensure that weight gain does not become a problem. Include adequate sodium and other nutrients while decreasing the number of calories.
8. Administer the medication with food if nausea becomes a problem.

■ CLIENT AND FAMILY EDUCATION RELATED TO MOOD-STABILIZING DRUGS

- Do not drive or operate dangerous machinery. Drowsiness or dizziness can occur.
- Do not stop taking the drug abruptly. Can produce serious withdrawal symptoms. The physician will administer orders for tapering the drug when therapy is to be discontinued.
- Report the following symptoms to the physician immediately. *Client taking anticonvulsant:* unusual bleeding, spontaneous bruising, sore throat, fever, malaise, dark urine, and yellow skin or eyes. *Client taking calcium channel blocker:* irregular heartbeat, shortness of breath, swelling of the hands and feet, pronounced dizziness, chest pain, profound mood swings, severe and persistent headache. *Client taking lithium:* ataxia, blurred vision, severe diarrhea, persistent nausea and vomiting, tinnitus, excessive urine output, increasing tremors, or mental confusion.
- For the client on lithium: Ensure that the diet contains adequate sodium. Drink 6 to 8 glasses of water each day. Avoid drinks that contain caffeine (they have a diuretic effect). Have serum lithium

level checked every 1 to 2 months or as advised by physician.

- Avoid consuming alcoholic beverages and nonprescription medications without approval from physician.
- Carry card at all times identifying the name of medications being taken.

INTERNET REFERENCES

- http://www.mentalhealth.com/fr30.html
- http://www.nimh.nih.gov/publicat/medicate.cfm
- http://www.fadavis.com/catalog/Nursing/Psychiatric%20and%20Mental%20Health%20Nursing/0483-monograph.htm

CHAPTER 27

Antipsychotic Agents

■ CHEMICAL CLASS: PHENOTHIAZINES

Indications

- Acute and chronic psychoses (including schizophrenia, schizoaffective disorder, psychotic depression, and drug-induced psychosis)
- Mania (while awaiting the effects of a mood stabilizer)
- Recurrent psychotic symptoms in dementia
- As an antiemetic (*chlorpromazine; perphenazine; prochlorperazine*)
- Intractable hiccups (*chlorpromazine; perphenazine*)
- Control of tics and vocal utterances in Tourette's disorder (*haloperidol; pimozide*).

Action

- These drugs are thought to work by blocking postsynaptic dopamine receptors in the basal ganglia, hypothalamus, limbic system, brain stem, and medulla
- Also demonstrate varying affinity for cholinergic, $alpha_1$-adrenergic, and histaminic receptors
- Antipsychotic effects may also be related to inhibition of dopamine-mediated transmission of neural impulses at the synapses.

Contraindications and Precautions

Contraindicated in:

- Hypersensitivity (cross-sensitivity may exist among phenothiazines)

- In comatose or severely CNS-depressed clients
- Poorly controlled seizure disorders
- Clients with blood dyscrasias
- Parkinson's disease
- Clients with liver, renal, or cardiac insufficiency.

Use Cautiously in:

- Severely ill or elderly clients
- Diabetic clients
- Clients with respiratory insufficiency
- Prostatic hypertrophy
- Safety in pregnancy and lactation has not been established.

Adverse Reactions and Side Effects

- Dry mouth
- Blurred vision
- Constipation
- Urinary retention
- Nausea
- Skin rash
- Sedation
- Orthostatic hypotension
- Photosensitivity
- Decreased libido
- Amenorrhea
- Retrograde ejaculation
- Gynecomastia
- Weight gain
- Reduction of seizure threshold
- Agranulocytosis
- Extrapyramidal symptoms
- Tardive dyskinesia
- Neuroleptic malignant syndrome.

Examples

Generic (Trade) Name	Half-Life (hr)	Daily Adult Dosage Range (mg)	Available Forms (mg)
Chlorpromazine (Thorazine)	8–35	40–800	**TABS:** 10, 25, 50, 100, 200 **CAPS (SR):** 30, 75, 150 **SYRUP:** 10/5 mL **CONC:** 30/mL, 100/mL **SUPP:** 25, 100 **INJECT:** 25/mL

Generic (Trade) Name	Half-Life (hr)	Daily Adult Dosage Range (mg)	Available Forms (mg)
Fluphenazine (Prolixin)	HCl: 15 ENANTHATE: 3.7 days DECANOATE: 6.8–9.6 days	1–40	**TABS:** 1, 2.5, 5, 10 **ELIXIR:** 2.5/5 mL; **CONC:** 5/mL **INJECT:** 2.5/mL **INJECT (ENANTHATE):** 25/mL **INJECT (DECANOATE):** 25/mL
Mesoridazine (Serentil)	24–48	30–400	**TABS:** 10, 25, 50, 100 **CONC:** 25/mL **INJECT:** 25/mL
Perphenazine (Trilafon)	8–21	12–64	**TABS:** 2, 4, 8, 16 **CONC:** 16/5 mL **INJECT:** 5/mL
Prochlorperazine (Compazine)	Unknown	15–150	**TABS:** 10, 25 **CAPS (SR):** 10, 15 **SUPP:** 2.5, 5, 25 **SYRUP:** 5/5 mL **INJECT:** 5/mL
Promazine (Sparine)	Unknown	40–1200	**TABS:** 25, 50 **INJECT:** 25/mL; 50/mL
Thioridazine (Mellaril)	9–30	150–800	**TABS:** 10, 15, 25, 50, 100, 150, 200 **CONC:** 30/mL; 100/mL **SUSP:** 25/5 mL; 100/5 mL
Trifluoperazine (Stelazine)	Unknown	4–40	**TABS:** 1, 2, 5, 10 **CONC:** 10/mL **INJECT:** 2/mL
Triflupromazine (Vesprin)	Unknown	60–150	**INJECT:** 10/mL; 20/mL

■ CHEMICAL CLASS: BENZISOXAZOLE

Indication

- Management of the manifestations of psychotic disorders.

Action

- Exerts antagonistic effects on dopamine type 2 (D_2), serotonin type 2 ($5\text{-}HT_2$), alpha$_1$- and alpha$_2$-adrenergic, and H_1 histaminergic receptors.

Contraindications and Precautions

Contraindicated in:

- Known hypersensitivity
- Comatose or severely depressed clients
- Clients with cardiac disease
- Lactation.

Use Cautiously in:

- Clients with hepatic or renal impairment
- Clients with history of seizures
- Clients exposed to temperature extremes
- Pregnancy (safety not established).

Adverse Reactions and Side Effects

- Anxiety
- Somnolence
- Extrapyramidal symptoms
- Dizziness
- Constipation
- Nausea
- Rhinitis
- Rash
- Tachycardia.

Example

Generic (Trade) Name	Half-Life (hr)	Daily Adult Dosage Range (mg)	Available Forms (mg)
Risperidone (Risperdal)	3–17 (drug) 21–30 (metabolite)	1–16	**TABS:** 1, 2, 3, 4 **ORAL SOLU:** 1/mL

■ CHEMICAL CLASS: BUTYROPHENONE

Indications

- Management of acute and chronic psychoses
- Control of tics and vocal utterances of Tourette's disorder
- Treating symptoms of dementia in the elderly
- Control of hyperactivity and severe behavior problems in children.

INVESTIGATIONAL USES:

- Antiemetic (doses smaller than those used to control psychotic behavior)
- Control in acute psychiatric situations
- Intractable hiccups
- Infantile autism.

Action

- Blocks postsynaptic dopamine receptors in the hypothalamus, limbic system, and reticular formation
- Demonstrates varying affinity for cholinergic, alpha$_1$-adrenergic, and histaminic receptors.

Contraindications and Precautions

Contraindicated in:

- Hypersensitivity to the drug
- In comatose or severely CNS-depressed clients
- Poorly controlled seizure disorders
- Clients with blood dyscrasias
- Parkinson's disease
- Clients with liver, renal, or cardiac insufficiency.

Use Cautiously in:

- Severely ill or elderly clients
- Diabetic clients
- Clients with respiratory insufficiency
- Prostatic hypertrophy
- Safety in pregnancy and lactation has not been established.

Adverse Reactions and Side Effects

- Refer to this section under "Phenothiazines."

Example

Generic (Trade) Name	Half-Life (hr)	Daily Adult Dosage Range (mg)	Available Forms (mg)
Haloperidol (Haldol)	13–35 (oral, IM lactate); 3 wk (IM decanoate)	1–100	TABS: 0.5, 1, 2, 5, 10, 20 CONC: 2/mL INJECT (LACTATE): 5/mL INJECT (DECANOATE): 50/mL; 100/mL

■ CHEMICAL CLASS: DIBENZOXAZEPINE

Indication

- Management of the manifestations of psychotic disorders.

Action

- Not fully understood
- Thought to act primarily in the reticular formation
- Reduces firing threshold of CNS neurons.

Contraindications and Precautions

Contraindicated in:

- Hypersensitivity
- Comatose or severe drug-induced depressed states
- Clients with blood dyscrasias
- Parkinson's disease
- Hepatic, renal, or cardiac insufficiency
- Severe hypotension or hypertension
- Children under 16
- Pregnancy and lactation (safety has not been established).

Use Cautiously in:

- Clients with history of seizures
- Respiratory insufficiency
- Prostatic hypertrophy
- Elderly or debilitated clients.

Adverse Reactions and Side Effects

- Refer to this section under "Phenothiazines."

Example

Generic (Trade) Name	Half-Life (hr)	Daily Adult Dosage Range (mg)	Available Forms (mg)
Loxapine (Loxitane)	INITIAL: 5 TERMINAL: 19	20–250	CAPS: 5, 10, 25, 50 CONC: 25/mL INJECT: 50/ml

■ CHEMICAL CLASS: DIBENZODIAZEPINE

Indication

- Management of severely ill schizophrenic clients who fail to respond adequately to standard antipsychotic drug treatment.

Action

- Exerts a strong antagonistic effect on dopamine D_1 and D_4 receptors and on serotonin 5-HT_2 receptors
- Has a low affinity for dopamine D_2 receptors
- Also acts as an antagonist at adrenergic, cholinergic, and histaminergic receptors.

Contraindications and Precautions

Contraindicated in:

- Myeloproliferative disorders
- History of clozapine-induced agranulocytosis or severe granulocytopenia
- Concomitant use with other drugs that have the potential to suppress bone marrow function
- Severe CNS depression or comatose states
- Uncontrolled epilepsy
- Lactation
- Children (safety not established).

Use Cautiously in:

- Clients with hepatic, renal, or cardiac insufficiency
- Diabetes mellitus
- Prostatic enlargement
- Narrow-angle glaucoma
- Pregnancy.

Adverse Reactions and Side Effects

- Agranulocytosis
- Seizures
- Salivation
- Sedation
- Tachycardia
- Constipation
- Fever

- Weight gain
- Orthostatic hypotension
- Neuroleptic malignant syndrome
- Hyperglycemia.

Example

Generic (Trade) Name	Half-Life (hr)	Daily Adult Dosage Range (mg)	Available Forms (mg)
Clozapine (Clozaril)	4–66	25–50 (initial therapy) 300–600 (target dose) 600–900 (may be required for some clients, depending on response)	TABS: 25, 100

■ CHEMICAL CLASS: DIBENZOTHIAZEPINE

Indication

- Management of the manifestations of psychotic disorders.

Action

- Antipsychotic activity is thought to be mediated through a combination of dopamine type 2 (D_2) and serotonin type 2 ($5\text{-}HT_2$) antagonism
- Other effects may be due to antagonism of histamine H_1 receptors and $alpha_1$-adrenergic receptors.

Contraindications and Precautions

Contraindicated in:
- Hypersensitivity
- Lactation
- Children (safety has not been established).

Use Cautiously in:
- Clients with hepatic or cardiovascular disease
- Clients with history of seizures
- Comatose or other CNS-depressed clients

- Clients at risk for aspiration pneumonia
- Pregnancy
- Elderly and debilitated clients.

Adverse Reactions and Side Effects

- Somnolence
- Dizziness
- Headache
- Constipation
- Dry mouth
- Dyspepsia
- Orthostatic hypotension
- Neuroleptic malignant syndrome
- Extrapyramidal symptoms
- Tardive dyskinesia
- Cataracts
- Lowered seizure threshold.

Example

Generic (Trade) Name	Half-Life (hr)	Daily Adult Dosage Range (mg)	Available Forms (mg)
Quetiapine (Seroquel)	6	INITIAL: 25–50 bid TARGET DOSE: 300–400	**TABS:** 25, 100, 200

■ CHEMICAL CLASS: DIHYDROINDOLONE

Indication

- Management of manifestations of psychotic disorders.

Action

- The exact mechanism of action is not fully understood
- It is thought that molindone exerts its effect on the ascending reticular activating system.

Contraindications and Precautions

Contraindicated in:

- Hypersensitivity
- Comatose or severely CNS-depressed clients
- Children under 12 (safety not established)
- Lactation
- Sensitivity to sulfites (contained in some preparations).

Use Cautiously in:

- Clients with history of seizures
- Respiratory, renal, hepatic, thyroid, or cardiovascular disorders
- Elderly or debilitated clients
- Pregnancy.

Adverse Reactions and Side Effects

- Refer to this section under "Phenothiazines."

Example

Generic (Trade) Name	Half-Life (hr)	Daily Adult Dosage Range (mg)	Available Forms (mg)
Molindone (Moban)	10–20	15–225	TABS: 5, 10, 25, 50, 100 CONC: 20/mL

■ CHEMICAL CLASS: THIENOBENZODIAZEPINE

Indication

- Management of the manifestations of psychotic disorders.

Action

- Antagonist of both 5-HT_2 and D_2 receptors, with preferential antagonism of the former
- Also shows antagonism for muscarinic, histaminic, and adrenergic receptors.

Contraindications and Precautions

Contraindicated in:

- Hypersensitivity

- Children (safety has not been established)
- Lactation.

Use Cautiously in:

- Clients with hepatic or cardiovascular disease
- Clients with history of seizures
- Comatose or other CNS-depressed clients
- Clients at risk for aspiration pneumonia
- Pregnancy
- Elderly and debilitated clients
- Conditions that may contribute to elevation in core body temperature.

Adverse Reactions and Side Effects

- Agitation
- Insomnia
- Headache
- Fever
- Somnolence
- Asthenia
- Dry mouth
- Constipation
- Weight gain
- Orthostatic hypotension
- Tachycardia
- Extrapyramidal symptoms (high dose–dependent)

Example

Generic (Trade) Name	Half-Life (hr)	Daily Adult Dosage Range (mg)	Available Forms (mg)
Olanzapine (Zyprexa)	30	10–15	TABS: 2.5, 5, 7.5, 10

■ CHEMICAL CLASS: THIOXANTHENE

Indication

- Manifestations of psychotic disorders.

Action

- Blocks postsynaptic dopamine receptors in the hypothalamus, limbic system, and reticular formation
- Demonstrates varying affinity for cholinergic, $alpha_1$-adrenergic, and histaminic receptors.

Contraindications and Precautions

Contraindicated in:

- Hypersensitivity
- Comatose or severely CNS-depressed clients
- Bone marrow depression or blood dyscrasias
- Parkinson's disease
- Severe hypotension or hypertension
- Children under age 12
- Pregnancy and lactation (safety not established).

Use Cautiously in:

- Patients with history of seizures
- Respiratory, renal, hepatic, thyroid, or cardiovascular disorders
- Elderly or debilitated clients
- Clients exposed to extreme environmental heat
- Clients taking atropine or atropine-like drugs.

Adverse Reactions and Side Effects

- Refer to this section under "Phenothiazines."

Example

Generic (Trade) Name	Half-Life (hr)	Daily Adult Dosage Range (mg)	Available Forms (mg)
Thiothixene (Navane)	34	6–60	CAPS: 1, 2, 5, 10, 20 CONC: 5/mL INJECT: 2/mL, 5/mL

■ NURSING DIAGNOSES RELATED TO ALL ANTIPSYCHOTIC AGENTS

1. Risk for violence directed at others related to panic anxiety and mistrust of others.
2. Risk for injury related to medication side effects of sedation, photosensitivity, reduction of seizure threshold, agranulocytosis, extrapyramidal symptoms, tardive dyskinesia, and/or neuroleptic malignant syndrome.
3. Risk for activity intolerance related to medication side effects of sedation, blurred vision, weakness.
4. Noncompliance with medication regimen related to suspiciousness and mistrust of others.

■ NURSING IMPLICATIONS FOR ANTIPSYCHOTIC AGENTS

The plan of care should include monitoring for the following side effects from antipsychotic medications. Nursing implications related to each side effect are designated by an asterisk (*).

1. **Anticholinergic Effects**
   a. ***Dry mouth***
      * Provide the client with sugarless candy or gum, ice, and frequent sips of water.
      * Ensure that client practices strict oral hygiene.

   b. ***Blurred Vision***
      * Explain that this symptom will most likely subside after a few weeks.
      * Advise client not to drive a car until vision clears.
      * Clear small items from pathways to prevent falls.

   c. ***Constipation***
      * Order foods high in fiber; encourage increase in physical activity and fluid intake if not contraindicated.

   d. ***Urinary Retention***
      * Instruct client to report any difficulty urinating; monitor intake and output.

2. **Nausea, Gastrointestinal Upset**
   * Tablets or capsules may be administered with food to minimize gastrointestinal upset.
   * Concentrates may be diluted and administered with fruit juice or other liquid; they should be mixed immediately before administration.

3. **Skin Rash**
   * Report appearance of any rash on skin to physician.
   * Avoid spilling any of the liquid concentrate on skin; contact dermatitis can occur.

4. **Sedation**
   * Discuss with physician possibility of administering drug at bedtime.
   * Discuss with physician possible decrease in dosage or order for less sedating drug.
   * Instruct client not to drive or operate dangerous equipment while experiencing sedation.

5. **Orthostatic Hypotension**
   * Instruct client to rise slowly from a lying or sitting

position; monitor blood pressure (lying and standing) each shift; document and report significant changes.

6. **Photosensitivity**
   * Ensure that client wears protective sunscreens, clothing, and sunglasses while spending time outdoors.
7. **Hormonal Effects**
   a. ***Decreased Libido, Retrograde Ejaculation, Gynecomastia (men)***
      * Provide explanation of the effects and reassurance of reversibility. If necessary, discuss with physician possibility of ordering alternate medication.

   b. ***Amenorrhea (women)***
      * Offer reassurance of reversibility; instruct client to continue use of contraception, because amenorrhea does not indicate cessation of ovulation.

   c. ***Weight Gain***
      * Weigh client every other day; order calorie-controlled diet; provide opportunity for physical exercise; provide diet and exercise instruction.
8. **Reduction of Seizure Threshold**
   * Closely observe clients with history of seizures.
   * NOTE: This is particularly important with clients taking clozapine (Clozaril). Reportedly, seizures affect 1 to 5 percent of individuals who take this drug, depending on the dosage (Pokalo, 1991).
9. **Agranulocytosis**
   * Potentially very serious side effect, but relatively rare with most of the antipsychotic drugs. It usually occurs within the first 3 months of treatment. Observe for symptoms of sore throat, fever, and malaise. A complete blood count should be monitored if these symptoms appear.
   * **EXCEPTION:** With clozapine (Clozaril), agranulocytosis occurs in 1 to 2 percent of all clients taking the drug (Pokalo, 1991). It is a potentially fatal blood disorder in which the client's white blood cell (WBC) count can drop to extremely low levels. Individuals receiving clozapine therapy are required to have blood levels drawn weekly for the first 6 months of therapy, followed by biweekly monitoring for patients with acceptable WBC counts. If the WBC count falls below 3000 mm^3 or the granulo-

cyte count falls below 1500 mm^3, clozapine therapy is discontinued. The disorder is reversible if discovered in the early stages; however, this additional required technology of weekly blood tests has made the cost of this drug prohibitive for some people.

10. **Salivation (with clozapine)**
    * A significant number of clients receiving clozapine (Clozaril) therapy experience extreme salivation. Offer support to the client, as this may be an embarrassing situation. It may even be a safety issue (e.g., risk of aspiration), if the problem is very severe.

11. **Extrapyramidal Symptoms (EPS)**
    * Observe for symptoms and report; administer antiparkinsonian drugs, as ordered.

    a. ***Pseudoparkinsonism (tremor, shuffling gait, drooling, rigidity)***
       * Symptoms may appear 1 to 5 days following initiation of antipsychotic medication; occurs most often in women, the elderly, and dehydrated clients.

    b. ***Akinesia (muscular weakness)***
       * Same as for pseudoparkinsonism.

    c. ***Akathisia (continuous restlessness and fidgeting)***
       * This occurs most frequently in women; symptoms may occur 50 to 60 days following initiation of therapy.

    d. ***Dystonia (involuntary muscular movements [spasms] of face, arms, legs, and neck)***
       * This occurs most often in men and in clients younger than 25 years of age.

    e. ***Oculogyric Crisis (uncontrolled rolling back of eyes)***
       * This may appear as part of the syndrome described as *dystonia*. It may be mistaken for seizure activity. Dystonia and oculogyric crisis should be treated as an emergency situation. The physician should be contacted; intravenous benztropine mesylate (Cogentin) is commonly administered. Stay with the client and offer reassurance and support during this frightening time.

12. ***Tardive Dyskinesia (bizarre facial and tongue movements, stiff neck, and difficulty swallowing)***
    * All clients receiving long-term (months or years) antipsychotic therapy are at risk.
    * Symptoms are potentially irreversible.

* Drug should be withdrawn at first sign, which is usually vermiform movements of the tongue; prompt action may prevent irreversibility.

13. **Neuroleptic Malignant Syndrome (NMS)**
   * This is a rare, but potentially fatal, complication of treatment with neuroleptic drugs. Routine assessments should include temperature and observation for parkinsonian symptoms.
   * Onset can occur within hours or even years after drug initiation, and progression is rapid over the following 24 to 72 hours.
   * Symptoms include severe parkinsonian muscle rigidity, hyperpyrexia up to 107°F, tachycardia, tachypnea, fluctuations in blood pressure, diaphoresis, and rapid deterioration of mental status to stupor and coma.
   * Discontinue neuroleptic medication immediately.
   * Monitor vital signs, degree of muscle rigidity, intake and output, and level of consciousness.
   * The physician may order bromocriptine (Parlodel) or dantrolene (Dantrium) to counteract the effects of NMS.

■ CLIENT AND FAMILY EDUCATION RELATED TO ALL ANTIPSYCHOTICS

- Use caution when driving or operating dangerous machinery. Drowsiness and dizziness can occur.
- Do not stop taking the drug abruptly after long-term use. To do so might produce withdrawal symptoms, such as nausea, vomiting, gastritis, headache, tachycardia, insomnia, or tremulousness.
- Use sunscreens and wear protective clothing when spending time outdoors. Skin is more susceptible to sunburn, which can occur in as little as 30 minutes.
- Report weekly (if receiving clozapine therapy) to have blood levels drawn and to obtain a weekly supply of the drug.
- Report occurrence of any of the following symptoms to the physician immediately: sore throat, fever, malaise, unusual bleeding, easy bruising, persistent nausea and vomiting, severe headache, rapid heart rate, difficulty urinating, muscle twitching, tremors, darkly colored urine, pale stools, yellow skin or eyes, muscular incoordination, or skin rash.

- Rise slowly from a sitting or lying position to prevent a sudden drop in blood pressure.
- Take frequent sips of water, chew sugarless gum, or suck on hard candy if experiencing a problem with dry mouth. Good oral care (frequent brushing, flossing) is very important.
- Consult the physician regarding smoking while taking this medication. Smoking increases the metabolism of some antipsychotics, possibly requiring an adjustment in dosage to achieve a therapeutic effect.
- Dress warmly in cold weather and avoid extended exposure to very high or low temperatures. Body temperature is harder to maintain with this medication.
- Do not drink alcohol while on antipsychotic therapy. These drugs potentiate each other's effects.
- Do not consume other medications (including over-the-counter products) without physician's approval. Many medications contain substances that interact with antipsychotics in a way that may be harmful.
- Be aware of possible risks of taking antipsychotic medication during pregnancy. Safe use during pregnancy and lactation has not been established. Antipsychotics are thought to readily cross the placental barrier; if so, a fetus could experience adverse effects of the drug. The client should inform the physician immediately if pregnancy occurs, is suspected, or is planned.
- Be aware of side effects of antipsychotic drugs. Refer to written materials furnished by health-care providers for safe self-administration.
- Continue to take medication, even if feeling well and as though it is not needed. Symptoms may return if medication is discontinued.
- Carry card or other identification at all times describing medication being taken.

INTERNET REFERENCES

- http://www.mentalhealth.com/fr30.html
- http://www.nimh.nih.gov/pubicat/medicate.cfm
- http://www.fadavis.com/catalog/Nursing/Psychiatric%20and%20Mental%20Health%20Nursing/0483-monograph.htm

CHAPTER 28

Antiparkinsonian Agents

■ CHEMICAL CLASS: ANTICHOLINERGICS

Indications

- Treatment of all forms of parkinsonism
- Relief of drug-induced extrapyramidal symptoms.

Action

- Block acetylcholine receptors to diminish excess cholinergic effects
- May also inhibit the reuptake and storage of dopamine at central dopamine receptors, thereby prolonging the action of dopamine.

Contraindications and Precautions

Contraindicated in:

- Hypersensitivity
- Angle-closure glaucoma
- Pyloric or duodenal obstruction
- Peptic ulcers
- Prostatic hypertrophy
- Megaesophagus
- Megacolon
- Myasthenia gravis.

Benztropine:

- Children <3 years of age.

Use Cautiously in:

- Tachycardia
- Cardiac arrhythmias
- Hypertension

- Hypotension
- Tendency toward urinary retention
- Clients exposed to high environmental temperatures.

Benztropine:

- Children >3 years of age
- Pregnancy and lactation (safety not established).

Adverse Reactions and Side Effects

- Dry mouth
- Blurred vision
- Constipation
- Paralytic ileus
- Urinary retention
- Tachycardia
- Decreased sweating
- Elevated temperature
- Nausea/vomiting
- Sedation
- Dizziness
- Exacerbation of psychoses
- Orthostatic hypotension.

Examples

Generic (Trade) Name	Half-Life (hr)	Daily Adult Dosage Range (mg)	Available Forms (mg)
Benztropine (Cogentin)	Unknown	0.5–6	**TABS:** 0.5, 1,2 **INJECT:** 1/mL
Biperiden (Akineton)	18.4–24.3	2–8	**TABS:** 2 **INJECT:** 5/mL
Ethopropazine (Parsidol)	Unknown	50–600	**TABS:** 10, 50
Procyclidine (Kemadrin)	11.5–12.6	5–20	**TABS:** 5
Trihexyphenidyl (Artane)	5.6–10.2	1–15	**TABS:** 2, 5 **CAPS (SR):** 5 **ELIXIR:** 2/5 mL

■ CHEMICAL CLASS: ANTIHISTAMINE

Indications

- Parkinsonism
- Drug-induced extrapyramidal reactions
- Motion sickness

- Allergy reactions
- Nighttime sedative
- Cough suppressant.

Action

- May decrease cholinergic activity and prolong dopamine action in the CNS to produce antiparkinsonian effects
- Blocks histamine release by competing with histamine for H_1 receptor sites. Decreased allergic response and somnolence are effected by diminished activity.

Contraindications and Precautions

Contraindicated in:

- Hypersensitivity to this drug, other antihistamines, or sulfites (contained in some preparations)
- Newborn or premature infants
- Concomitant use with monoamine oxidase inhibitors
- Lactation.

Use Cautiously in:

- Narrow-angle glaucoma
- Peptic ulcer
- Prostatic hypertrophy
- Asthmatic attack
- Bladder neck obstruction
- Pyloroduodenal obstruction
- Elderly or debilitated clients
- Pregnancy
- Seizure disorders
- Hypertension.

Adverse Reactions and Side Effects

- Refer to this section under "Anticholinergics."

Example

Generic (Trade) Name	Half-Life (hr)	Daily Adult Dosage Range (mg)	Available Forms (mg)
Diphenhydramine (Benadryl)	4–15	75–200	**TABS & CAPS:** 25, 50 **ELIXIR:** 12.5/5 mL **INJECT:** 50/mL

■ CHEMICAL CLASS: DOPAMINERGIC AGONISTS

Indications

- Treatment of all forms of parkinsonism

Amantadine:

- Relief of drug-induced extrapyramidal symptoms

Bromocriptine:

- Neuroleptic malignant syndrome
- Acromegaly
- Hyperprolactinemia-associated dysfunctions
- Cocaine addiction.

Action

- Increase the content of dopamine in the brain directly by stimulation of dopamine receptors or indirectly by blocking neuronal reuptake of dopamine.

Contraindications and Precautions

Contraindicated in:

Amantadine:

- Hypersensitivity to the drug; safe use in pregnancy, lactation, and in children under 1 year not established.

Bromocriptine:

- Hypersensitivity to this drug, other ergot alkaloids, or sulfites (contained in some preparations)
- Patients with severe peripheral vascular disease
- Pregnancy and lactation
- Children under 15 (safety not established).

Use Cautiously in:

- Hepatic or renal impairment
- Uncontrolled psychiatric disturbances
- History of congestive heart failure, myocardial infarction, or ventricular arrhythmia
- Elderly or debilitated clients
- Orthostatic hypotension.

Amantadine:

- Clients with a history of seizures, recurrent eczematoid dermatitis, concurrent use of CNS stimulants.

Bromocriptine:

- Clients with acromegaly.

Adverse Reactions and Side Effects

- Refer to this section under "Anticholinergics."

Examples

Generic (Trade) Name	Half-Life (hr)	Daily Adult Dosage Range (mg)	Available Forms (mg)
Amantadine (Symmetrel)	15	75–200	**TABS & CAPS:** 25, 50 **ELIXIR:** 12.5/5 mL **INJECT:** 50/mL
Bromocriptine (Parlodel)	6–8	2.5–100	**TABS:** 2.5 **CAPS:** 5

■ NURSING DIAGNOSES RELATED TO ANTIPARKINSONIAN AGENTS

1. Risk for injury related to symptoms of Parkinson's disease or drug-induced EPS.
2. Hyperthermia related to anticholinergic effect of decreased sweating.
3. Activity intolerance related to side effects of drowsiness, dizziness, ataxia, weakness, confusion.
4. Knowledge deficit related to medication regimen.

■ NURSING IMPLICATIONS FOR ANTIPARKINSONIAN AGENTS

The plan of care should include monitoring for the following side effects from antiparkinsonian medications. Nursing implications related to each side effect are designated by an asterisk (*).

1. **Anticholinergic Effects:** These side effects are identical to those produced by antipsychotic drugs. Taking both medications compounds these effects. For this reason, the physician may elect to prescribe an antiparkinsonian agent only at the onset of EPS, rather than as routine adjunctive therapy.
   a. ***Dry Mouth***
      * Offer sugarless candy or gum, ice, and frequent sips of water.
      * Ensure that client practices strict oral hygiene.
   b. ***Blurred Vision***

* Explain that symptom will most likely subside after a few weeks.
* Offer to assist with tasks requiring visual acuity.

c. ***Constipation***
   * Order foods high in fiber; encourage increase in physical activity and fluid intake, if not contraindicated.

d. ***Paralytic Ileus***
   * A rare, but potentially very serious side effect of anticholinergic drugs. Monitor for abdominal distention, absent bowel sounds, nausea, vomiting, and epigastric pain.
   * Report any of these symptoms to physician immediately.

e. ***Urinary Retention***
   * Instruct client to report any difficulty urinating; monitor intake and output.

f. ***Tachycardia, Decreased Sweating, Elevated Temperature***
   * Assess vital signs each shift; document and report significant changes to physician.
   * Ensure that client remains in cool environment, because the body is unable to cool itself naturally with this medication.

2. **Nausea, Gastrointestinal Upset**
   * May administer tablets or capsules with food to minimize gastrointestinal upset.
3. **Sedation, Drowsiness, Dizziness**
   * Discuss with physician possibility of administering drug at bedtime.
   * Discuss with physician possible decrease in dosage or order for less sedating drug.
   * Instruct client not to drive or use dangerous equipment while experiencing sedation or dizziness.
4. **Exacerbation of Psychoses**
   * Assess for signs of loss of contact with reality.
   * Intervene during a hallucination, talk about real people and real events, and reorient client to reality.
   * Stay with client during period of agitation and delirium; remain calm and reassure client of his or her safety.
   * Discuss with physician possible decrease in dosage or change in medication.
5. **Orthostatic Hypotension**
   * Instruct client to rise slowly from a lying or sitting position; monitor blood pressure (lying and stand-

ing) each shift and document and report significant changes.

■ CLIENT AND FAMILY EDUCATION RELATED TO ALL ANTIPARKINSONIAN AGENTS

- Take the medication with food if gastrointestinal upset occurs.
- Use caution when driving or operating dangerous machinery. Drowsiness and dizziness can occur.
- Do not stop taking the drug abruptly. To do so might produce unpleasant withdrawal symptoms.
- Report occurrence of any of the following symptoms to the physician immediately: pain or tenderness in area in front of ear, extreme dryness of mouth, difficulty urinating, abdominal pain, constipation, fast pounding heart beat, rash, visual disturbances, and mental changes.
- Rise slowly from a sitting or lying position to prevent a sudden drop in blood pressure.
- Stay inside in air-conditioned room when weather is very hot. Perspiration is decreased with antiparkinsonian agents, and the body cannot cool itself as well. There is greater susceptibility to heat stroke. Inform physician if air-conditioned housing is not available.
- Take frequent sips of water, chew sugarless gum, or suck on hard candy if dry mouth is a problem. Good oral care (frequent brushing, flossing) is very important.
- Do not drink alcohol while on antiparkinsonian therapy.
- Do not consume other medications (including over-the-counter products) without physician's approval. Many medications contain substances that interact with antiparkinsonian agents in a way that may be harmful.
- Be aware of possible risks of taking antiparkinsonian agents during pregnancy. Safe use during pregnancy and lactation has not been fully established. It is thought that antiparkinsonian agents readily cross the placental barrier; if so, fetus could experience adverse effects of the drug. Inform physician immediately if pregnancy occurs, is suspected, or is planned.

- Be aware of side effects of antiparkinsonian agents. Refer to written materials furnished by health-care providers for safe self-administration.
- Continue to take medication, even if feeling well and as though it is not needed. Symptoms may return if medication is discontinued.
- Carry card or other identification at all times describing medications being taken.

■ INTERNET REFERENCES

- http://www.mentalhealth.com/fr30.html
- http://www.nimh.nih.gov/publicat/medicate.cfm
- http://www.fadavis.com/catalog/Nursing/Psychiatric%20and%20Mental%20Health%20Nursing/0483-monograph.htm

CHAPTER 29

Sedative-Hypnotics

■ CHEMICAL CLASS: BENZODIAZEPINES

Indications

- Insomnia characterized by difficulty in falling asleep, frequent nocturnal awakenings, or early morning awakening
- Can be used for recurring insomnia or poor sleeping habits and in acute or chronic medical situations requiring restful sleep.

Action

- Potentiate gamma-aminobutyric acid (GABA) neuronal inhibition
- The sedative effects involve GABA receptors in the limbic, neocortical, and mesencephalic reticular systems.

Contraindications and Precautions

Contraindicated in:

- Hypersensitivity to these or other benzodiazepines
- Pregnancy and lactation.

Quazepam:

- Established or suspected sleep apnea.

Triazolam:

- Concurrent use with ketoconazole, itraconazole, or nefazodone, medications that impair the metabolism of triazolam by cytochrome P450 3A (CYP3A).

Flurazepam:

- Children under age 15.

Estazolam; quazepam; temazepam; triazolam:

- Children under age 18.

Use Cautiously in:

- Elderly and debilitated clients
- Hepatic or renal dysfunction
- Clients with history of drug abuse and dependence
- Depressed or suicidal clients
- Respiratory depression and sleep apnea.

Adverse Reactions and Side Effects

- Drowsiness
- Headache
- Confusion
- Lethargy
- Tolerance
- Physical and psychological dependence
- Potentiates the effects of other CNS depressants
- May aggravate symptoms in depressed persons
- Palpitations, tachycardia, hypotension
- Paradoxical excitement
- Dry mouth
- Nausea and vomiting
- Blood dyscrasias.

Examples

Generic (Trade) Name	Controlled Categories	Half-Life (hr)	Daily Adult Dosage Range (mg)	Available Forms (mg)
Estazolam (ProSom)	C-IV	8–28	0.5–2	**TABS:** 1, 2
Flurazepam (Dalmane)	C-IV	2–3 (active metabolite, 47–100)	15–30	**CAPS:** 15, 30
Quazepam (Doral)	C-IV	41 (active metabolite, 47–100)	7.5–15	**TABS:** 7.5, 15
Temazepam (Restoril)	C-IV	9–15	15–30	**CAPS:** 7.5, 15, 30
Triazolam (Halcion)	C-IV	1.5–5.5	0.125–0.5	**TABS:** 0.125, 0.25

■ CHEMICAL CLASS: BARBITURATES

Indications

- Short-term treatment of insomnia

- Anxiety states
- Preoperative sedation.

Mephobarbital; phenobarbital:

- Anticonvulsant.

Action

- Depresses the CNS
- Interferes with transmission through the reticular formation, which is concerned with arousal
- Action on neurotransmitters is not well defined
- All levels of CNS depression can occur, from mild sedation to hypnosis to coma to death.

Contraindications and Precautions

Contraindicated in:

- Hypersensitivity to barbiturates
- Severe hepatic, renal, cardiac, or respiratory disease
- Individuals with history of drug abuse or dependence
- Porphyria
- Intra-arterial or subcutaneous administration.

Use Cautiously in:

- Elderly and debilitated clients
- Clients with hepatic, renal, cardiac, or respiratory impairment
- Depressed or suicidal clients
- Children
- Pregnancy and lactation.

Adverse Reactions and Side Effects

- Refer to this section under "Benzodiazepines."

Examples

Generic (Trade) Name	Controlled Categories	Half-Life (hr)	Daily Adult Dosage Range (mg)	Available Forms (mg)
Amobarbital (Amytal)	C-II	16–40	60–200	**POWDER FOR INJ:** 250/vial, 500/vial
Aprobarbital (Alurate)	C-III	14–34	40–160	**ELIXIR:** 40/5 mL
Butabarbital (Butisol)	C-III	66–140	45–100	**TABS:** 15, 30, 50, 100 **ELIXIR:** 30/5 mL

Generic (Trade) Name	Controlled Categories	Half-Life (hr)	Daily Adult Dosage Range (mg)	Available Forms (mg)
Mephobarbital (Mebaral)	C-IV	11–67	96–400 (sedative) 400–600 (epilepsy)	**TABS:** 32, 50, 100
Pentobarbital (Nembutal)	C-II	15–50	60–200	**CAPS:** 50, 100 **SUPP:** 30, 60, 120, 200 **INJECT:** 50/mL
Phenobarbital (Luminal)	C IV	53–118	30–320	**TABS:** 15,16, 30, 60, 100 **CAPS:** 16 **ELIXIR:** 15/5 mL; 20/5 mL **INJECT (MG/ML):** 30, 60, 65, 130
Secobarbital (Seconal)	C-II	15–40	100–300	**CAPS:** 100 **INJECT:** 50/mL

■ CHEMICAL CLASS: MISCELLANEOUS

Indications

- Short-term treatment of insomnia
- In anxiety states and/or for preoperative sedation (all except zolpidem).

Action

Zolpidem:
- Binds to GABA receptors in the CNS; appears to be selective for the omega$_1$-receptor subtype

Chloral hydrate; ethchlorvynol; glutethimide:
- Unknown
- They produce a calming effect through depression of the CNS.

Contraindications and Precautions

Contraindicated in:
- Hypersensitivity
- In combination with other CNS depressants
- Pregnancy and lactation

Glutethimide; ethchlorvynol:
- Porphyria

Zolpidem; glutethimide; ethchlorvynol:
- Children.

Chloral hydrate:
- Severe hepatic, renal, or cardiac impairment
- Esophagitis, gastritis, or peptic ulcer disease (oral form).

Use cautiously in:
- Elderly or debilitated clients
- Depressed or suicidal clients
- Clients with history of drug abuse or dependence
- Clients with hepatic, renal or respiratory dysfunction.

Adverse Reactions and Side Effects

- Refer to this section under "Benzodiazepines."

Examples

Generic (Trade) Name	Controlled Categories	Half-Life (hr)	Daily Adult Dosage Range (mg)	Available Forms (mg)
Chloral hydrate (Noctec)	C-IV	7–10	500–1000	**CAPS:** 500 **SYRUP:** 250/5 mL, 500/5 mL **SUPP:** 324, 500, 648
Ethchlorvynol (Placidyl)	C-IV	10–20	500–1000	**CAPS:** 200, 500, 750
Glutethimide (Doriden)	C-II	10–12	250–500	**TABS:** 250
Zolpidem (Ambien)	C-IV	2–3	5–10	**TABS:** 5, 10

■ NURSING DIAGNOSES RELATED TO ALL SEDATIVE-HYPNOTICS

1. Risk for injury related to abrupt withdrawal from long-term use or decreased mental alertness caused by residual sedation.
2. Sleep pattern disturbance related to situational crises, physical condition, or severe level of anxiety.
3. Risk for activity intolerance related to side effects of lethargy, drowsiness, dizziness.
4. Risk for acute confusion related to action of the medication on the central nervous system.

■ NURSING IMPLICATIONS FOR SEDATIVE-HYPNOTICS

The nursing care plan should include monitoring for the following side effects from sedative-hypnotics. Nursing implications related to each side effect are designated by an asterisk (*):

1. **Drowsiness, Confusion, Lethargy (most common side effects)**
   * Instruct client not to drive or operate dangerous machinery while taking the medication.
2. **Tolerance, Physical and Psychological Dependence**
   * Instruct client receiving long-term therapy not to quit taking the drug abruptly. Abrupt withdrawal can be life-threatening. Symptoms include depression, insomnia, increased anxiety, abdominal and muscle cramps, tremors, vomiting, sweating, convulsions, and delirium.
3. **Potentiates the Effects of Other CNS Depressants**
   * Instruct client not to drink alcohol or take other medications that depress the CNS while taking this medication.
4. **May Aggravate Symptoms in Depressed Persons**
   * Assess mood daily.
   * Take necessary precautions for potential suicide.
5. **Orthostatic Hypotension, Palpitations, Tachycardia**
   * Monitor lying and standing blood pressure and pulse every shift.
   * Instruct client to arise slowly from a lying or sitting position.
   * Monitor pulse rate and rhythm and report any significant change to the physician.
6. **Paradoxical Excitement**
   * Withhold drug and notify the physician.
7. **Dry mouth**
   * Have client take frequent sips of water, ice chips, suck on hard candy, or chew sugarless gum.
8. **Nausea and Vomiting**
   * Have client take drug with food or milk.
9. **Blood Dyscrasias**
   * Symptoms of sore throat, fever, malaise, easy bruising, or unusual bleeding should be reported to the physician immediately.

■ CLIENT AND FAMILY EDUCATION RELATED TO ALL SEDATIVE-HYPNOTICS

- Do not drive or operate dangerous machinery. Drowsiness and dizziness can occur.
- Do not stop taking the drug abruptly. Can produce serious withdrawal symptoms, such as depression, insomnia, anxiety, abdominal and muscle cramps, tremors, vomiting, sweating, convulsions, and delirium.
- Do not consume other CNS depressants (including alcohol).
- Do not take nonprescription medications without approval from physician.
- Rise slowly from the sitting or lying position to prevent a sudden drop in blood pressure.
- Report to physician immediately symptoms of sore throat, fever, malaise, easy bruising, unusual bleeding, or motor restlessness.
- Be aware of the risks of taking these drugs during pregnancy. (Congenital malformations have been associated with use during the first trimester.) If pregnancy is suspected or planned, notify the physician of the desirability to discontinue the drug.
- Be aware of possible side effects. Refer to written materials furnished by health-care providers regarding the correct method of self-administration.
- Carry card or piece of paper at all times stating names of medications being taken.

■ INTERNET REFERENCES

- http://www.mentalhealth.com/fr30.html
- http://www.nimh.nih.gov/publicat/medicate.cfm
- http://www.fadavis.com/catalog/Nursing/Psychiatric%20and%20Mental%20Health%20Nursing/0483-monograph.htm

CHAPTER 30

Central Nervous System Stimulants

■ CHEMICAL CLASS: AMPHETAMINES

Indications

- Narcolepsy
- Attention-deficit disorder with hyperactivity in children
- Adjunctive therapy to caloric restriction in the treatment of exogenous obesity.

Action

- CNS stimulation is mediated by release of norepinephrine from central noradrenergic neurons in cerebral cortex, reticular activating system, and brain stem
- At higher doses, dopamine may be released in the mesolimbic system.

Contraindications and Precautions

Contraindicated in:

- Hypersensitivity to sympathomimetic amines
- Advanced arteriosclerosis
- Symptomatic cardiovascular disease
- Moderate to severe hypertension
- Hyperthyroidism
- Hypersensitivity or idiosyncrasy to the sympathomimetic amines
- Glaucoma
- Moderate to severe hypertension

- Agitated states
- History of drug abuse
- During or within 14 days following administration of monoamine oxidase inhibitors (MAOIs) (hypertensive crisis may occur)
- Children under 3 years of age
- Pregnancy and lactation.

Use Cautiously in:

- Psychotic children
- Tourette's disorder
- Clients with mild hypertension
- Anorexia
- Insomnia
- Elderly, debilitated, or asthenic clients
- Clients with suicidal or homicidal tendencies.

Adverse Reactions and Side Effects

- Overstimulation
- Restlessness
- Insomnia
- Headache
- Palpitations
- Tachycardia
- Anorexia
- Weight loss
- Dry mouth
- Tolerance
- Physical and psychological dependence
- Hypertension.

Examples

Generic (Trade) Name	Controlled Categories	Half-Life (hr)	Daily Dosage Range (mg)	Available Forms (mg)
Amphetamine sulfate	C-II	7–33	5–60	**TABS:** 5, 10
Dextroamphetamine sulfate (Dexedrine; Dextrostat)	C-II	7–33	5–60	**TABS:** 5, 10 **CAPS (SR):** 5, 10, 15
Methamphetamine HCl (Desoxyn)	C-II	4–5	5–25	**TABS:** 5 **TABS (LA):** 5, 10, 15

■ CHEMICAL CLASS: ANOREXIGENICS

Indication

- Management of exogenous obesity, in conjunction with a reduced-calorie diet.

Action

- The exact mechanism of action is unclear
- It is thought that appetite suppression is produced by a direct stimulant effect on the satiety center in the hypothalamic and limbic regions.

Diethylpropion; phentermine:

- Act primarily on adrenergic pathways.

Mazindol:

- Acts on both adrenergic and dopaminergic pathways.

Sibutramine:

- Inhibits the reuptake of norepinephrine, serotonin, and dopamine.

Contraindications and Precautions

Contraindicated in:

- Hypersensitivity
- Cardiovascular disease (including arrhythmias)
- Hypertension
- Glaucoma
- Agitated states
- History of drug abuse
- During or within 14 days following administration of MAOIs
- Coadministration with other CNS stimulants
- Pregnancy and lactation
- Children under 12 years of age.

Sibutramine:

- Anorexia nervosa
- Severe renal impairment
- Children under 16 years of age
- Concomitantly with other serotonin reuptake inhibitors (may cause serotonin syndrome).

Use cautiously in:

- Mild hypertension
- Diabetes mellitus
- Elderly or debilitated clients
- Clients with a history of seizures.

Adverse Reactions and Side Effects

- Refer to this section under "Amphetamines."

Examples

Generic (Trade) Name	Controlled Categories	Half-Life (hr)	Daily Adult Dosage Range (mg)	Available Forms (mg)
Benzphetamine (Didrex)	C-III	7–33	25–150	**TABS:** 25, 50
Diethylpropion (Tenuate)	C-IV	1–3.5	75–100	**TABS:** 25 **TABS (SR):** 75
Mazindol (Mazanor)	C-IV	Not well established	1–3	**TABS:** 1, 2
Phendimetrazine (Bontril PDM; Prelu-2)	C-III	1.9–9.8	35–105	**TABS & CAPS:** 35 **CAPS (SR):** 105
Phentermine (Adipex-P, Fastin, Ionamin, Zantryl)	C-IV	Not well established	15–37.5	**TABS:** 8, 30, 37.5 **CAPS:** 15, 18.75, 30, 37.5
Sibutramine (Meridia)	C-IV	1.1	5–15	**CAPS:** 5, 10, 15

■ CHEMICAL CLASS: MISCELLANEOUS

Indications

- Attention-deficit disorder with hyperactivity in children
- Narcolepsy.

Methylphenidate

- Treatment of depression in elderly, cancer, and poststroke clients.

Action

- CNS stimulant with actions similar to amphetamines
- Exact mechanism of action is unknown
- Pemoline is thought to act through dopaminergic mechanisms.

Contraindications and Precautions

Contraindicated in:

- Hypersensitivity

- History of tics or Tourette's disorder
- Pregnancy, lactation, and children under 6 years of age (safety has not been established).

Methylphenidate:

- Marked anxiety, tension, or agitation
- Glaucoma
- Severe depression
- Treatment of normal fatigue states.

Use Cautiously in:

- Clients with history of seizure disorder and/or electroencephalogram abnormalities
- Hypertension
- History of drug or alcohol dependence
- Emotionally unstable clients
- Renal or hepatic insufficiency.

Adverse Reactions and Side Effects

- Refer to this section under "Amphetamines."

Examples

Generic (Trade) Name	Controlled Categories	Half-Life (hr)	Daily Dosage Range (mg)	Available Forms (mg)
Methylphenidate (Ritalin)	C-II	1–3	10–60	TABS: 5, 10, 20 TABS (SR): 20
Pemoline (Cylert)	C-IV	~12	37.5–112.5	TABS: 18.75, 37.5, 75

■ NURSING DIAGNOSES RELATED TO CENTRAL NERVOUS SYSTEM STIMULANTS

1. Risk for injury related to overstimulation and hyperactivity.
2. Risk for self-directed violence related to abrupt withdrawal after extended use.
3. Alteration in nutrition, less than body requirements, related to side effects of anorexia and weight loss.
4. Alteration in nutrition, more than body requirements, related to excess intake in relation to metabolic needs.
5. Sleep pattern disturbance related to overstimulation resulting from use of the medication.

■ NURSING IMPLICATIONS FOR CENTRAL NERVOUS SYSTEM STIMULANTS

The plan of care should include monitoring for the following side effects from CNS stimulants. Nursing implications related to each side effect are designated by an asterisk (*).

1. **Overstimulation, Restlessness, Insomnia**
   * Assess mental status for changes in mood, level of activity, degree of stimulation, and aggressiveness.
   * Ensure that the client is protected from injury.
   * Keep stimuli low and environment as quiet as possible to discourage overstimulation.
   * To prevent insomnia, administer the last dose at least 6 hours before bedtime. Administer sustained-release forms in the morning.
2. **Palpitations, Tachycardia**
   * Monitor and record vital signs at regular intervals (two or three times a day) throughout therapy. Report significant changes to the physician immediately.
3. **Anorexia, Weight Loss**
   * If this drug is being taken by children with behavior disorders (and not as an anorexigenic): To reduce anorexia, the medication may be administered immediately after meals. The client should be weighed regularly (at least weekly) during hospitalization and at home while receiving therapy with CNS stimulants because of the potential for anorexia and weight loss as well as temporary interruption of growth and development.
4. **Tolerance, Physical and Psychological Dependence**
   * Tolerance develops rapidly. If anorexigenic effects begin to diminish, the client should notify the physician immediately. The client should be on a reduced-calorie diet and a program of regular exercise in addition to the medication.
   * In children with behavior disorders, a drug "holiday" should be attempted periodically under direction of the physician to determine the effectiveness of the medication and the need for continuation.
   * The drug should not be withdrawn abruptly. To do so could initiate the following syndrome of symptoms: nausea, vomiting, abdominal cramping,

suicidal ideation, increased dreaming, and psychotic behavior.

■ CLIENT AND FAMILY EDUCATION RELATED TO ALL CENTRAL NERVOUS SYSTEM STIMULANTS

- Use caution in driving or operating dangerous machinery. Drowsiness, dizziness, and blurred vision can occur.
- Do not stop taking the drug abruptly. To do so could produce serious withdrawal symptoms.
- Avoid taking medication late in the day to prevent insomnia. Take no later than 6 hours before bedtime.
- Do not take other medications (including over-the-counter drugs) without physician's approval. Many medications contain substances that, in combination with CNS stimulants, can be harmful.
- Diabetic clients should monitor blood sugar two or three times a day or as instructed by the physician. Be aware of the need for possible alteration in insulin requirements owing to changes in food intake, weight, and activity.
- Avoid consumption of large amounts of caffeinated products (coffee, tea, colas, chocolate), as they may enhance the stimulant effect of these medications.
- Follow a reduced-calorie diet provided by the dietitian, as well as a program of regular exercise. Do not exceed the recommended dose if the appetite suppressant effect diminishes. Contact the physician.
- Notify physician if restlessness, insomnia, anorexia, or dry mouth becomes severe or if rapid, pounding heartbeat becomes evident.
- Be aware of possible risks of taking CNS stimulants during pregnancy. Safe use during pregnancy and lactation has not been established. Inform the physician immediately if pregnancy is suspected or planned.
- Be aware of potential side effects of CNS stimulants. Refer to written materials furnished by health-care providers for safe self-administration.
- Carry a card or other identification at all times describing medications being taken.

■ INTERNET REFERENCES

- http://www.mentalhealth.com/fr30.html
- http://www.nimh.nih.gov/publicat/medicate.cfm
- http://www.fadavis.com/catalog/Nursing/Psychiatric%20and%20Mental%20Health%20Nursing/0483-monograph.htm

Bibliography

Abel, EL: Psychoactive Drugs and Sex. Plenum, New York, 1985.

Abel, GG: Paraphilias. In Kaplan, HI, and Sadock, BJ (eds): Comprehensive Textbook of Psychiatry, Vol 1, ed 5. Williams & Wilkins, Baltimore, 1989.

Abrams, R: Electroconvulsive Therapy. Oxford University Press, New York, 1988.

Ackerman, S: The management of obesity. Hosp Pract 18(3): 117–135, 1983.

Aguilera, DC: Crisis intervention: Theory and methodology, ed 8. CV Mosby, St. Louis, 1998.

Aguilera, DC, and Messick, JM: Crisis Intervention: Theory and Methodology, ed 4. CV Mosby, St. Louis, 1982.

Aleksandrowicz, DR: Psychoanalytic studies of mania. In Bel maker, RH, and vanPraag, HM (eds): Mania: An evolving concept. Spectrum Publications, Jamaica, NY, 1980.

Alexander, F: Psychosomatic Medicine. WW Norton, New York, 1950.

American Heart Association: Blood pressure statistics. [Online]. Available: http://www.amhrt.org, 1999.

American Hospital Association: A Patient's Bill of Rights. American Hospital Association, Chicago, 1975.

American Medical Association (AMA): Strategies for the treatment and prevention of sexual assault. [Online]. Available: http://www.ama-assn.org/public/releases/assault/saguide.htm, 1999.

American Nurses Association: Nursing: A Social Policy Statement. American Nurses Association, Kansas City, MO, 1980.

American Nurses Association: Standards of Clinical Nursing Practice, ed 2. American Nurses Association, Kansas City, MO, 1998.

American Psychiatric Association: Diagnostic and Statistical Manual of Mental Disorders, ed 3—revised. American Psychiatric Association, Washington, DC, 1987.

American Psychiatric Association: Diagnostic and Statistical Manual of Mental Disorders, ed 4. American Psychiatric Association, Washington, DC, 1994.

Andreasen, NC, and Wasek, P: Adjustment disorders in adolescents and adults. Arch Gen Psychiatry 37:1166–1170, 1980.

Barsky, AJ: Somatoform disorders. In Kaplan, HI, and Sadock, BJ (eds): Comprehensive Textbook of Psychiatry, Vol 1, ed 5. Williams & Wilkins, Baltimore, 1989.

Bartlett, JG, and Finkbeiner, AK: The Guide to Living With HIV Infection, ed 3. Johns Hopkins University Press, Baltimore, 1996.

Beck, A, et al. Cognitive Theory of Depression. Guilford Press, New York, 1979.

Becker, JV: Impact of sexual abuse on sexual functioning. In Leiblum, SR, and Rosen, RC (eds): Principles and Practice of Sex Therapy: Update for the 1990s, ed 2. Guilford Press, New York, 1989.

Becker, JV, and Kavoussi, RJ: Sexual disorders. In Talbot, JA, Hales, RE, and Yudofsky, SC (eds): Textbook of Psychiatry. The American Psychiatric Press, Washington, DC, 1988.

Bennett, G, and Woolf, DS: Substance Abuse: Pharmacologic, Developmental, and Clinical Perspectives, ed 2. John Wiley & Sons, New York, 1991.

Bernier, SL: Mental health issues and nursing in corrections. In McFarland, GK, and Thomas, MD (eds): Psychiatric mental health nursing: Application of the nursing process. JB Lippincott, Philadelphia, 1991.

Birchwood, MJ, et al.: Schizophrenia: An Intergrated Approach to Research and Treatment. New York University Press, New York, 1989.

Black, DW, and Andreasen, NC: Schizophrenia, schizophreniform disorder, and delusional (paranoid) disorder. In Hales, RE, Yudofsky, SC, and Talbott, JA (eds): Textbook of Psychiatry, ed 2. The American Psychiatric Press, Washington, DC, 1994.

Booth, GK: Disorders of impulse control. In Goldman, HH (ed): Review of General Psychiatry. Lange Medical Publications, Los Altos, CA, 1984.

Bowen, M: Family Therapy in Clinical Practice. Jason Aronson, New York, 1978.

Bowlby, J: Attachment and Loss: Separation, Anxiety, and Anger. Basic Books, New York, 1973.

Bradford, JM, and McLean, D: Sexual offenders, violence, and testosterone: A clinical study. Can J Psychiatry 29:335–343, 1984.

Bruch, H: Eating disorders in adolescence. Proc Am Psychopathol Assoc 59:181–202, 1970.

Bruch, H: Psychotherapy in anorexia nervosa and developmental obesity. In Goodstein, RK (ed): Eating and Weight Disorders. Springer, New York, 1983.

Burgess, AW: Intra-familial sexual abuse. In Campbell, J, and Humphreys, J (eds): Nursing Care of Victims of Family Violence. Reston Publishing, Reston, VA, 1984.

Burgess, AW: Psychiatric Nursing in the Hospital and the Community, ed 5. Appleton & Lange, Norwalk, CT, 1990.

Cadoret, R: Antisocial personality. In Winokur, G, and Clayton, PJ (eds): The Medical Basis of Psychiatry. WB Saunders, Philadelphia, 1994.

Caplan, G: Principles of Preventive Psychiatry. Basic Books, New York, 1964.

Carpenito, LJ: Nursing Diagnosis: Application to Clinical Practice, ed 5. JB Lippincott, Philadelphia, 1993.

Carroll-Johnson, RM: Classification of Nursing Diagnoses: Proceedings of the Eighth National Conference. JB Lippincott, Philadelphia, 1989.

Case, J (ed): Special Focus: Psychiatric services. Hospital Home Health, 10(5), 61–68, 1993.

Casey, V, and Dwyer, JT: Premenstrual syndrome: Theories and evidence. Nutrition Today (Nov/Dec):4–12, 1987.

Celano, MP: Activities and games for group psychotherapy with sexually abused children. Int J Group Psychother 40(4):419–428, 1990.

Chess, S, Thomas, A, and Birch, H: The origins of personality. Sci Am 223:102, 1970.

Christ, GH, Siegel, K, and Moynihan, RT: Psychosocial issues: Prevention and treatment. In DeVita, VT, Hellman, S, and Rosenberg, SA (eds): AIDS: Etiology, diagnosis, treatment, and prevention, ed 2. JB Lippincott, Philadelphia, 1988.

Clunn, P: Child Psychiatric Nursing. Mosby-Year Book, St. Louis, MO, 1991.

Cohen, MB, et al.: An intensive study of twelve cases of manic-depressive psychosis. Psychiatry, 17, 103–138, 1954.

Complementary and alternative medicine: Complementary & Alternative Medicine Newsletter, V(2). Office of Alternative Medicine Clearinghouse, Silver Spring, MD, 1998.

Coniglione, T: Our doctors must begin looking at the total person. InBalance. The Balanced Healing Medical Center, Oklahoma City, OK, 1998.

Credit, LP, Hartunian, SG, and Nowak, MJ: Your guide to complementary medicine. Avery Publishing Group, Garden City Park, NY, 1998.

Cutting, J: The Psychology of Schizophrenia. Livingstone Churchill, New York, 1985.

Dato, C, and Rafferty, M: The homeless mentally ill. International Nursing Review, 32(6), 170–173, 1985.

Deglin, JH, and Vallerand, AH: Davis's Drug Guide for Nurses, ed 6. FA Davis, Philadelphia, 1999.

DeWitt, KN: Adjustment disorder. In Goldman, HH (ed): Review of General Psychiatry. Lange Medical Publications, Los Altos, CA, 1984.

Doenges, M, Moorhouse, M: Nurse's Pocket Guide: Nursing Diagnoses with Interventions, ed 6. FA Davis, Philadelphia, 1998.

Doenges, M, Townsend, M, and Moorhouse, M: Psychiatric Care Plans: Guidelines for Client Care, ed 3. FA Davis, Philadelphia, 1998.

Drug Enforcement Administration: Drug Abuse, Drug Enforcement. U.S. Department of Justice, Washington, DC, 1979.

Duespohl, TA: Nursing Diagnosis Manual for the Well and Ill Client. WB Saunders, Philadelphia, 1986.

Duffey, JM, and Miller, MP: Toward resolving the issue: In-home psychiatric nursing. Journal of the American Psychiatric Nurses Association, 2(3), 104–106, 1996.

Dunbar, HF: Emotions and Bodily Changes. Columbia University Press, New York, 1954.

Eckert, ED, and Mitchell, JE: Anorexia nervosa and bulimia nervosa. In Winokur, G, and Clayton, PJ (eds): The medical basis of psychiatry, ed 2. WB Saunders, Philadelphia, 1994.

Egeland, JA, et al.: Amish study: Lithium-sodium countertransport and catechol *O*-methyltransferase in pedigrees of bipolar probands. Am J Psychiatry 141:1049, 1984.

Engel, G: Grief and grieving. Am J Nurs 64:93, 1964.

Erikson, EH: Childhood and Society. WW Norton, New York, 1963.

Estes, NJ, and Heinemann, ME: Alcoholism: Development, Consequences, and Interventions, ed 2. CV Mosby, St. Louis, MO, 1982.

Estes, NJ, Smith-DiJulio, K, and Heinemann, ME: Nursing Diagnosis of the Alcoholic Person. CV Mosby, St. Louis, MO, 1980.

Finkelman, AW: Psychiatric home care. Aspen Publications, Gaithersburg, MD, 1997.

Freeman, CP, et al.: ECT: Patients who complain. Br J Psychiatry 137:17–25, 1980.

Freud, S: Collected Papers of Sigmund Freud. (Ernest Jones, ed). Basic Books, New York, 1959.

Freud, S: The neuro-psychoses of defense (1894). In Strachey, J (ed): Standard Edition of the Complete Psychological Works of Sigmund Freud, Vol 3. Hogarth Press (original work published 1894), London, 1962.

Freud, S: New introductory lectures on psychoanalysis and other works. In Strachey, J (ed): The Standard Edition of the Complete Psychological Works of Sigmund Freud, Vol 22. Hogarth Press, London, 1964.

Friedmann, E, and Thomas, SA: Pet ownership, social support, and one-year survival after acute myocardial infarction in the cardiac arrhythmia suppression trial. Am J Cardiol, 76(17):1213, 1995.

Gibbons, JL: Total body sodium and potassium in depressive illness. Clin Sci 19:133, 1960.

Gibson, RW, et al.: On the dynamics of the manic-depresive personality. Am J Psychiatry, 115, 1101–1107, 1959.

Gordon, M: Nursing Diagnosis: Process and Application, ed 2. McGraw-Hill, New York,1987.

Grace, HK, and Camilleri, D: Mental Health Nursing: A Sociopsychological Approach, ed 2. WC Brown, Dubuque, IA, 1981.

Green, R: One hundred and ten feminine and masculine boys: Behavioral contrasts and demographic similarities. Arch Sex Behav 5:425–446, 1976.

Green, R: Gender identity in childhood and later sexual orienta-

tion: Follow up of 78 males. Am J Psychiatry 142:339–341, 1985.
Guinness, AE (ed): Family guide to natural medicine. The Reader's Digest Association, Pleasantville, NY, 1993.
Hamilton, DB: Psychiatric nursing: Content review and tests. In Beare, PG (ed): Davis's NCLEX-RN Review. FA Davis, Philadelphia, 1991.
Hartmann, H: Contributions to the metapsychology of schizophrenia. In Hartmann, H (ed): Essays on Ego Psychology. International Universities Press, New York, 1964.
Hays, JS, and Larson, KH: Interacting with Patients. Macmillan, New York, 1963.
Hellwig, K: Psychiatric home care nursing: Managing patients in the community setting. Journal of Pyschosocial Nursing 31(12), 21–24, 1993.
Hollandsworth, JG: The Physiology of Psychological Disorders. Plenum Press, New York, 1990.
Horney, K: New ways in Psychoanalysis. WW Norton, New York, 1939.
Hufft, A, and Peternelj-Taylor, C: Forensic nursing: An emerging speciality. In Catalano, JT (ed): 1999 Contemporary Professional Nursing Update. FA Davis, Philadelphia, 1999.
Hunter, JK: Making a difference for homeless patients. RN, December 1992.
Hyde, JS: Understanding Human Sexuality, ed 3. McGraw-Hill, New York, 1986.
Institute for Natural Resources: Alternative medicine: An objective view, ed 2. INR, Berkeley, CA, 1998.
International Association of Forensic Nurses (IAFN) and American Nurses' Association (ANA): Scope and standards of forensic nursing practice. American Nurses Publishing. Washington, DC, 1997.
Janowsky, DS, et al.: Neurochemistry of depression and mania. In Georgotas, A, and Cancro, R (eds): Depression and Mania. Elsevier Science Publishing, New York, 1988.
Johnson, C, and Dorman, B: What is autism? Autism Society of America. [Online}. Available: http://www.autism-society.org/autism.html, 1998.
Kanner, L: To what extent is early infantile autism determined by constitutional inadequacies? Childhood Psychosis: Initial Studies and New Insights. VH Winston, Washington, DC, 1973.
Kansas Child Abuse Prevention Council (KCAPC): A Guide About Child Abuse and Neglect. National Committee for Prevention of Child Abuse and Parents Anonymous, Wichita, KS, 1992.
Kaplan, HI: History of psychosomatic medicine. In Kaplan, HI, and Sadock, BJ (eds): Comprehensive Textbook of Psychiatry. Williams & Wilkins, Baltimore, 1989.
Kaplan, HI, and Sadock, BJ: Modern Synopsis of Comprehensive Textbook of Psychiatry, ed 4. Williams & Wilkins, Baltimore, 1985.
Kaplan, HI, and Sadock, BJ: Modern Synopsis of Comprehen-

sive Textbook of Psychiatry, ed 5. Williams & Wilkins, Baltimore, 1989.

Kaplan, HI, and Sadock, BJ: Synopsis of Psychiatry: Behavioral sciences/clinical psychiatry, ed 8. Williams & Wilkins, Baltimore, 1998.

Kaplan, HI, and Sadock, BJ, and Grebb, JA: Kaplan and Sadock's Synopsis of Psychiatry, ed 7. Williams & Wilkins, Baltimore, 1994.

Kelsoe, JR: Molecular genetics of mood disorders. Journal of California Alliance for the Mentally Ill, 2(4), 20–22, 1991.

Kicey, C: Catecholamines and depression: A physiological theory of depression. Am J Nurs 74:2018, 1974.

Kim, MJ, McFarland, GK, and McLane, AM: Classification of Nursing Diagnoses: Proceedings of the Fifth National Conference. CV Mosby, St. Louis, MO, 1984.

Klein, M: Mourning and its relation to manic-depressive states. In Kline, M (ed): Contributions to psychoanalysis, 1921–1945. Hogarth Press, London, 1948.

Kluft, RP: Multiple personality in childhood. Psychiatr Clin North Am 7:121–134, 1984.

Koegel, P, Burnam, MA, and Baumohl, J: The causes of homelessness. In Baumohl, J (ed): Homelessness in America. Oryx Press, Phoenix, AZ, 1996.

Kohlberg, L: Moral development. International Encyclopedia of Social Science. Macmillan, New York, 1968.

Kolb, LC: Modern Clinical Psychiatry, ed 9. WB Saunders, Philadelphia, 1977.

Kolodny, RC, Masters, WH, and Johnson, VE: Textbook of Sexual Medicine. Little, Brown, Boston, 1979.

Kübler-Ross, E: On Death and Dying. Macmillan, New York, 1969.

Kuhn, MA: Pharmacotherapeutics: A Nursing Process Approach, ed 4. FA Davis, Philadelphia, 1998.

Leahy, RL, and Beck, AT: Cognitive therapy of depression and mania. In Georgotas, A, and Cancro, R (eds): Depression and Mania. Elsevier Science Publishing, New York, 1988.

Ledray, LE, and Arndt, S: Examining the sexual assault victim: A new model for nursing care. Journal of Psychosocial Nursing, 32(2), 7–12, 1994.

Lego, S: Book review: "Live from death row." Journal of the American Psychiatric Nurses Association, 1(5), 171–174, 1995.

Leigh, G: Psychosocial factors in the etiology of substance abuse. In Bratter, TE, and Forrest, GG (eds): Alcoholism and Substance Abuse: Strategies for Clinical Intervention. The Free Press, New York, 1985.

Leon, GR, and Dinklage, D: Obesity and anorexia nervosa. In Ollendick, TH, and Hersen, M (eds): Handbook of Child Psychopathology, ed 2. Plenum Press, New York, 1989.

Lutz, CA, and Przytulski, KR: Nutrition and diet therapy. FA Davis, Philadelphia, 1994.

Lynch, VA: Clinical forensic nursing: A new perspective in the management of crime victims from trauma to trial. Critical

Care Nursing Clinics of North America, 7(3), 489–507, 1995.

Mahler, M, et al.: Psychological Birth of the Human Infant: Symbiosis and Individuation. Basic Books, New York, 1975.

Marciniak, RD: Other psychiatric disorders. In Walker, JI (ed): Essentials of Clinical Psychiatry. JB Lippincott, Philadelphia, 1985.

Mark, B: Hospital treatment of borderline patients: Toward a better understanding of problematic issues. J Psychosoc Nurs Ment Health Serv 18(8):25–31, 1980.

Martin, M: Battered women. In Hutchings, N (ed): The Violent Family: Victimization of Women, Children, and Elders. Human Sciences Press, New York, 1988.

Masters, JC, and Spitler, R: Neuroleptic malignant syndrome. Journal of Psychosocial Nursing 24(9):11–16, 1986.

Matthysse, S, and Kety, SS: Catecholamines and Schizophrenia. Pergamon Press, Elmsford, NY, 1975.

McCracken, JT: Somatoform disorders. In Walker, JI (ed): Essentials of Clinical Psychiatry. JB Lippincott, Philadelphia, 1985.

Minuchin, S, et al.: Family organization and family therapy. Arch Gen Psychiatry 32:1031–1038, 1975.

Minuchin, S, Rosman, B, and Baker, L: Psychosomatic Families. Harvard University Press, Cambridge, MA, 1978.

Money World: Hocus pocus comes of age, November 1997, p17.

National Association for Home Care (NAHC): How to choose a home care provider. [Online]. Available:http://www.nahc.org/Consumer/wihc.html, 1996.

National Association for Home Care (NAHC): Basic statistics about home care. [Online]. Available: http://www.nahc.org/Consumer/hcstats.html, 1999.

National Clearinghouse on Child Abuse and Neglect (NCCAN). What is child maltreatment? [Online]. Available: http://www.calib.com/nccanch/pubs/, 1994.

National Coalition for the Homeless (NCH): How many people experience homelessness? [Online]. Available: http://nch.ari.net/numbers.html, 1999.

National Institutes of Health: NIH consensus report on acupuncture, 15(5), 1997.

Nemiah, JC: Dissociative disorders (hysterical neuroses, dissociative type). In Kaplan, HI, and Sadock, BJ (eds): Comprehensive Textbook of Psychiatry, Vol 1, ed 5. Williams & Wilkins, Baltimore, 1989.

North American Nursing Diagnosis Association: Nursing Diagnoses: Definitions and Classification, 1999–2000. NANDA, Philadelphia, 1999.

Pasquali, EA, Arnold, HM, DeBasio, N, and Alesi, EG: Mental Health Nursing: A Holistic Approach, ed 3. CV Mosby, St. Louis, 1989.

Pauls, DL, and Leckman, JF: The inheritance of Gilles de la Tourette's syndrome and associated behaviors. N Engl J Med 315:993–997, 1986.

Pauly, IB: Female transsexualism. Arch Sex Behav 3:487–526, 1974.

PDR for Herbal Medicines. Medical Economics, Montvale, NJ, 1998.

Pelletier, LR: Psychiatric home care. Journal of Psychosocial Nursing, 26(3), 22–27, 1988.

Peplau, HE: Interpersonal techniques: The crux of psychiatric nursing. Am J Nurs 62(6):50–54, 1962.

Peplau, HE: Interpersonal Relations in Nursing. Springer, New York, 1991.

Peschel, E, and Peschel, R: Neurobiological disorders. J California Alliance for the Mentally Ill 2(4):4, 1991.

Piaget, J, and Inhelder, B: The Psychology of the Child. Basic Books, New York, 1969.

Platt-Koch, LM: Borderline personality disorder: A therapeutic approach. Am J Nurs 83(12):1666–1671, 1983.

Plomin, R: Childhood temperament. In Lahey, BB, and Kazdin, AE (eds): Advances in Clinical Child Psychology, Vol 6. Plenum Press, New York, 1983.

Pokalo, CL: Clozapine: Benefits and controversies. Journal of Psychosocial Nursing 29(2):33–36, 1991.

Popkin, MK: Adjustment disorder and impulse control disorder. In Kaplan, HI, and Sadock, BJ (eds): Comprehensive Textbook of Psychiatry, Vol 2, ed 5. Williams & Wilkins, Baltimore, 1989.

Popper, CW, and Steingard, RJ: Disorders usually first diagnosed in infancy, childhood, or adolescence. In Hales, RE, Yudofsky, SC, and Talbott, JA (eds): The American Psychiatric Press Textbook of Psychiatry, ed 2. The American Psychiatric Press, Washington, DC, 1994.

Reynolds, JI, and Logsdon, JB: Assessing your patient's mental status. Nursing 79, 9(8):26–33, 1979.

Rice, ME, Harris, GT, and Quinsey, VL: Treatment for forensic patients. In Sales, BD, and Shah, SA (eds): Mental Health and Law: Research, Policy and Services. Carolina Academic Press, Durham, NC, 1996.

Richie, R, and Lusky, K: Psychiatric home health nursing: A new role in community mental health. Community Mental Health Journal 23(3):229–235, 1987.

Robinson, L: Psychiatric Nursing as a Human Experience, ed 3. WB Saunders, Philadelphia, 1983.

Rosen, AC, Rekers, GA, and Bentler, PM: Ethical issues in the treatment of children. J Soc Issues 32:84, 1978.

Rosner, TA, and Pollice, SA: Tourette's syndrome. Journal of Psychosocial Nursing 29(1):4–9, 1991.

Sadock, VA: Normal human sexuality and sexual disorders. In Kaplan, HI, and Sadock, BJ (eds): Comprehensive Textbook of Psychiatry, Vol 1, ed 5. Williams & Wilkins, Baltimore, 1989.

Scanlon, VC, and Sanders, T: Essentials of Anatomy and Physiology, ed 2. FA Davis, Philadelphia, 1995.

Scheibel, A: Schizophrenia: Cells in disarray. Journal of the California Alliance for the Mentally Ill, 2(4):9–10, 1991.

Schieber, SC: The psychiatric interview, psychiatric history, and mental status examination. In Hales, RE, Yudofsky, SC, and Talbott, JA (eds): Textbook of Psychiatry, ed 2. American Psychiatric Press, Washington, DC, 1994.

Schmitt, K: Development, administration, and scoring of the NCLEX-RN. In Beare, PG, (ed): Davis's NCLEX-RN Review, ed 2, 1996.

Schoenen, J, Jacquy, J, and Lenaerts, M: Effectiveness of high-dose riboflavin in migraine prophylaxis: A randomized controlled trial. Neurology, 50:466–469, 1998.

Schultz, JM, and Dark, SL: Manual of Psychiatric Nursing Care Plans, ed 3. Scott, Foresman and Company, Glenview, IL, 1990.

Segraves, RT: Hormones and libido. In Leiblum, SR, and Rosen, RC (eds): Sexual Desire Disorders. The Guilford Press, New York, 1988.

Seligman, M: Depression and learned helplessness. In Friedman, R, and Katz, M (eds): The Psychology of Depression: Contemporary Theory and Research. VH Winston & Sons, Washington, DC, 1974.

Selye, H: The Stress of life. McGraw-Hill, New York, 1956.

Silver, JM, and Yudofsky, S: Violence and aggression. In Kass, FI, Oldham, JM, and Pardes, H (eds): The Columbia University College of Physicians and Surgeons Complete Home Guide to Mental Health. Henry Holt and Company, New York, 1992.

Skinner, K: The therapeutic milieu: Making it work. Journal of Psychiatric Nursing and Mental Health Services, 38–44, August, 1979.

Smith, LS: Sexual assault: The nurse's role. AD Nurse 2(2):24–28, 1987a.

Smith, LS: Battered women: The nurse's role. AD Nurse 2(5):21–24, 1987b.

Smith, SF, Karasik, DA, and Meyer, BJ: Psychiatric and Psychosocial Nursing: A Review for NCLEX in the Nursing Process. National Nursing Review, Los Altos, CA, 1984.

Sobel, DS, and Ornstein, R: The healthy mind, healthy body handbook. DR_x, Los Altos, CA, 1996.

Stoudemire, GA: Somatoform disorders, factitious disorders, and malingering. In Talbott, JA, Hales, RE, and Yudofsky, SC (eds): Textbook of Psychiatry. American Psychiatric Press, Washington, DC, 1988.

Sullivan, HS: The Interpersonal Theory of Psychiatry. WW Norton, New York, 1953.

Sullivan, HS: Clinical Studies in Psychiatry. WW Norton, New York, 1956.

Sullivan, HS: Schizophrenia as a Human Process. WW Norton, New York, 1962.

The Sunday Oklahoman: Accent on today's woman: Sugar blues. Oklahoma Publishing Co., Aug. 2, 1998.

Sundel, M, and Sundel, SS: Behavior Modification in the Human Services: A Systematic Introduction to Concepts and Applications, ed 2. Prentice-Hall, Englewood Cliffs, NJ, 1982.
Swearingen, PL: Manual of Nursing Therapeutics. Addison-Wesley, Menlo Park, CA, 1986.
Tardiff, K: Violence. In Hales, RE, Yudofsky, SC, and Talbott, JA (eds): Textbook of Psychiatry, ed 2. The American Psychiatric Press, Washington, DC, 1994.
Townsend, MC: Psychiatric Mental Health Nursing: Concepts of Care. FA Davis, Philadelphia, 1993.
Townsend, MC: Drug Guide for Psychiatric Nursing, ed 2. FA Davis, Philadelphia, 1995.
Townsend, MC: Psychiatric Mental Health Nursing: Concepts of Care, ed 2. FA Davis, Philadelphia, 1996.
Townsend, MC: Essentials of Psychiatric/Mental Health Nursing, FA Davis, Philadelphia, 1999.
Townsend, MC: Psychiatric Mental Health Nursing: Concepts of Care, ed 3. FA Davis, Philadelphia, 2000.
U.S. Conference of Mayors (USCM): A status report on hunger and homelessness in America's cities: 1998. U.S. Conference of Mayors, Washington, DC, 1998.
U.S. Department of Agriculture and U.S. Department of Health and Human Services: Nutrition and your Health: Dietary Guidelines for Americans, ed 4. USDA and USDHHS, Washington, DC, 1995.
Vande Vusse, L, and Simandl, G: Sexuality patterns, altered. In Gettrust, KV, and Brabec, PD (eds): Nursing Diagnosis in Clinical Practice: Guides for Care Planning. Delmar, Albany, NY, 1992.
Wallsten, SM: Geriatric mental health: A portrait of homelessness. Journal of Psychosocial Nursing, 30(9), 20–24, 1992.
Wark, D: Prison violence: Homicide, assault, and rape. [Online]. Available: http://oak.cats.ohiou.edu/~dw101094/esp/soc4661.html/, 1998.
West, DJ: Sex offenses and offending. In Tonry, M, and Morris, N (eds): Crime and Justice: An Annual Review of Research. University of Chicago Press, Chicago, 1983.
Wheeler, K: Psychiatric clinical pathways in home care. In Dykes, PC (ed): Psychiatric clinical pathways: An interdisciplinary approach. Aspen Publishers, Gaithersburg, MD, 1998.
Wise, MG, and Gray, KF: Delirium, dementia, and amnestic disorders. In Hales, RE, Yudofsky, SC, and Talbott, JA (eds): The American Psychiatric Press Textbook of Psychiatry, ed 2. American Psychiatric Press, Washington, DC, 1994.
Wolpe, J: The Practice of Behavior Therapy, ed 2. Pergamon Press, New York, 1973.
Wolters Kluwer: Drug Facts and Comparisons, ed 54. Wolters Kluwer, St. Louis, 2000.
Yalom, IE: The Theory and Practice of Group Psychotherapy, ed 3. Basic Books, New York, 1985.
Yeager, S: New Foods for Healing. Rodale Press, Emmaus, PA, 1998.

APPENDIX A

Comparison of Developmental Theories

Age	Stage	Major Developmental Tasks
	S. Freud's Stages of Psychosexual Development	
Birth–18 months	Oral	Relief from anxiety through oral gratification of needs
18 months–3 years	Anal	Learning independence and control, with focus on the excretory function
3–6 years	Phallic	Identification with parent of same sex; development of sexual identity; focus on genital organs
6–12 years	Latency	Sexuality repressed; focus on relationships with same-sex peers
13–20 years	Genital	Libido reawakened as genital organs mature; focus on relationships with members of the opposite sex

Table continued on following page

Age	Stage	Major Developmental Tasks
	Stages of Development in H.S. Sullivan's Interpersonal Theory	
Birth–18 months	Infancy	Relief from anxiety through oral gratification of needs
18 months–6 years	Childhood	Learning to experience a delay in personal gratification without undo anxiety
6–9 years	Juvenile	Learning to form satisfactory peer relationships
9–12 years	Preadolescence	Learning to form satisfactory relationships with persons of the same sex; initiation of feelings of affection for another person
12–14 years	Early adolescence	Learning to form satisfactory relationships with persons of the opposite sex; developing a sense of identity
14–21 years	Late adolescence	Establishing self-identity; experiencing satisfying relationships; working to develop a lasting, intimate opposite-sex relationship
	Stages of Development in Eric Erikson's Psychosocial Theory	
Infancy (birth–18 months)	Trust vs. mistrust	To develop a basic trust in the mothering figure and be able to generalize it to others
Early childhood (18 months–3 years)	Autonomy vs. shame and doubt	To gain some self-control and independence within the environment
Late childhood (3–6 years)	Initiative vs. guilt	To develop a sense of purpose and the ability to initiate and direct own activities
School age (6–12 years)	Industry vs. inferiority	To achieve a sense of self-confidence by learning, competing, performing successfully, and receiving

		recognition from significant others, peers, and acquaintances
Adolescence (12–20 years)	Identity vs. role confusion	To integrate the tasks mastered in the previous stages into a secure sense of self
Young adulthood (20–30 years)	Intimacy vs. isolation	To form an intense, lasting relationship or a commitment to another person, a cause, an institution, or a creative effort
Adulthood (30–65 years)	Generativity vs. stagnation	To achieve the life goals established for oneself, while also considering the welfare of future generations
Old age (65 years–death)	Ego integrity vs. despair	To review one's life and derive meaning from both positive and negative events, while achieving a positive sense of self-worth

Stages of Development in M. Mahler's Theory of Object Relations

Birth–1 month	I. Normal autism	Fulfillment of basic needs for survival and comfort
1–5 months	II. Symbiosis	Developing awareness of external source of need fulfillment
	III. Separation-individuation	
5–10 months	a. Differentiation	Commencement of a primary recognition of separateness from the mothering figure
10–16 months	b. Practicing	Increased independence through locomotor functioning; increased sense of separateness of self
16–24 months	c. Rapprochement	Acute awareness of separateness of self; learning to seek "emotional refueling" from mothering figure to maintain feeling of security

Table continued on following page

Age	Stage	Major Developmental Tasks
	Stages of Development in M. Mahler's Theory of Object Relations	
24–36 months	d. Consolidation	Sense of separateness established; on the way to object constancy: able to internalize a sustained image of loved object/person when it is out of sight; resolution of separation anxiety
	J. Piaget's Stages of Cognitive Development	
Birth–2 years	Sensorimotor	With increased mobility and awareness, develops a sense of self as separate from the external environment; the concept of object permanence emerges as the ability to form mental images evolves
2–6 years	Preoperational	Learning to express self with language; develops understanding of symbolic gestures; achieves object permanence
6–12 years	Concrete operations	Learning to apply logic to thinking; develops understanding of reversibility and spatiality; learning to differentiate and classify; increased socialization and application of rules
12–15+ years	Formal operations	Learning to think and reason in abstract terms; makes and tests hypotheses; logical thinking and reasoning ability expand and refined; cognitive maturity achieved
	L. Kohlberg's Stages of Moral Development	

Preconventional (common from ages 4–10 years)	1. Punishment and obedience orientation	Behavior motivated by fear of punishment
	2. Instrumental relativist orientation	Behavior motivated by egocentrism and concern for self
Conventional (common from ages 10–13 years and into adulthood)	3. Interpersonal concordance orientation	Behavior motivated by the expectations of others; strong desire for approval and acceptance
	4. Law and order orientation	Behavior motivated by respect for authority
Postconventional (can occur from adolescence on)	5. Social contract legalistic orientation	Behavior motivated by respect for universal laws and moral principles and guided by an internal set of values
	6. Universal ethical principle orientation	Behavior motivated by internalized principles of honor, justice, and respect for human dignity and guided by the conscience

Stages of Development in H. Peplau's Interpersonal Theory

Infancy	Learning to count on others	Learning to communicate in various ways to the primary caregiver to have comfort needs fulfilled
Toddlerhood	Learning to delay gratification	Learning the satisfaction of pleasing others by delaying self-gratification in small ways
Early childhood	Identifying oneself	Learning appropriate roles and behaviors by acquiring the ability to perceive the expectations of others
Late childhood	Developing skills in participation	Learning the skills of compromise, competition, and cooperation with others; establishment of a more realistic view of the world and a feeling of one's place in it.

Adapted from Townsend, 2000, pp 34, 36, 39, 40, 41, 45.

APPENDIX B

Ego Defense Mechanisms

Defense Mechanisms	Example	Defense Mechanisms	Example
Compensation: Covering up a real or perceived weakness by emphasizing a trait one considers more desirable	A physically handicapped boy who is unable to participate in football compensates by becoming a great scholar	**Projection:** Attributing feelings or impulses unacceptable to one's self to another person	Sue feels a strong sexual attraction to her track coach. She tells her friend, "He's coming on to me!"

Denial: Refusing to acknowledge the existence of a real situation or the feelings associated with it	A woman who drinks alcohol every day and cannot stop fails to acknowledge that she has a problem.	**Rationalization:** Attempting to make excuses or formulate logical reasons to justify unacceptable feelings or behaviors	John tells the rehab nurse, "I drink because it's the only way I can deal with my bad marriage and my worse job."
Displacement: The transfer of feelings from one target to another that is considered less threatening or neutral	A client is angry at his physician, does not express it, but becomes verbally abusive with the nurse.	**Reaction formation:** Preventing unacceptable or undesirable thoughts or behaviors from being expressed by exaggerating opposite thoughts or types of behaviors	Jane hates nursing. She attended nursing school to please her parents. During career day, she speaks to prospective students about the excellence of nursing as a career.
Identification: An attempt to increase self-worth by acquiring certain attributes and characteristics of an individual one admires	A teenager who required lengthy rehabilitation after an accident decides to become a physical therapist as a result of his experiences.	**Regression:** Retreating in response to stress to an earlier level of development and the comfort measures associated with that level of functioning	When 2–year-old Jay is hospitalized for tonsilitis, he will drink only from a bottle, even though his Mom states he has been drinking from a cup for 6 months.

Table continued on following page

Defense Mechanisms	Example	Defense Mechanisms	Example
Intellectualization: An attempt to avoid expressing actual emotions associated with a stressful situation by using the intellectual processes of logic, reasoning, and analysis	S's husband is being transferred with his job to a city far away from her parents. She hides her anxiety by explaining to her parents the advantages associated with the move.	**Repression:** The involuntary blocking of unpleasant feelings and experiences from one's awareness	An accident victim can remember nothing about his accident.
		Sublimation: Rechanneling of drives or impulses that are personally or socially unacceptable into activities that are constructive	A mother whose son was killed by a drunk driver channels her anger and energy into being the president of Mothers Against Drunk Drivers.
Introjection: Integrating the beliefs and values of another	Children integrate their parents' value system into	**Suppression:** The voluntary blocking of unpleasant feelings	Scarlet O'Hara says, "I don't want to think about that

individual into one's own ego structure	the process of conscience formation. Child says to friend, "Don't cheat. It's wrong."	and experiences from one's awareness	now. I'll think about that tomorrow."
Isolation: Separating a thought or memory from the feeling tone or emotion associated with it	A young woman describes being attacked and raped without showing any emotion.	**Undoing:** Symbolically negating or cancelling out an experience that one finds intolerable	Joe was nervous about his new job and yelled at his wife. On his way home he stops and buys her some flowers.

From Townsend, 2000, p 20, with permission.

APPENDIX C

Levels of Anxiety

Level	Perceptual Field	Ability to Learn	Physical Characteristics	Emotional/Behavioral Characteristics
Mild	Heightened perception (e.g., noises may seem louder; details within the environment are cleaner) Increased awareness Increased alertness	Learning is enhanced.	Restlessness Irritability	May remain superficial with others Rarely experienced as distressful Motivation increased
Moderate	Reduction in perceptual field Less alert to environmental events (e.g., someone talking may not be	Learning still occurs, but not at optimal ability. Decreased attention span.	Increased restlessness Increased heart and respiration rate Increased perspiration Gastric discomfort	A feeling of discontent May lead to a degree of impairment in interpersonal relationships as individual begins to

	heard; part of the room may not be noticed)	Decreased ability to concentrate.	Increased muscular tension Increase in speech rate, volume, and pitch	focus on self and the need to relieve personal discomfort
Severe	Greatly diminished Only extraneous details perceived, or fixation on a single detail may occur May not take notice of an event even when attention is directed by another	Extremely limited attention span. Unable to concentrate or problem-solve. Effective learning cannot occur.	Headaches Dizziness Nausea; diarrhea Trembling Insomnia Palpitations Tachycardia Hyperventilation Urinary frequency	Feelings of dread, loathing, horror Total focus on self and intense desire to relieve the anxiety
Panic	Unable to focus on even one detail within the environment Misperceptions of the environment common (e.g., a perceived detail may be elaborated and out of proportion)	Learning cannot occur. Unable to concentrate. Unable to comprehend even simple directions.	Dilated pupils Labored breathing Severe trembling Sleeplessness Palpitations Diaphoresis and pallor Muscular incoordination Immobility or purposeless hyperactivity Incoherence or inability to verbalize	Sense of impending doom Terror Bizarre behavior, including shouting, screaming, running about wildly, clinging to anyone or anything from which a sense of safety and security is derived Hallucinations; delusions Extreme withdrawal into the self

From Townsend, 2000, p 19, with permission.

APPENDIX D

Stages of Grief

A Comparison of Models by Elisabeth Kübler-Ross, John Bowlby, and George Engel

Stages				
Kübler-Ross	**Bowlby**	**Engel**	**Possible Time Dimension**	**Behaviors**
I. Denial	I. Numbness/ protest	I. Shock/disbelief	Occurs immediately on experiencing the loss Usually lasts no more than 2 weeks	Individual refuses to acknowledge that the loss has occurred.
II. Anger	II. Disequilibrium	II. Developing awareness	In most cases begins within hours of the loss Peaks within 2 to 4 weeks	Anger is directed toward self or others. Ambivalence and guilt may be felt toward the lost object.

III. Bargaining				The individual fervently seeks alternatives to improve current situation.
		III. Restitution		Attends to various rituals associated with the culture in which the loss has occurred.
IV. Depression	III. Disorganization and despair	IV. Resclution of the loss	A year or more	The actual work of grieving. Preoccupation with the lost object. Feelings of helplessness and loneliness occur in response to realization of the loss. Feelings associated with the loss are confronted.
V. Acceptance	IV. Reorganization	V. Recovery		Resolution is complete. The bereaved person experiences a reinvestment in new relationships and new goals. In the case of the terminally ill person, he or she expresses a readiness to die.

From Townsend, 2000, p 430, with permission.

APPENDIX E

Relationship Development and Therapeutic Communication

■ PHASES OF A THERAPEUTIC NURSE-CLIENT RELATIONSHIP

Psychiatric nurses use interpersonal relationship development as the primary intervention with clients in various psychiatric and mental health settings. This is congruent with Peplau's (1962) identification of *counseling* as the major subrole of nursing in psychiatry. If Sullivan's (1953) belief is true, that is, that all emotional problems stem from difficulties with interpersonal relationships, then this role of the nurse in psychiatry becomes especially meaningful and purposeful. It becomes an integral part of the total therapeutic regimen.

The therapeutic interpersonal relationship is the means by which the nursing process is implemented. Through the relationship, problems are identified and resolution is sought. Tasks of the relationship have been categorized into four phases: the preinteraction phase, the orientation (introductory) phase, the working phase, and the termination phase. Although each phase is presented as specific and distinct from the others, there may be some overlapping of tasks, particularly when the interaction is limited.

The Preinteraction Phase

The preinteraction phase involves preparation for the first encounter with the client. Tasks include the following:

1. Obtaining available information about the client from the chart, significant others, or other health-team members. From this information, the initial assessment is begun. From this initial information, the nurse may also become aware of personal responses to knowledge about the client.
2. Examining one's feelings, fears, and anxieties about working with a particular client. For example, the nurse may have been reared in an alcoholic family and have ambivalent feelings about caring for a client who is alcohol dependent. All individuals bring attributes and feelings from prior experiences to the clinical setting. The nurse needs to be aware of how these preconceptions may affect his or her ability to care for individual clients.

The Orientation (Introductory) Phase

During the orientation phase, the nurse and client become acquainted. Tasks include the following:

1. Creating an environment for the establishment of trust and rapport.
2. Establishing a contract for intervention that details the expectations and responsibilities of both the nurse and client.
3. Gathering assessment information to build a strong client database.
4. Identifying the client's strengths and limitations.
5. Formulating nursing diagnoses.
6. Setting goals that are mutually agreeable to the nurse and client.
7. Developing a plan of action that is realistic for meeting the established goals.
8. Exploring feelings of both the client and the nurse in terms of the introductory phase. Introductions are often uncomfortable, and the participants may experience some anxiety until a degree of rapport has been established. Interactions may remain on a superficial level until anxiety subsides. Several interactions may be required to fulfill the tasks associated with this phase.

Thc Working Phase

The therapeutic work of the relationship is accomplished during this phase. Tasks include the following:

1. Maintaining the trust and rapport that was established during the orientation phase.
2. Promoting the client's insight and perception of reality.
3. Problem-solving in an effort to bring about change in the client's life.
4. Overcoming resistance behaviors on the part of the client as the level of anxiety rises in response to discussion of painful issues.
5. Continuously evaluating progress toward goal attainment.

The Termination Phase

Termination of the relationship may occur for a variety of reasons: The mutually agreed-upon goals may have been reached, the client may be discharged from the hospital, or in the case of a student nurse, it may be the end of a clinical rotation. Termination can be a difficult phase for both the client and nurse. Tasks include the following:

1. Bringing a therapeutic conclusion to the relationship. This occurs when
   a. Progress has been made toward attainment of mutually set goals.
   b. A plan for continuing care or for assistance during stressful life experiences is mutually established by the nurse and client.
   c. Feelings about termination of the relationship are recognized and explored. Both the nurse and client may experience feelings of sadness and loss. The nurse should share his or her feelings with the client. Through these interactions, the client learns that it is acceptable to undergo these feelings at a time of separation. Through this knowledge, the client experiences growth during the process of termination.
   NOTE: When the client feels sadness and loss, behaviors to delay termination may become evident. If the nurse experiences the same feelings, he or she may allow the client's behaviors to delay termination. For therapeutic closure, the nurse must establish the reality of the separation and resist being manipulated into repeated delays by the client.

Therapeutic Communication Techniques

Technique	Explanation/Rationale	Examples
Using silence	Gives the client the opportunity to collect and organize thoughts, to think through a point, or to consider introducing a topic of greater concern than the one being discussed.	
Accepting	Conveys an attitude of reception and regard.	"Yes, I understand what you said." Eye contact; nodding.
Giving recognition	Acknowledging; indicating awareness. Better than complimenting, which reflects the nurse's judgment.	"Hello, Mr. J. I notice that you made a ceramic ashtray in OT." "I see you made your bed."
Offering self	Making oneself available on an unconditional basis increases client's feelings of self-worth.	"I'll stay with you a while." "We can eat our lunch together." "I'm interested in you."
Giving broad openings	Allows the client to take the initiative in introducing the topic. Emphasizes the importance of the client's role in the interaction.	"What would you like to talk about today?" "Tell me what you are thinking."
Offering general leads	Offers the client encouragement to continue.	"Yes, I see" "Go on." "And after that?"

Table continued on following page

Therapeutic Communication Techniques

Technique	Explanation/Rationale	Examples
Placing the event in time or sequence	Clarifies the relationship of events in time so that the nurse and client can view them in perspective.	"What seemed to lead up to . . . ?" "Was this before or after . . . ?" "When did this happen?"
Making observations	Verbalizing what is observed or perceived. This encourages the client to recognize specific behaviors and compare perceptions with the nurse.	"You seem tense." "I notice you are pacing a lot." "You seem uncomfortable when you . . ."
Encouraging description of perceptions	Asking the client to verbalize what is being perceived. Often used with clients experiencing hallucinations.	"Tell me what is happening now." "Are you hearing the voices again?" "What do the voices seem to be saying?"
Encouraging comparison	Asking the client to compare similarities and differences in ideas, experiences, or interpersonal relationships. Helps the client recognize life experiences that tend to recur as well as those aspects of life that are changeable.	"Was this something like . . . ?" "How does this compare to the time when . . . ?" "What was your response the last time this situation occurred?"
Restating	The main idea the client has expressed is repeated. Lets the client know whether an expressed statement has been understood and gives him or her the chance to continue, or to clarify, if necessary.	Pt. "I can't study. My mind keeps wandering." Ns: "You have difficulty concentrating." Pt: "I can't take that new job. What if I can't do it?" Ns: "You're afraid you will fail in this new position."

Reflecting	Questions and feelings are referred back to the client so that they may be recognized and accepted and so that the client may recognize that his or her point of view has value. A good technique to use when the client asks the nurse for advice.	Pt: "What do you think I should do about my wife's drinking problem?" Ns: "What do *you* think you should do?" Pt: "My sister won't help a bit toward my mother's care. I have to do it all!" Ns: "You feel angry when she doesn't help."
Focusing	Taking notice of a single idea or even a single word. Works especially well with a client who is moving rapidly from one thought to another. This technique is *not* therapeutic, however, with the client who is very anxious. Focusing should not be pursued until the anxiety level has subsided.	"This point seems worth looking at more closely. Perhaps you and I can discuss it together."
Exploring	Delving further into a subject, idea, experience, or relationship. Especially helpful with clients who tend to remain on a superficial level of communication. However, if the client chooses not to disclose further information, the nurse should refrain from pushing or probing in an area that obviously creates discomfort.	"Please explain that situation in more detail." "Tell me more about that particular situation."

Table continued on following page

Therapeutic Communication Techniques

Technique	Explanation/Rationale	Examples
Seeking clarification and validation	Striving to explain that which is vague or incomprehensible and searching for mutual understanding. Clarifying the meaning of what has been said facilitates and increases understanding for both client and nurse.	"I'm not sure that I understand. Would you please explain?" "Tell me if my undertanding agrees with yours." "Do I under stand correctly that you said . . . ?"
Presenting reality	When the client has a misperception of the environment, the nurse defines reality or indicates his or her perception of the situation for the client.	"I understand that the voices seem real to you, but I do not hear any voices." "There is no one else in the room but you and me."
Voicing doubt	Expressing uncertainty as to the reality of the client's perceptions. Often used with clients experiencing delusional thinking.	"I find that hard to believe." "That seems rather doubtful to me."
Verbalizing the implied	Putting into words what the client has only implied or said indirectly. Can also be used with the client who is mute or is otherwise experiencing impaired verbal communication. Clarifies that which is *implicit* rather than *explicit*.	Pt: "It's a waste of time to be here. I can't talk to you or anyone." Ns: "Are you feeling that no one understands?" Pt: (Mute) Ns: "It must have been very difficult for you when your husband died in the fire."
Attempting to translate words into feelings	When feelings are expressed indirectly, the nurse tries to "desymbolize" what	Pt: "I'm way out in the ocean." Ns: "You must be feeling very lonely now."

	has been said and find clues to the underlying true feelings.	
Formulating a plan of action	When a client has a plan in mind for dealing with what is considered to be a stressful situation, it may serve to prevent anger or anxiety from escalating to an unmanageable level.	"What could you do to let your anger out harmlessly?" "Next time this comes up, what might you do to handle it more appropriately?"

Nontherapeutic Communication Techniques

Technique	**Explanation/Rationale**	**Examples**
Giving reassurance	Indicates to the client that there is no cause for anxiety, thereby devaluing the client's feelings. May discourage the client from further expression of feelings if he or she believes they will only be downplayed or ridiculed.	"I wouldn't worry about that if I were you." "Everything will be all right." **Better to say:** "We will work on that together."
Rejecting	Refusing to consider or showing contempt for the client's ideas or behavior. This may cause the client to discontinue interaction with the nurse for fear of further rejection.	"Let's not discuss . . ." "I don't want to hear about . . ." **Better to say:** "Let's look at that a little closer."

Table continued on following page

Nontherapeutic Communication Techniques

Technique	Explanation/Rationale	Examples
Giving approval or disapproval	Sanctioning or denouncing the client's ideas or behavior. Implies that the nurse has the right to pass judgment on whether the client's ideas or behaviors are "good" or "bad" and that the client is expected to please the nurse. The nurse's acceptance of the client is then seen as conditional, depending upon the client's behavior.	"That's good. I'm glad that you . . ." "That's bad. I'd rather you wouldn't . . ." **Better to say:** Let's talk about how your behavior invoked anger in the other clients at dinner."
Agreeing/disagreeing	Indicating accord with or opposition to the client's ideas or opinions. Implies that the nurse has the right to pass judgment on whether the client's ideas or opinions are "right" or "wrong." Agreement prevents the client from later modifying his or her point of view without admitting error. Disagreement implies inaccuracy, provoking the need for defensiveness on the part of the client.	"That's right. I agree." "That's wrong. I disagree." "I don't believe that." **Better to say:** "Let's discuss what you feel is unfair about the new community rules."
Giving advice	Telling the client what to do or how to behave implies that the nurse knows what	"I think you should . . ." "Why don't you . . ."

	is best and that the client is incapable of any self-direction. Nurtures the client in the dependent role by discouraging independent thinking.	**Better to say:** "What do you think you should do?"
Probing	Persistent questioning of the client. Pushing for answers to issues the client does not wish to discuss. Causes the client to feel used and valued only for what is shared with the nurse. Places the client on the defensive.	"Tell me how your mother abused you when you were a child." "Tell me how you feel toward your mother now that she is dead." "Now tell me about . . ." **Better Technique:** The nurse should be aware of the client's response and discontinue the interaction at the first sign of discomfort.
Defending	Attempting to protect someone or something from verbal attack. To defend what the client has criticized is to imply that he or she has no right to express ideas, opinions, or feelings. Defending does not change the client's feelings and may cause the client to think the nurse is taking sides with those being criticized and against the client.	"No one here would lie to you." "You have a very capable physician. I'm sure he only has your best interests in mind." **Better to say:** "I will try to answer your questions and clarify some issues regarding your treatment."

Table continued on following page

Nontherapeutic Communication Techniques

Technique	Explanation/Rationale	Examples
Requesting an explanation	Asking the client to provide the reasons for thoughts, feelings, behavior, and events. Asking "Why?" a client did something or feels a certain way can be very intimidating and implies that the client must defend his or her behavior or feelings.	"Why did you think that?" "Why do you feel this way?" "Why did you do that?" **Better to say:** "Describe what you were feeling just before that happened."
Indicating the existence of an external source of power.	Attributing the source of thoughts, feelings, and behavior to others or to outside influences. This encourages the client to project blame for his or her thoughts or behaviors on others rather than accepting the responsibility personally.	"What makes you say that?" "What made you do that?" "What made you so angry last night?" **Better to say:** "You became angry when your brother insulted your wife."
Belittling expressed feelings	When the nurse misjudges the degree of the client's discomfort, a lack of empathy and understanding may be conveyed. The nurse may tell the client to "perk up" or "snap out of it." This causes the client to feel insignificant or unimportant. When one is experiencing discomfort, it	Pt: "I have nothing to live for. I wish I were dead." Ns: "Everybody gets down in the dumps at times. I feel that way myself sometimes." **Better to say:** "You must be very upset. Tell me what you are feeling right now."

	is no relief to hear that others are or have been in similar situations.	
Making stereotyped comments	Clichés and trite expressions are meaningless in a nurse-client relationship. For the nurse to make empty conversation is to encourage a like response from the client.	"I'm fine, and how are you?" "Hang in there. It's for your own good." "Keep your chin up." **Better to say:** "The therapy must be difficult for you at times. How do you feel about your progress at this point?"
Using denial	When the nurse denies that a problem exists, he or she blocks discussion with the client and avoids helping the client identify and explore areas of difficulty.	Pt: "I'm nothing." Ns: "Of course you're something. Everybody is somebody." **Better to say:** "You're feeling like no one cares about you right now."
Interpreting	With this technique the therapist seeks to make conscious that which is unconscious, to tell the client the meaning of his experience.	"What you really mean is . . ." "Unconsciously you're saying . . ." **Better technique:** The nurse must leave interpretation of the client's behavior to the psychiatrist. The nurse has not been prepared to perform this technique and, in attempting to do so, may endanger other nursing roles with the client.

Table continued on following page

Nontherapeutic Communication Techniques

Technique	Explanation/Rationale	Examples
Introducing an unrelated topic	Changing the subject causes the nurse to take over the direction of the discussion. This may occur to get to something that the nurse wants to discuss with the client or to get away from a topic that he or she would prefer not to discuss.	Pt: "I don't have anything to live for." Ns: "Did you have visitors this weekend?" **Better technique:** The nurse must remain open and free to hear the client, to take in all that is being conveyed, both verbally and nonverbally.

Adapted from Hays and Larson, 1963.

APPENDIX F

Psychosocial Therapies

GROUP THERAPY

Group therapy is a type of psychosocial therapy with a number of clients at one time. The group is founded in a specific theoretical framework, with the goal being to encourage improvement in interpersonal functioning.

Nurses often lead "therapeutic groups," which are based to a lesser degree in theory. The focus of therapeutic groups is more on group relations, interactions among group members, and the consideration of a selected issue.

Types of groups include *task groups,* in which the function is to accomplish a specific outcome or task; *teaching groups,* in which knowledge or information is conveyed to a number of individuals; *supportive-therapeutic groups,* which help prevent future upsets by teaching participants effective ways of dealing with emotional stress arising from situational or developmental crises; and *self-help groups* of individuals with similar problems who meet to help each other with emotional distress associated with those problems.

Yalom (1985) identified 11 curative factors that individuals can achieve through interpersonal interactions within the group. They include the following:

1. The instillation of hope.
2. Universality (individuals come to understand that they are not alone in the problems they experience).
3. The imparting of information.
4. Altruism (mutual sharing and concern for each other).
5. The corrective recapitulation of the primary family group.

6. The development of socializing techniques.
7. Imitative behavior.
8. Interpersonal learning.
9. Group cohesiveness.
10. Catharsis (open expression of feelings).
11. Existential factors (the group is able to help individual members take direction of their own lives and to accept responsibility for the quality of their existence).

■ PSYCHODRAMA

Psychodrama is a specialized type of therapeutic group that employs a dramatic approach in which clients become "actors" in life-situation scenarios.

The group leader is called the *director,* group members are the *audience,* and the *set,* or *stage,* may be specially designed or may be just any room or part of a room selected for this purpose. Actors are members from the audience who agree to take part in the "drama" by role playing a situation about which they have been informed by the director. Usually the situation is an issue with which one individual client has been struggling. The client plays the role of himself or herself and is called the *protagonist.* In this role, the client is able to express true feelings toward individuals (represented by group members) with whom he or she has unresolved conflicts.

In some instances, the group leader may ask for a client to volunteer to be the protagonist for that session. The client may choose a situation he or she wishes to enact and select the audience members to portray the roles of others in the life situation.

The psychodrama setting provides the client with a safer and less threatening atmosphere than the real situation in which to express true feelings. Resolution of interpersonal conflicts is facilitated.

When the drama has been completed, group members from the audience discuss the situation they have observed, offer feedback, express their feelings, and relate their own similar experiences. In this way, all group members benefit from the session, either directly or indirectly.

Nurses often serve as actors, or role players, in psychodrama sessions. Leaders of psychodrama have graduate degrees in psychology, social work, nursing, or medicine with additional training in group therapy and specialty preparation to become a psychodramatist.

■ FAMILY THERAPY

In family therapy, the nurse-therapist works with the family as a group to improve communication and interaction patterns. Areas of assessment include communication, manner of self-concept reinforcement, family members' expectations, handling differences, family interaction patterns, and the "climate" of the family (a blend of feelings and experiences that are the result of sharing and interacting).

The Family as a System: General systems theory is a way of organizing thought according to the holistic perspective. A system is considered greater than the sum of its parts. A family can be viewed as a system composed of various subsystems. The systems approach to family therapy is composed of eight major concepts: (1) differentiation of self, (2) triangles, (3) nuclear family emotional process, (4) family projection process, (5) multigenerational transmission process, (6) sibling position profiles, (7) emotional cutoff, and (8) societal regression. The goal is to increase the level of differentiation of self while remaining in touch with the family system.

The Structural Model: In this model, the family is viewed as a social system within which the individual lives and to which the individual must adapt. The individual both contributes to and responds to stresses within the family. Major concepts include systems, subsystems, transactional patterns, and boundaries. The goal of therapy is to facilitate change in the family structure. The therapist does this by joining the family, evaluating the family system, and restructuring the family.

The Strategic Model: This model uses the interactional or communications approach. Functional families are open systems within which clear and precise messages, congruent with the situation, are sent and received. Healthy communication patterns promote nurturance and individual self-worth. In dysfunctional families, viewed as partially closed systems, communication is vague, and messages are often inconsistent and incongruent with the situation. Destructive patterns of communication tend to inhibit healthful nurturing and decrease individual feelings of self-worth. Concepts of this model include double-bind communication, pseudomutuality and pseudohostility, marital schism, and marital skew. The goal of therapy is to create change in destructive behavior and communication patterns among family members. This is accomplished by using paradoxical intervention (prescribing the symptom) and reframing (changing the setting or viewpoint in relation to which a situation is experienced and placing it in another, more positive frame of reference).

■ MILIEU THERAPY

In psychiatry, milieu therapy, or a therapeutic community, constitutes a manipulation of the environment in an effort to create behavioral changes and to improve the psychological health and functioning of the individual. The goal of therapeutic community is for the client to learn adaptive coping, interaction, and relationship skills that can be generalized to other aspects of his or her life. The community environment itself serves as the primary tool of therapy.

According to Skinner (1979), a therapeutic community is based on seven basic assumptions:

1. The health in each individual is to be realized and encouraged to grow.
2. Every interaction is an opportunity for therapeutic intervention.
3. The client owns his own environment.
4. Each client owns his behavior.
5. Peer pressure is a useful and a powerful tool.
6. Inappropriate behaviors are dealt with as they occur.
7. Restrictions and punishment are to be avoided.

Because the goals of milieu therapy relate to helping the client learn to generalize that which is learned to other aspects of his or her life, the conditions that promote a therapeutic community in the hospital setting are similar to the types of conditions that exist in real-life situations. They include the following:

1. The fulfillment of basic physiological needs.
2. Physical facilities that are conducive to the achievement of the goals of therapy.
3. The existence of a democratic form of self-government.

4. The assignment of unit responsibilities according to client capabilities.
5. A structured program of social and work-related activities.
6. The inclusion of community and family in the program of therapy in an effort to facilitate discharge from the hospital.

The program of therapy on the milieu unit is conducted by the interdisciplinary treatment (IDT) team. The team includes some, or all, of the following disciplines and may include others that are not specified here: psychiatrist, clinical psychologist, psychiatric clinical nurse specialist, psychiatric nurse, mental health technician, psychiatric social worker, occupational therapist, recreational therapist, art therapist, music therapist, psychodramatist, dietitian, and chaplain.

Nurses play a crucial role in the management of a therapeutic milieu. They are involved in the assessment, diagnosis, outcome identification, planning, implementation, and evaluation of all treatment programs. They have significant input into the IDT plans that are developed for all clients. They are responsible for ensuring that clients' basic needs are fulfilled, for continual assessment of physical and psychosocial status, for medication administration, for the development of trusting relationships, for setting limits on unacceptable behaviors, for client education, and, ultimately, for helping clients, within the limits of their capability, become productive members of society.

■ CRISIS INTERVENTION

A *crisis* is a situation that produces "psychological disequilibrium in a person who confronts a hazardous circumstance that for him constitutes an important problem, which he can for the time being neither escape nor solve with his customary problem-solving resources" (Caplan, 1964). All individuals experience crises at one time or another. This does not necessarily indicate psychopathology.

Crises are precipitated by specific, identifiable events and are determined by an individual's personal perception of the situation. They are acute, not chronic, and generally last no more than 4 to 6 weeks.

Crises occur when an individual is exposed to a stressor and previous problem-solving techniques are ineffective. This causes the level of anxiety to rise. Panic may ensue when new techniques are employed and resolution fails to occur.

Six types of crises have been identified. They include dispositional crises, crises of anticipated life transitions, crises resulting from traumatic stress, maturational or developmental crises, crises reflecting psychopathology, and psychiatric emergencies. The type of crisis determines the method of intervention selected.

Crisis intervention is designed to provide rapid assistance for individuals who have an urgent need. Aguilera and Messick (1982) have identified the minimum therapeutic goal of crisis intervention as "psychological resolution of the individual's immediate crisis and restoration to at least the level of functioning that existed before the crisis period. A maximum goal is improvement in functioning above the precrisis level."

Nurses regularly respond to individuals in crisis in all types of settings. Nursing process is the vehicle by which nurses assist individuals in crisis with a short-term problem-solving approach to change. A four-phase technique is used: assessment/analysis, planning of therapeutic intervention, intervention, and evaluation of crisis resolution and anticipatory planning. Through this structured method of assistance, nurses assist individuals in crisis to develop more adaptive coping strategies for dealing with stressful situations in the future.

■ RELAXATION THERAPY

Stress is a part of our everyday lives. It can be positive or negative, but it cannot be eliminated. Keeping stress at a manageable level is a lifelong process.

Individuals under stress respond with a physiological arousal that can be dangerous over long periods. Indeed, the stress response has been shown to be a major contributor, either directly or indirectly, to coronary heart disease, cancer, lung ailments, accidental injuries, cirrhosis of the liver, and suicide—six of the leading causes of death in the United States.

Relaxation therapy is an effective means of reducing the stress response in some individuals. The degree of anxiety that an individual experiences in response to stress is related to certain predisposing factors, such as characteristics of temperament with which he or she was born, past experiences resulting in learned patterns of responding, and existing conditions, such as health status, coping strategies, and adequate support systems.

Deep relaxation can counteract the physiological and behavioral manifestations of stress. Various methods of relaxation include the following:

Deep-Breathing Exercises: Tension is released when the lungs are allowed to breathe in as much oxygen as possible. Deep-breathing exercises involve inhaling slowly and deeply through the nose, holding the breath for a few seconds, then exhaling slowly through the mouth, pursing the lips as if trying to whistle.

Progressive Relaxation: This method of deep-muscle relaxation is based on the premise that the body responds to anxiety-provoking thoughts and events with muscle tension. Each muscle group is tensed for 5 to 7 seconds and then relaxed for 20 to 30 seconds, during which time the individual concentrates on the difference in sensations between the two conditions. Soft, slow background music may facilitate relaxation. A modified version of this technique (called passive progressive relaxation) involves relaxation of the muscles by concentrating on the feeling of relaxation within the muscle, rather than the actual tensing and relaxing of the muscle.

Meditation: The goal of meditation is to gain mastery over attention. It brings on a special state of consciousness as attention is concentrated solely on one thought or object. During meditation, as the individual becomes totally preoccupied with the selected focus, the respiration rate, heart rate, and blood pressure decrease. The overall metabolism declines, and the need for oxygen consumption is reduced.

Mental Imagery: Mental imagery uses the imagination in an effort to reduce the body's response to stress. The frame of reference is very personal, based on what each individual considers to be a relaxing environment. The relaxing scenario is most useful when taped and played back at a time when the individual wishes to achieve relaxation.

Biofeedback: Biofeedback is the use of instrumentation to become aware of processes in the body that usually go unnoticed and to help bring them under voluntary control. Biological conditions, such as muscle tension, skin surface temperature, blood pressure, and heart rate, are monitored by the biofeedback equipment. With special training, the individual learns to use relaxation and voluntary control to modify the biological condition, in turn indicating a modification of the autonomic function it represents. Biofeedback is often used together with other relaxation techniques such as deep breathing, progressive relaxation, and mental imagery.

ASSERTIVENESS TRAINING

Assertive behavior helps individuals feel better about themselves by encouraging them to stand up for their own basic human rights. These rights have equal representation for all individuals. But along with rights comes an equal number of responsibilities. Part of being assertive includes living up to these responsibilities.

Assertive behavior increases self-esteem and the ability to develop satisfying interpersonal relationships. This is accomplished through honesty, directness, appropriateness, and respecting one's own rights, as well as the rights of others.

Individuals develop patterns of responding in various ways, such as through role modeling, by receiving positive or negative reinforcement, or by conscious choice. These patterns can take the form of nonassertiveness, assertiveness, aggressiveness, or passive-aggressiveness.

Nonassertive individuals seek to please others at the expense of denying their own basic human rights. *Assertive* individuals stand up for their own rights while protecting the rights of others. Those who respond *aggressively* defend their own rights by violating the basic rights of others. Individuals who respond in a passive-aggressive manner defend their own rights by expressing resistance to social and occupational demands.

Some important behavioral considerations of assertive behavior include eye contact, body posture, personal distance, physical contact, gestures, facial expression, voice, fluency, timing, listening, thoughts, and content. Various techniques have been developed to assist individuals in the process of becoming more assertive.

1. **Standing up for one's basic human rights**

   Example: "I have the right to express my opinion."
2. **Assuming responsibility for one's own statements**

   Example: "I *don't want to* go out with you tonight," instead of "I *can't* go out with you tonight." The latter implies a lack of power or ability.
3. **Responding as a "broken record":** Persistently repeating in a calm voice what is wanted.

   Example:

Telephone salesperson:	"I want to help you save money by changing long-distance services."
Assertive response:	"I don't want to change my long-distance service."
Telephone salesperson:	"I can't believe you don't want to save money!"
Assertive response:	"I don't want to change my long-distance service."

4. **Agreeing assertively:** Assertively accepting negative aspects about oneself. Admitting when an error has been made.

   Example:

Ms. Jones:	"You sure let that meeting get out of hand. What a waste of time."
Ms. Smith:	"Yes, I didn't do a very good job of conducting the meeting today."

5. **Inquiring assertively:** Seeking additional information about critical statements.

   Example:

Male board member:	"You made a real fool of yourself at the board meeting last night."
Female board member:	"Oh, really? Just what about my behavior offended you?"
Male board member:	"You were so damned pushy!"
Female board member:	"Were you offended that I spoke up for my beliefs, or was it because my beliefs are in direct opposition to yours?"

6. **Shifting from content to process:** Changing the focus of the communication from discussing the topic at hand to analyzing what is actually going on in the interaction.

   Example:

Wife:	"Would you please call me if you will be late for dinner?"
Husband:	"Why don't you just get off my back! I always have to account for every minute of my time with you!"
Wife:	"Sounds to me like we need to discuss some other things here. What are you *really* angry about?"

7. **Clouding/fogging:** Concurring with the critic's argument without becoming defensive and without agreeing to change.

   Example:

Nurse No. 1:	"You make so many mistakes. I don' know how you ever got this job!"
Nurse No. 2:	"You're right. I have made some mistakes since I started this job."

8: **Defusing:** Putting off further discussion with an angry individual until he or she is calmer.

   Example:
   "You are very angry right now. I don't want to discuss this matter with you while you are so upset. I will discuss it with you in my office at 3 o'clock this afternoon."

9. **Delaying assertively:** Putting off further discussion with another individual until one is calmer.

   Example:
   "That's a very challenging position you have taken, Mr. Brown. I'll need time to give it some thought. I'll call you later this afternoon."

10. **Responding assertively with irony**

   Example:

Man:	"I bet you're one of them so-called 'women's libbers,' aren't you?"
Woman:	"Yes, thank you for noticing."

■ COGNITIVE THERAPY

Cognitive therapy, developed by Aaron Beck, is commonly used in the treatment of mood disorders. In cognitive therapy, the individual is taught to control thought distortions that are considered to be a factor in the development and maintenance of mood disorders. In the cognitive model, depression is characterized by a triad of negative distortions related to expectations of the environment, self, and future. The environment and activities within it are viewed as unsatisfying, the self is unrealistically devalued, and the future is perceived as hopeless. In the same model, mania is characterized by a positive cognitive triad—the self is seen as highly valued and powerful, experiences within the environment are viewed as overly positive, and the future is seen as one of unlimited opportunity (Leahy and Beck, 1988).

The general goals in cognitive therapy are to obtain symptom relief as quickly as possible, to assist the client in identifying dysfunctional patterns of thinking and behaving, and to guide the client to evidence and logic that effectively test the validity of the dysfunctional thinking. Therapy focuses on changing "automatic thoughts" that occur spontaneously and contribute to the distorted affect. Examples of "automatic thoughts" in depression include the following:

1. **Personalizing:** "I'm the only one who failed."
2. **All or nothing:** "I'm a complete failure."
3. **Mind reading:** "He thinks I'm foolish."
4. **Discounting positives:** "The other questions were so easy. Any dummy could have gotten them right."

Examples of "automatic thoughts" in mania include the following:

1. **Personalizing:** "She's this happy only when she's with me."
2. **All or nothing:** "Everything I do is great."
3. **Mind reading:** "She thinks I'm wonderful."
4. **Discounting negatives:** "None of those mistakes are really important."

The client is asked to describe evidence that both supports and disputes the automatic thought. The logic underlying the inferences is then reviewed with the client. Another technique involves evaluating what would most likely happen if the client's automatic thoughts were true. Implications of consequences are then discussed.

Clients should not become discouraged if one technique seems not to be working. There is no single technique that works with all clients. He or she should be reassured that there are a number of techniques that may be used, and both therapist and client may explore these possibilities. Cognitive therapy has been shown to be an effective treatment for mood disorders, particularly in conjunction with psychopharmacological intervention.

APPENDIX G

Electroconvulsive Therapy

DEFINED

Electroconvulsive therapy (ECT) is a type of somatic treatment in which electric current is applied to the brain through electrodes placed on the temples. The current is sufficient to induce a grand mal seizure, from which the desired therapeutic effect is achieved.

INDICATIONS

ECT is used primarily in the treatment of severe depression. It is sometimes administered in conjunction with antidepressant medication, but most physicians prefer to perform this treatment only after an unsuccessful trial of drug therapy.

ECT may also be used as a fast-acting treatment for very hyperactive manic clients in danger of physical exhaustion and for individuals who are extremely suicidal.

ECT was originally attempted in the treatment of schizophrenia, but with little success in most instances. There has been evidence, however, of its effectiveness in the treatment of acute psychoses and catatonia and schizophrenia that is accompanied by affective symptomatology (Kaplan and Sadock, 1998).

CONTRAINDICATIONS

ECT should not be used if there is increased intracranial pressure (from brain tumor, recent cardiovascular accident, or other cerebrovascular lesion). Other conditions, although not considered absolute contraindications, may render clients at high risk for the treatment. These conditions are largely cardiovascular in nature and include myocardial infarction or cerebrovascular accident within the preceding 3 months, aortic or cerebral aneurysm, severe underlying hypertension, and congestive heart failure.

■ MECHANISM OF ACTION

The exact mechanism of action is unknown. However, it is thought that ECT produces biochemical changes in the brain—an increase in the levels of norepinephrine, serotonin, and dopamine—similar to the effects of antidepressant medications.

■ SIDE EFFECTS AND NURSING IMPLICATIONS

Temporary Memory Loss and Confusion

- These are the most common side effects of ECT. It is important for the nurse to be present when the client awakens in order to alleviate the fears that accompany this loss of memory.
- Provide reassurance that memory loss is only temporary
- Describe to client what has occurred.
- Reorient client to time and place.
- Allow client to verbalize fears and anxieties related to receiving ECT.
- To minimize confusion, provide a good deal of structure for client's routine activities.

■ RISKS INVOLVED

1. **Death:** The mortality rate from ECT falls in the range of 0.01 to 0.04 percent (Abrams, 1988). The major cause is cardiovascular complications, such as acute myocardial infarction or cardiac arrest.
2. **Brain Damage:** Brain damage is considered to be a risk, but evidence is largely unsubstantiated.
3. **Permanent Memory Loss:** Prolonged or permanent

memory loss has been reported by some individuals (Freeman et al., 1980).

Although the potential for these effects appears to be minimal, the client must be made aware of the risks involved before consenting to treatment.

POTENTIAL NURSING DIAGNOSES ASSOCIATED WITH ECT

1. Risk for injury related to certain risks associated with ECT.
2. Risk for aspiration related to altered level of consciousness immediately following treatment.
3. Decreased cardiac output related to vagal stimulation occurring during the ECT.
4. Altered thought processes related to side effects of temporary memory loss and confusion.
5. Knowledge deficit related to necessity for, and side effects and risks of, ECT.
6. Anxiety (moderate to severe) related to impending therapy.
7. Self-care deficit related to incapacitation during postictal stage.
8. Risk for activity intolerance related to post-ECT confusion and memory loss.

NURSING INTERVENTIONS FOR CLIENT RECEIVING ECT

1. Ensure that physician has obtained informed consent and that a signed permission form is on the chart.
2. Ensure that most recent laboratory reports (complete blood count [CBC], urinalysis) and results of electrocardiogram (ECG) and x-ray examination are available.
3. Client should receive nothing by mouth (NPO) on the morning of the treatment.
4. Prior to the treatment, client should void, dress in nightclothes (or other loose clothing), and remove dentures and eyeglasses or contact lenses. Bed rails should be raised.
5. Take baseline vital signs and blood pressure.

6. Administer cholinergic blocking agent (atropine sulfate, glycopyrrolate) approximately 30 minutes before treatment, as ordered by the physician, to decrease secretions and increase heart rate (which is suppressed in response to vagal stimulation caused by the ECT).
7. Assist physician and/or anesthesiologist as necessary in the administration of intravenous medications. A short-acting anesthetic, such as methohexital sodium (Brevital Sodium), is given along with the muscle relaxant succinylcholine chloride (Anectine).
8. Administer oxygen and provide suctioning as required.
9. After the procedure, take vital signs and blood pressure every 15 minutes for the first hour. Position client on side to prevent aspiration.
10. Stay with client until he or she is fully awake.

APPENDIX H

Medication Assessment Tool

Date__________ Client's name______________________________ Age__________

Marital status__________ Children______________________ Occupation__________

Presenting symptoms (subjective and objective)______________________________

Diagnosis (*DSM-IV*) ____

Current vital signs: Blood pressure sitting _____/_____ Standing _____/_____ Pulse ______ Respirations ______

CURRENT/PAST USE OF PRESCRIPTION DRUGS (Indicate with c or p beside name of drug whether current or past use):

Name	Dosage	How Long Used	Why Prescribed	By Whom	Side Effects/Results

CURRENT/PAST USE OF OVER-THE-COUNTER DRUGS (Indicate with c or p beside name of drug whether current or past use):

Name	Dosage	How Long Used	Why Prescribed	By Whom	Side Effects/Results

CURRENT/PAST USE OF STREET DRUGS, ALCOHOL, NICOTINE, AND/OR CAFFEINE:

Name	Amount Used	How Often Used	When Last Used	Effects Produced

Any allergies to food or drugs? ______________________

Any special diet considerations? ______________________

Do you have (or have you ever had) any of the following? If yes, provide explanation on the back of this sheet.

	Yes	No
1. Difficulty swallowing	___	___
2. Delayed wound healing	___	___
3. Constipation problems	___	___
4. Urination problems	___	___
5. Recent change in elimination patterns	___	___
6. Weakness or tremors	___	___
7. Seizures	___	___
8. Headaches	___	___
13. Blood clots/pain in legs	___	___
14. Fainting spells	___	___
15. Swollen ankles/legs/hands		
16. Asthma	___	___
17. Varicose veins	___	___
18. Numbness/tingling (state location)	___	___
19. Ulcers	___	___
23. Sexual dysfunction	___	___
24. Lumps in your breasts	___	___
25. Blurred or double vision	___	___
26. Ringing in the ears	___	___
27. Insomnia	___	___
28. Skin Rashes	___	___
29. Diabetes	___	___

9. Dizziness	___	___	20. Nausea/vomiting	___	___	30. Hepatitis (or other liver disease)	___	___
10. High blood pressure	___	___	21. Problems with diarrhea	___	___	31. Kidney disease	___	___
11. Palpitations	___	___	22. Shortness of breath	___	___	32. Glaucoma	___	___
12. Chest pain	___	___						

Are you pregnant or breastfeeding? ________ Date of last menses ________ Type of contraception used __________

Describe any restrictions/limitations that might interfere with your use of medication for your current problem. __________

Prescription orders:

Patient teaching related to medications prescribed:

Laboratory work ordered:

Nurse's Signature

Client's Signature

From Townsend, 2000, p 259, with permission.

APPENDIX I

Cultural Assessment Tool

Client's name ______________________ Ethnic origin ______________________

Address ______________________ Birth date ______________________

Name of significant other ______________________ Relationship ______________________

Primary language spoken ______________________ Second language spoken ______________________

How does client usually communicate with people who speak a different language? ______________________

Is an interpreter required? ______________________ Available? ______________________

Highest level of education achieved ______________________ Occupation ______________________

Presenting problem ______________________

Has this problem ever occurred before? ______________________

If so, in what manner was it handled previously? ______________________

What is client's usual manner of coping with stress? ______________________

Who is(are) the client's main support system(s)? ______________________

Describe the family living arrangements ______________________

Who is the major decision maker in the family? ______

Describe client's/family members' role within the family ______

______

Describe religious beliefs and practices ______

Are there any religious requirements or restrictions that place limitations on the client's care? ______

If so, describe ______

Who in the family takes responsibility for health concerns? ______

Describe any special health beliefs and practices ______

From whom does family usually seek medical assistance in time of need? ______

Describe client's usual emotional/behavioral response to:

Anxiety ______

Anger ______

Loss/change/failure ______

Pain ______

Fear ______

Describe any topics that are particularly sensitive or that the client is unwilling to discuss (because of cultural taboos) ______

______

Describe any activities in which the client is unwilling to participate (because of cultural customs or taboos) ______

______

What are the client's personal feelings regarding touch? ______

What are the client's personal feelings regarding eye contact? ______

What is the client's personal orientation to time? (past, present, future) ______

Describe any particular illnesses to which the client may be bioculturally susceptible ______
(e.g., hypertension and sickle cell anemia in African-Americans)

Describe any nutritional deficiencies to which the client may be bioculturally susceptible ____________________
(e.g., lactose intolerance in Native-Americans and Asian-Americans)

Describe client's favorite foods ____________________

Are there any foods the client requests or refuses because of cultural beliefs related to this illness? ____________________
(e.g., "hot" and "cold" foods for Hispanic-Americans and Asian-Americans). If so, please describe. ____________________

____

____

Describe client's perception of the problem and expectations of health care ____________________

____

____

____

From Townsend, 2000, p 790, with permission.

APPENDIX J

The DSM-IV *Multiaxial Evaluation System*

The APA endorses case evaluation on a multiaxial system "to facilitate comprehensive and systematic evaluation with attention to the various mental disorders and general medical conditions, psychosocial and environmental problems, and level of functioning that might be overlooked if the focus were on assessing a single presenting problem." Each individual is evaluated on five axes. They are defined by the *DSM-IV* in the following manner:

Axis I: Clinical Disorders and Other Conditions That May Be a Focus of Clinical Attention

This includes all mental disorders (except personality disorders and mental retardation).

Axis II: Personality Disorders and Mental Retardation

These disorders usually begin in childhood or adolescence and persist in a stable form into adult life.

Axis III: General Medical Conditions

These include any current general medical condition that is potentially relevant to the understanding or management of the individual's mental disorder.

Axis IV: Psychosocial and Environmental Problems

These are problems that may affect the diagnosis, treatment, and prognosis of mental disorders named on axes I and II. These include problems related to primary support group, social environment, education, occupation, housing, economics, access to health-care services, interaction with the legal system or crime, and other types of psychosocial and environmental problems.

Axis V: Global Assessment of Functioning

This allows the clinician to rate the individual's overall functioning on the Global Assessment of Functioning (GAF) Scale. This scale represents in global terms a single measure of the individual's psychological, social, and occupational functioning. A copy of the GAF Scale appears in Appendix K.

APPENDIX K

Global Assessment of Functioning Scale

Consider psychological, social, and occupational functioning on a hypothetical continuum of mental health-illness. Do not include impairment in functioning due to physical (or environment) limitations.

Code (**Note:** Use intermediate codes when appropriate, e.g., 45, 68, 72)

100 **Superior functioning in a wide range of activities, life's problems never seem to get out of hand, is sought out by others because of his or her many positive qualities. No symp-**
91 **toms.**

90 **Absent or minimal symptoms** (e.g., mild anxiety before an exam), **good functioning in all areas, interested and involved in a wide range of activities, socially effective, generally satisfied with life, no more than everyday problems or concerns** (e.g., an occasional
81 argument with family members).

80 **If symptoms are present, they are transient and expectable reactions to psychosocial stressors** (e.g., difficulty concentrating after family argument); **no more than slight impairment in social, occupational, or school functioning** (e.g., temporarily falling behind in
71 schoolwork).

70 **Some mild symptoms** (e.g., depressed mood and mild insomnia) **OR some difficulty in social, occupational, or school functioning**

(e.g., occasional truancy, or theft within the
household), **but generally functioning pretty
well, has some meaningful interpersonal re-**
61 **lationships.**

60 **Moderate symptoms** (e.g., flat affect and cir-
cumstantial speech, occasional panic attacks)
**OR moderate difficulty in social, occupa-
tional, or school functioning** (e.g., few friends,
51 conflicts with peers or co-workers).

50 **Serious symptoms** (e.g., suicidal ideation, severe obsessional rituals, frequent shoplifting)
**OR any serious impairment in social, occu-
pational, or school functioning** (e.g., no
41 friends, unable to keep a job).

40 **Some impairment in reality testing or communication** (e.g., speech is at times illogical,
obscure, or irrelevant) **OR major impairment
in several areas, such as work or school,
family relations, judgment, thinking, or
mood** (e.g., depressed man avoids friends, ne-
glects family, and is unable to work; child frequently beats up younger children, is defiant at
31 home, and is failing at school).

30 **Behavior is considerably influenced by delusions or hallucinations OR serious impairment in communication or judgment** (e.g.,
sometimes incoherent, acts grossly inappropriately, suicidal preoccupation) **OR inability to
function in almost all areas** (e.g., stays in bed
21 all day; no job, home, or friends).

20 **Some degree of hurting self or others** (e.g.,
suicide attempts without clear expectation of
death; frequently violent; manic excitement)
**OR occasionally fails to maintain minimal
personal hygiene (e.g., smears feces) OR
gross impairment in communication** (e.g.,
11 largely incoherent or mute).

10 **Persistent danger of severely hurting self or
others** (e.g., recurrent violence) **OR persistent
inability to maintain minimal personal hygiene OR serious suicidal act with clear ex-**
1 **pectation of death.**

0 **Inadequate information.**

APPENDIX L*

DSM-IV *Classification: Axes I and II Categories and Codes*

■ DISORDERS USUALLY FIRST DIAGNOSED IN INFANCY, CHILDHOOD, OR ADOLESCENCE

Mental Retardation

317 Mild Mental Retardation
318.0 Moderate Retardation
318.1 Severe Retardation
318.2 Profound Mental Retardation
319 Mental Retardation, Severity Unspecified

Learning Disorders

315.00 Reading Disorder
315.1 Mathematics Disorder
315.2 Disorder of Written Expression
315.9 Learning Disorder Not Otherwise Specified (NOS)

Motor Skills Disorder

315.4 Developmental Coordination Disorder

Communication Disorders

315.31 Expressive Language Disorder
315.31 Mixed Receptive/Expressive Language Disorder

*Reprinted with permission from the *Diagnostic and Statistical Manual of Mental Disorders, Fourth Edition.* Copyright 1994 American Psychiatric Association.

315.39 Phonological Disorder
370.0 Stuttering
315.39 Communication Disorders NOS

Pervasive Developmental Disorders

299.00 Autistic Disorder
299.80 Rett's Disorder
299.10 Childhood Disintegrative Disorders
299.80 Asperger's Disorder
299.80 Pervasive Developmental Disorder NOS

Attention-Deficit and Disruptive Behavior Disorders

314.xx Attention-Deficit/Hyperactivity Disorder
314.01 Combined type
314.00 Predominantly inattentive type
314.01 Predominantly hyperactive-impulsive type
314.9 Attention-Deficit/Hyperactivity Disorder NOS
312.8 Conduct Disorder
Specify Childhood- or Adolescent-Onset Type
313.81 Oppositional Defiant Disorder
312.9 Disruptive Behavior Disorder NOS

Feeding and Eating Disorders of Infancy or Early Childhood

307.52 Pica
307.53 Rumination Disorder
307.59 Feeding Disorder of Infancy or Early Childhood

Tic Disorders

307.23 Tourette's Disorder
307.22 Chronic Motor or Vocal Tic Disorder
307.21 Transient Tic Disorder
307.20 Tic Disorder NOS

Elimination Disorders

— Encopresis
787.6 With constipation and overflow incontinence
307.7 Without constipation and overflow incontinence
307.6 Enuresis (Not Due to a General Medical Condition)

Other Disorders of Infancy, Childhood, or Adolescence

309.21 Separation Anxiety Disorder
313.23 Selective Mutism

313.89	Reactive Attachment Disorder of Infancy or Early Childhood
307.3	Sterotypic Movement Disorder
313.9	Disorder of Infancy, Childhood, or Adolescence NOS

■ DELIRIUM, DEMENTIA, AMNESTIC AND OTHER COGNITIVE DISORDERS

Delirium

293.0	Delirium Due to (indicate the general medical condition)
—	Substance Intoxication Delirium (refer to Substance-Related Disorders for substance-specific codes)
—	Substance Withdrawal Delirium (refer to Substance-Related Disorders for substance-specific codes)
—	Delirium Due to Multiple Etiologies (code each of the specific etiologies)
780.09	Delirium NOS

Dementia

290.xx	Dementia of the Alzheimer's Type With Early Onset: if onset at age 65 or below
290.10	Uncomplicated
290.11	With delirium
290.12	With delusions
290.13	With depressed mood
290.xx	Dementia of the Alzheimer's Type With Late Onset: if onset after age 65
290.00	Uncomplicated
290.3	With delirium
290.20	With delusions
290.21	With depressed mood
290.xx	Vascular Dementia
290.40	Uncomplicated
290.41	With delirium
290.42	With delusions
290.43	With depressed mood
294.9	Dementia Due to Human Immunodeficiency Virus (HIV) Disease
294.1	Dementia Due to Head Trauma
294.1	Dementia Due to Parkinson's Disease
294.1	Dementia Due to Huntington's Disease

290.10	Dementia Due to Pick's Disease
290.10	Dementia Due to Creutzfeldt-Jakob Disease
294.1	Dementia Due to (indicate the general medical condition not listed above)
—	Substance-Induced Persisting Dementia (refer to Substance-Related Disorders for substance-specific codes)
—	Dementia Due to Multiple Etiologies (code each of the specific etiologies)
294.8	Dementia NOS

Amnestic Disorders

294.0	Amnestic Disorder Due to (indicate the general medical condition)
—	Substance-Induced Persisting Amnestic Disorder (refer to specific substance for code)
294.8	Amnestic Disorder NOS

Other Cognitive Disorders

294.9	Cognitive disorder NOS

■ MENTAL DISORDERS DUE TO A GENERAL MEDICAL CONDITION NOT ELSEWHERE CLASSIFIED

293.89	Catatonic Disorder Due to (indicate the general medical condition)
310.1	Personality Change Due to (indicate the general medical condition)
293.9	Mental Disorder NOS Due to (indicate the general medical condition)

■ SUBSTANCE-RELATED DISORDERS

Alcohol-Related Disorders

Alcohol Use Disorders

303.90	Alcohol Dependence
305.00	Alcohol Abuse

Alcohol-Induced Disorders

303.00	Alcohol Intoxication
291.8	Alcohol Withdrawal
291.0	Alcohol Intoxication Delirium
291.0	Alcohol Withdrawal Delirium
291.2	Alcohol-Induced Persisting Dementia

291.1	Alcohol-Induced Persisting Amnestic Disorder
291.x	Alcohol-Induced Psychotic Disorder
291.5	With Delusions
291.3	With Hallucinations
291.8	Alcohol-Induced Mood Disorder
291.8	Alcohol-Induced Anxiety Disorder
292.8	Alcohol-Induced Sexual Dysfunction
292.89	Alcohol-Induced Sleep Disorder
291.9	Alcohol Related Disorder NOS

Amphetamine (or Amphetamine-like)-Related Disorders

Amphetamine Use Disorders

304.40	Amphetamine Dependence
305.70	Amphetamine Abuse

Amphetamine-Induced Disorders

292.89	Amphetamine Intoxication
292.0	Amphetamine Withdrawal
292.81	Amphetamine Intoxication Delirium
292.xx	Amphetamine-Induced Psychotic Disorder
292.11	With Delusions
292.12	With Hallucinations
292.84	Amphetamine-Induced Mood Disorder
292.89	Amphetamine-Induced Anxiety Disorder
292.89	Amphetamine-Induced Sexual Dysfunction
292.89	Amphetamine-Induced Sleep Disorder
292.9	Amphetamine-Related Disorder NOS

Caffeine-Related Disorders

Caffeine-Induced Disorders

305.90	Caffeine Intoxication
292.89	Caffeine-Induced Anxiety Disorder
292.89	Caffeine-Induced Sleep Disorder
292.9	Caffeine-Related Disorder NOS

Cannabis-Related Disorders

Cannabis Use Disorders

304.30	Cannabis Dependence
305.20	Cannabis Abuse

Cannabis-Induced Disorders

292.89	Cannabis Intoxication
292.81	Cannabis Intoxication Delirium
292.xx	Cannabis-Induced Psychotic Disorder

292.11	With Delusions
292.12	With Hallucinations
292.89	Cannabis-Induced Anxiety Disorder
292.9	Cannabis-Related Disorder NOS

Cocaine-Related Disorders

Cocaine Use Disorders

304.20	Cocaine Dependence
305.60	Cocaine Abuse

Cocaine-Induced Disorders

292.89	Cocaine Intoxication
292.0	Cocaine Withdrawal
292.81	Cocaine Intoxication Delirium
292.xx	Cocaine-Induced Psychotic Disorder
292.11	With Delusions
292.12	With Hallucinations
292.84	Cocaine-Induced Mood Disorder
292.89	Cocaine-Induced Anxiety Disorder
292.89	Cocaine-Induced Sexual Dysfunction
292.89	Cocaine-Induced Sleep Disorder
292.9	Cocaine-Related Disorder NOS

Hallucinogen-Related Disorders

Hallucinogen Use Disorders

304.50	Hallucinogen Dependence
305.30	Hallucinogen Abuse

Hallucinogen-Induced Disorders

292.89	Hallucinogen Intoxication
292.89	Hallucinogen Persisting Perception Disorder (Flashbacks)
292.81	Hallucinogen Intoxication Delirium
292.xx	Hallucinogen-Induced Psychotic Disorder
292.11	With Delusions
292.12	With Hallucinations
292.84	Hallucinogen-Induced Mood Disorder
292.89	Hallucinogen-Induced Anxiety Disorder
292.9	Hallucinogen-Related Disorder NOS

Inhalant-Related Disorders

Inhalant Use Disorders

304.60	Inhalant Dependence
305.90	Inhalant Abuse

Inhalant-Induced Disorders

292.89	Inhalant Intoxication
292.81	Inhalant Intoxication Delirium
292.82	Inhalant-Induced Persisting Dementia
292.xx	Inhalant-Induced Psychotic Disorder
292.11	With Delusions
292.12	With Hallucinations
292.84	Inhalant-Induced Mood Disorder
292.89	Inhalant-Induced Anxiety Disorder
292.9	Inhalant-Related Disorder NOS

Nicotine-Related Disorders

Nicotine Use Disorders

305.10	Nicotine Dependence

Nicotine-Induced Disorders

292.0	Nicotine Withdrawal
292.9	Nicotine-Related Disorder NOS

Opioid-Related Disorders

Opioid Use Disorders

304.00	Opioid Dependence
305.50	Opioid Abuse

Opioid-Induced Disorders

292.89	Opioid Intoxication
292.0	Opioid Withdrawal
292.81	Opioid Intoxication Delirium
292.xx	Opioid-Induced Psychotic Disorder
292.11	With Delusions
292.12	With Hallucinations
292.84	Opioid-Induced Mood Disorder
292.89	Opioid-Induced Sexual Dysfunction
292.89	Opioid-Induced Sleep Disorder
292.9	Opioid-Related Disorder NOS

Phencyclidine (or Phencyclidine-like)-Related Disorders

Phencyclidine Use Disorders

304.90	Phencyclidine Dependence
305.90	Phencyclidine Abuse

Phencyclidine-Induced Disorders

292.89	Phencyclidine Intoxication

292.81 Phencyclidine Intoxication Delirium
292.xx Phencyclidine-Induced Psychotic Disorder
292.11 With Delusions
292.12 With Hallucinations
292.84 Phencyclidine-Induced Mood Disorder
292.89 Phencyclidine-Induced Anxiety Disorder
292.9 Phencyclidine-Related Disorder NOS

Sedative-, Hypnotic-, or Anxiolytic-Related Disorders

Sedative, Hypnotic, or Anxiolytic Substance Use Disorders

304.10 Sedative, Hypnotic, or Anxiolytic Dependence
305.40 Sedative, Hypnotic, or Anxiolytic Abuse

Sedative-, Hypnotic-, or Anxiolytic-Induced Disorders

292.89 Sedative, Hypnotic, or Anxiolytic Intoxication
292.0 Sedative, Hypnotic, or Anxiolytic Withdrawal
292.81 Sedative, Hypnotic, or Anxiolytic Intoxication Delirium
292.81 Sedative, Hypnotic, or Anxiolytic Withdrawal Delirium
292.82 Sedative-, Hypnotic-, or Anxiolytic-Induced Persisting Dementia
292.83 Sedative-, Hypnotic-, or Anxiolytic-Induced Persisting Amnestic Disorder
292.xx Sedative-, Hypnotic-, or Anxiolytic-Induced Psychotic Disorder
292.11 With Delusions
292.12 With Hallucinations
292.84 Sedative-, Hypnotic-, or Anxiolytic-Induced Mood Disorder
292.89 Sedative-, Hypnotic-, or Anxiolytic-Induced Anxiety Disorder
292.89 Sedative-, Hypnotic-, or Anxiolytic-Induced Sexual Dysfunction
292.89 Sedative-, Hypnotic-, or Anxiolytic-Induced Sleep Disorder
292.9 Sedative-, Hypnotic-, or Anxiolytic-Related Disorder NOS

Polysubstance-Related Disorder

304.80 Polysubstance Dependence

Other (or Unknown) Substance-Related Disorders

Other (or Unknown) Substance Use Disorders

304.90 Other (or Unknown) Substance Dependence
305.90 Other (or Unknown) Substance Abuse

Other (or Unknown) Substance-Induced Disorders

292.89 Other (or Unknown) Substance Intoxication
292.0 Other (or Unknown) Substance Withdrawal
292.81 Other (or Unknown) Substance-Induced Delirium
292.82 Other (or Unknown) Substance-Induced Persisting Dementia
292.83 Other (or Unknown) Substance-Induced Persisting Amnestic Disorder
292.xx Other (or Unknown) Substance-Induced Psychotic Disorder
292.11 With Delusions
292.12 With Hallucinations
292.84 Other (or Unknown) Substance-Induced Mood Disorder
292.89 Other (or Unknown) Substance-Induced Anxiety Disorder
292.89 Other (or Unknown) Substance-Induced Sexual Dysfunction
292.89 Other (or Unknown) Substance-Induced Sleep Disorder
292.9 Other (or Unknown) Substance-Related Disorder NOS

■ SCHIZOPHRENIA AND OTHER PSYCHOTIC DISORDERS

295.xx Schizophrenia
295.30 Paranoid type
295.10 Disorganized type
295.20 Catatonic type
295.90 Undifferentiated type
295.60 Residual type
295.40 Schizophreniform Disorder
295.70 Schizoaffective Disorder
297.1 Delusional Disorder
298.8 Brief Psychotic Disorder
297.3 Shared Psychotic Disorder (Folie à Deux)

293.xx	Psychotic Disorder Due to a General Medical Condition
293.81	With Delusions
293.82	With Hallucinations
—	Substance-Induced Psychotic Disorder (refer to Substance-Related Disorders for substance-specific codes)
298.9	Psychotic Disorder NOS

■ MOOD DISORDERS

(Code current state of Major Depressive Disorder or Bipolar Disorder in fifth digit: 0 = unspecified; 1 = mild; 2 = moderate; 3 = severe, without psychotic features; 4 = severe, with psychotic features; 5 = in partial remission; 6 = in full remission.)

Depressive Disorders

296.xx	Major Depressive Disorder
296.2x	Single episode
296.3x	Recurrent
300.4	Dysthymic Disorder
311	Depressive Disorder NOS

Bipolar Disorders

296.xx	Bipolar I Disorder
296.0x	Single manic episode
296.40	Most recent episode hypomanic
296.4x	Most recent episode manic
296.6x	Most recent episode mixed
296.5x	Most recent episode depressed
296.7	Most recent episode unspecified
296.89	Bipolar II Disorder (specify current or most recent episode: Hypomanic or Depressed)
301.13	Cyclothymic Disorder
296.80	Bipolar Disorder NOS
293.83	Mood Disorder Due to (indicate the general medical condition)
—	Substance-Induced Mood Disorder (refer to Substance-Related Disorders for substance-specific codes)
296.90	Mood Disorder NOS

■ ANXIETY DISORDERS

300.01	Panic Disorder Without Agoraphobia
300.21	Panic Disorder With Agoraphobia

300.22 Agoraphobia Without History of Panic Disorder
300.29 Specific Phobia
300.23 Social Phobia
300.3 Obsessive-Compulsive Disorder
309.81 Posttraumatic Stress Disorder
308.3 Acute Stress Disorder
300.02 Generalized Anxiety Disorder
293.89 Anxiety Disorder Due to (indicate the general medical condition)
— Substance-Induced Anxiety Disorder (refer to Substance-Related Disorders for substance-specific codes)
300.00 Anxiety Disorder NOS

■ SOMATOFORM DISORDERS

300.81 Somatization Disorder
300.11 Undifferentiated Somatoform Disorder
300.7 Conversion Disorder
300.7 Pain Disorder
307.xx Associated with Psychological Factors
307.80 Associated with Both Psychological Factors and a General Medical Condition
307.89 Hypochondriasis
300.81 Body Dysmorphic Disorder
300.81 Somatoform Disorder NOS

■ FACTITIOUS DISORDERS

300.xx Factitious Disorder
300.16 With predominantly psychological signs and symptoms
300.19 With predominantly physical signs and symptoms
300.19 With combined psychological and physical signs and symptoms
300.19 Factitious Disorder NOS

■ DISSOCIATIVE DISORDERS

300.12 Dissociative Amnesia
300.13 Dissociative Fugue

300.14 Dissociative Identity Disorder
300.6 Depersonalization Disorder
300.15 Dissociative Disorder NOS

■ SEXUAL AND GENDER IDENTITY DISORDERS

Sexual Dysfunctions

Sexual Desire Disorders

302.71 Hypoactive Sexual Desire Disorder
302.79 Sexual Aversion Disorder

Sexual Arousal Disorders

302.72 Female Sexual Arousal Disorder
302.72 Male Erectile Disorder

Orgasmic Disorders

302.73 Female Orgasmic Disorder
302.74 Male Orgasmic Disorder
302.75 Premature Ejaculation

Sexual Pain Disorders

302.76 Dyspareunia (Not Due to a General Medical Condition)
306.51 Vaginismus (Not Due to a General Medical Condition)

Sexual Dysfunctions Due to a General Medical Condition

625.8 Female Hypoactive Sexual Desire Disorder Due to (indicate the general medical condition)
608.89 Male Hypoactive Sexual Desire Disorder Due to (indicate the general medical condition)
607.84 Male Erectile Disorder Due to (indicate the general medical condition)
625.0 Female Dyspareunia Due to (indicate the general medical condition)
608.89 Male Dyspareunia Due to (indicate the general medical condition)
625.8 Other Female Sexual Dysfunction Due to (indicate the general medical condition)
608.89 Other Male Sexual Dysfunction Due to (indicate the general medical condition)
— Substance-Induced Sexual Dysfunction (re-

fer to Substance-Related Disorders for substance-specific codes)

302.70	Sexual Dysfunction NOS

Paraphilias

302.4	Exhibitionism
302.81	Fetishism
302.89	Frotteurism
302.2	Pedophilia
302.83	Sexual Masochism
302.84	Sexual Sadism
302.3	Transvestic Fetishism
302.82	Voyeurism
302.9	Paraphilia NOS

Gender Identity Disorders

302.xx	Gender Identity Disorder
302.6	In Children
302.85	In Adolescents or Adults
302.6	Gender Identity Disorder NOS

302.9	Sexual Disorder NOS

■ EATING DISORDERS

307.1	Anorexia Nervosa
307.51	Bulimia Nervosa
307.50	Eating Disorder NOS

■ SLEEP DISORDERS

Primary Sleep Disorders

Dyssomnias

307.42	Primary Insomnia
307.44	Primary Hypersomnia
347	Narcolepsy
780.59	Breathing-Related Sleep Disorder
307.45	Circadian Rhythm Sleep Disorder
307.47	Dyssomnia NOS

Parasomnias

307.47	Nightmare Disorder
307.46	Sleep Terror Disorder

307.46	Sleepwalking Disorder
307.47	Parasomnia NOS

Sleep Disorders Related to Another Mental Disorder

307.42	Insomnia Related to (indicate the Axis I or Axis II disorder)
307.44	Hypersomnia Related to (indicate the Axis I or Axis II disorder)

Other Sleep Disorders

780.xx	Sleep Disorder Due to (indicate the general medical condition)
780.52	Insomnia type
780.54	Hypersomnia type
780.59	Parasomnia type
780.59	Mixed type
—	Substance-Induced Sleep Disorder (refer to Substance-Related Disorders for substance-specific codes)

■ IMPULSE CONTROL DISORDERS NOT ELSEWHERE CLASSIFIED

312.34	Intermittent Explosive Disorder
312.32	Kleptomania
312.33	Pyromania
312.31	Pathological Gambling
312.39	Trichotillomania
312.30	Impulse Control Disorder NOS

■ ADJUSTMENT DISORDERS

309.xx	Adjustment Disorder
309.0	With Depressed Mood
309.24	With Anxiety
309.28	With Mixed Anxiety and Depressed Mood
309.3	With Disturbance of Conduct
309.4	With Mixed Disturbance of Emotions and Conduct
309.9	Unspecified

PERSONALITY DISORDERS

NOTE: These are coded on Axis II.

301.0	Paranoid Personality Disorder
301.20	Schizoid Personality Disorder
301.22	Schizotypal Personality Disorder
301.7	Antisocial Personality Disorder
301.83	Borderline Personality Disorder
301.50	Histrionic Personality Disorder
301.81	Narcissistic Personality Disorder
301.82	Avoidant Personality Disorder
301.6	Dependent Personality Disorder
301.4	Obsessive-Compulsive Personality Disorder
301.9	Personality Disorder NOS

OTHER CONDITIONS THAT MAY BE A FOCUS OF CLINICAL ATTENTION

(Psychological Factors) Affecting Medical Condition

316 *Choose name based on nature of factors:*
- Mental Disorder Affecting Medical Condition
- Psychological Symptoms Affecting Medical Condition
- Personality Traits or Coping Style Affecting Medical Condition
- Maladaptive Health Behaviors Affecting Medical Condition
- Stress-Related Physiological Response Affecting Medical Condition
- Other or Unspecified Psychological Factors Affecting Medical Condition

Medication-Induced Movement Disorders

332.1	Neuroleptic-Induced Parkinsonism
333.92	Neuroleptic Malignant Syndrome
333.7	Neuroleptic-Induced Acute Dystonia
333.99	Neuroleptic-Induced Acute Akathisia
333.82	Neuroleptic-Induced Tardive Dyskinesia
333.1	Medication-Induced Postural Tremor
333.90	Medication-Induced Movement Disorder NOS

Other Medication-Induced Disorder

995.2 Adverse Effects of Medication NOS

Relational Problems

V61.9	Relational Problem Related to a Mental Disorder or General Medical Condition
V61.20	Parent-Child Relational Problem
V61.1	Partner Relational Problem
V61.8	Sibling Relational Problem
V62.81	Relational Problem NOS

Problems Related to Abuse or Neglect

V61.21	Physical Abuse of Child
V61.21	Sexual Abuse of Child
V61.21	Neglect of Child
V61.1	Physical Abuse of Adult
V61.1	Sexual Abuse of Adult

Additional Conditions That May Be a Focus of Clinical Attention

V15.81	Noncompliance with Treatment
V65.2	Malingering
V71.01	Adult Antisocial Behavior
V71.02	Childhood or Adolescent Antisocial Behavior
V62.89	Borderline Intellectual Functioning (coded on Axis II)
780.9	Age-Related Cognitive Decline
V62.82	Bereavement
V62.3	Academic Problem
V62.2	Occupational Problem
313.82	Identity Problem
V62.89	Religious or Spiritual Problem
V62.4	Acculturation Problem
V62.89	Phase of Life Problem

■ ADDITIONAL CODES

300.9	Unspecified Mental Disorder (nonpsychotic)
V71.09	No Diagnosis or Condition on Axis I
799.9	Diagnosis or Condition Deferred on Axis I
V71.09	No Diagnosis on Axis II
799.9	Diagnosis Deferred on Axis II

■ *DSM-IV* CRITERIA SETS AND AXES PROVIDED FOR FURTHER STUDY

Text and criteria for these disorders will be provided to facilitate systematic clinical research:

Postconcussional disorder
Mild neurocognitive disorder
Caffeine withdrawal
Alternative dimensional descriptors for schizophrenia
Postpsychotic depression of schizophrenia
Simple schizophrenia
Minor depressive disorder
Alternative criteria B for dysthymic disorder
Recurrent brief depressive disorder
Premenstrual dysphoric disorder
Mixed anxiety-depressive disorder
Factitious disorder by proxy
Dissociative trance disorder
Binge eating disorder
Depressive personality disorder
Passive-aggressive personality disorder (negativistic personality disorder)
Medication-induced movement disorders
Defensive Functioning Scale
Global Assessment of Relational Functioning (GARF) Scale
Social and Occupational Functioning Assessment Scale (SOFAS)

APPENDIX M*

Mental Status Assessment

Gathering the correct information about the client's mental status is essential to the development of an appropriate plan of care. The mental status examination is a description of all the areas of the client's mental functioning (Scheiber, 1994). The following are the components that are considered critical in the assessment of a client's mental status.

■ IDENTIFYING DATA

1. Name
2. Gender
3. Age
4. Race/culture
5. Occupational/financial status
6. Educational Level
7. Significant other
8. Living arrangements
9. Religious preference
10. Allergies
11. Special diet considerations
12. Chief complaint
13. Medical diagnosis

■ GENERAL DESCRIPTION

Appearance

1. Grooming and dress
2. Hygiene

---

*From Townsend, 2000, pp 861–862, with permission.

3. Posture
4. Height and weight
5. Level of eye contact
6. Hair color and texture
7. Evidence of scars, tattoos, or other distinguishing skin marks
8. Evaluation of client's appearance compared with chronological age

Motor Activity

1. Tremors
2. Tics or other stereotypical movements
3. Mannerisms and gestures
4. Hyperactivity
5. Restlessness or agitation
6. Aggressiveness
7. Rigidity
8. Gait patterns
9. Echopraxia
10. Psychomotor retardation
11. Freedom of movement (range of motion)

Speech Patterns

1. Slowness or rapidity of speech
2. Pressure of speech
3. Intonation
4. Volume
5. Stuttering or other speech impairments
6. Aphasia

General Attitude

1. Cooperative/uncooperative
2. Friendly/hostile/defensive
3. Uninterested/apathetic
4. Attentive/interested
5. Guarded/suspicious

■ EMOTIONS

Mood

1. Sad
2. Depressed

3. Despairing
4. Irritable
5. Anxious
6. Elated
7. Euphoric
8. Fearful
9. Guilty
10. Labile

Affect

1. Congruent with mood
2. Constricted or blunted (diminished amount/range and intensity of emotional expression)
3. Flat (absence of emotional expression)
4. Appropriate or inappropriate (defines congruence of affect with the situation or with the client's behavior)

■ THOUGHT PROCESSES

Form of Thought

1. Flight of ideas
2. Associative looseness
3. Circumstantiality
4. Tangentiality
5. Neologisms
6. Concrete thinking
7. Clang associations
8. Word salad
9. Perseveration
10. Echolalia
11. Mutism
12. Poverty of speech (restriction in the amount of speech)
13. Ability to concentrate
14. Attention span

Content of Thought

1. Delusions
   a. Persecutory
   b. Grandiose
   c. Reference
   d. Control or influence
   e. Somatic

   f. Nihilistic
2. Suicidal or homicidal ideas
3. Obsessions
4. Paranoia/suspiciousness
5. Magical thinking
6. Religiosity
7. Phobias
8. Poverty of content (vague, meaningless responses)

■ PERCEPTUAL DISTURBANCES

1. Hallucinations
   a. Auditory
   b. Visual
   c. Tactile
   d. Olfactory
   e. Gustatory
2. Illusions
3. Depersonalization (altered perception of the self)
4. Derealization (altered perception of the environment)

■ SENSORIUM AND COGNITIVE ABILITY

1. Level of alertness/consciousness
2. Orientation
   a. Time
   b. Place
   c. Person
   d. Circumstances
3. Memory
   a. Recent
   b. Remote
   c. Use of confabulation
4. Capacity for abstract thought

■ IMPULSE CONTROL

1. Ability to control impulses related to the following:
   a. Aggression
   b. Hostility
   c. Fear
   d. Guilt

  e. Affection
  f. Sexual feelings

JUDGMENT AND INSIGHT

1. Ability to solve problems
2. Ability to make decisions
3. Knowledge about self
   a. Awareness of limitations
   b. Awareness of consequences of actions
   c. Awareness of illness
4. Adaptive/maladaptive use of coping strategies and ego defense mechanisms

APPENDIX N

Assigning Nursing Diagnoses to Client Behaviors

Following is a list of client behaviors. Beside each behavior is the NANDA nursing diagnosis that corresponds to the behavior and that may be used in planning care for the client exhibiting the specific behavioral symptom.

Behavior	*NANDA Nursing Diagnosis(es)*
Aggression; hostility	Risk for injury; Risk for violence, directed at others
Anorexia or refusal to eat	Altered nutrition: less than body requirements
Anxious behavior	Anxiety (specify level)
Confusion; memory loss	Confusion, acute/chronic; Altered thought processes
Delusions	Altered thought processes
Denial of problems	Ineffective denial
Depressed mood or anger turned inward	Dysfunctional grieving
Detoxification; withdrawal from substances	Risk for injury
Difficulty making important life decisions	Decisional conflict (specify)
Difficulty with interpersonal relationships	Impaired social interaction
Disruption in capability to perform usual responsibilities	Altered role performance

Dissociative behaviors (depersonalization; derealization)	Sensory-perceptual alteration (kinesthetic)
Expresses feelings of disgust about body or body part	Body image disturbance
Expresses lack of control over personal situation	Powerlessness
Flashbacks, nightmares, obsession with traumatic experience	Posttrauma response
Hallucinations	Sensory-perceptual alteration (auditory; visual)
Highly critical of self or others	Self-esteem disturbance
HIV-positive; altered immunity	Altered protection
Inability to meet basic needs	Self-care deficit (specify)
Insomnia or hypersomnia	Sleep pattern disturbance
Loose associations or flight of ideas	Impaired verbal communication
Manic hyperactivity	Risk for injury
Manipulative behavior	Ineffective individual coping
Multiple personalities; gender identity disturbance	Personal identity disturbance
Orgasm, problems with; lack of sexual desire	Sexual dysfunction
Overeating, compulsive	Altered nutrition: (Risk for) more than body requirements
Phobias	Fear
Physical symptoms as coping behavior	Ineffective individual coping
Projection of blame; rationalization of failures; denial of personal responsibility	Defensive coping
Ritualistic behaviors	Anxiety (severe); ineffective individual coping
Seductive remarks; inappropriate sexual behaviors	Impaired social interaction

Self-mutilative behaviors	Risk for self-mutilation
Sexual behaviors (difficulty, limitations, or changes in; reported dissatisfaction)	Altered sexuality patterns
Stress from caring for chronically ill person	Caregiver role strain
Stress from locating to new environment	Relocation stress syndrome
Substance use as a coping behavior	Ineffective individual coping
Substance use (denies use is a problem)	Ineffective denial
Suicidal	Risk for violence, directed at self; risk for suicide
Suspiciousness	Altered thought processes; ineffective individual coping
Vomiting, excessive, self-induced	Risk for fluid volume deficit
Withdrawn behavior	Social isolation

From Townsend, 2000, pp 871–872.

Subject Index

Numbers followed by an "f" indicate figures; numbers followed by a "t" indicate tabular material

Drug Index

Numbers followed by a "t" indicate tabular material. Trade names appear in bold.

Index of Nursing Diagnoses